Advanced Principles of Critical Care

Advanced Principles of Critical Care

Edited by Eduardo Raymond

hayle
medical

New York

Hayle Medical,
750 Third Avenue, 9th Floor,
New York, NY 10017, USA

Visit us on the World Wide Web at:
www.haylemedical.com

ISBN: 978-1-63241-591-2

Cataloging-in-Publication Data

Advanced principles of critical care / edited by Eduardo Raymond.
    p. cm.
Includes bibliographical references and index.
ISBN 978-1-63241-591-2
1. Critical care medicine. 2. Emergency medicine. 3. Intensive care units.
I. Raymond, Eduardo.
RC86.7 .A38 2019
616.025--dc23

Table of Contents

Preface

This book has been an outcome of determined endeavour from a group of educationists in the field. The primary objective was to involve a broad spectrum of professionals from diverse cultural background involved in the field for developing new researches. The book not only targets students but also scholars pursuing higher research for further enhancement of the theoretical and practical applications of the subject.

In healthcare, an important treatment for patients with severe life-threatening conditions and injuries is provided by critical and intensive care units. A combination of close monitoring, constant care, life support using specialized equipment, and specific medications help to ensure health and normal bodily functions. Patients are generally treated for trauma, sepsis, multiple organ failure and acute respiratory distress syndrome. Patients who have undergone highly invasive surgical procedures and are at risk of complications, or patients with rapidly deteriorating health conditions are eligible for critical care. Dedicated nursing is integral to critical care. Performing assessment of critical conditions, operating and maintaining life support systems, providing intensive therapy and medications, ensuring adequate tissue and organ perfusion are crucial aspects of critical care nursing. This book brings forth some of the most innovative practices and elucidates the unexplored aspects of critical care. The various studies that are constantly contributing towards advancing technologies and evolution of this field are examined in detail. Those in search of information to further their knowledge will be greatly assisted by this book.

It was an honour to edit such a profound book and also a challenging task to compile and examine all the relevant data for accuracy and originality. I wish to acknowledge the efforts of the contributors for submitting such brilliant and diverse chapters in the field and for endlessly working for the completion of the book. Last, but not the least; I thank my family for being a constant source of support in all my research endeavours.

Editor

Rituximab—A Drug with Many Facets and Cures: A Treatment for Acute Refractory Hypoxemic Respiratory Failure Secondary to Severe Granulomatosis with Polyangiitis

Braden Powers, Aditya Uppalapati, Sindhura Gogineni, and Zafar Akram Jamkhana

Division of Pulmonary, Critical Care and Sleep Medicine, Saint Louis University 1402 South Grand Avenue, MC/SLUH/7 FDT, St. Louis, MO 63110-0250, USA

Correspondence should be addressed to Aditya Uppalapati; doctoraditya@yahoo.com

Academic Editors: C. Diez, M. Doganay, C. Lazzeri, G. Pichler, A. J. Reddy, and K. S. Waxman

Granulomatosis with Polyangiitis (GPA) is a rare systemic anti neutrophil cytoplasmic antibody (ANCA-) associated granulomatous vasculitis of the small and medium sized blood vessels. Diffuse alveolar hemorrhage (DAH) is a rare life-threatening complication of GPA. In our patient, cyclophosphamide was held secondary to complications of acute kidney injury, hematuria, and concern for a possible hemorrhagic cystitis. However, during the workup for hematuria the patient acutely developed respiratory failure and was found to have DAH. The patient was initially supported with mechanical ventilation volume control mode, steroids, and plasma exchange. With no improvement of oxygenation, the mode of ventilation was changed to airway pressure release ventilation (APRV) and the patient was started on rituximab. The patient clinically improved over the next few days, was able to be extubated, and was transferred out of the intensive care unit.

1. Introduction

Granulomatosis with polyangiitis (GPA) is a necrotizing vasculitis that affects small and medium sized blood vessels with granuloma formation. It typically produces granulomatous inflammation of the upper, lower respiratory tracts and necrotizing glomerulonephritis in the kidneys. It is associated with ANCA. Its current incidence is unknown; however, its prevalence is believed to be 3/100,000 people in the USA. Diffuse alveolar hemorrhage (DAH) is identified in 25% of the patients with severe GPA [1]. We report a case of GPA with refractory hypoxemia secondary to diffuse alveolar hemorrhage that was treated with rituximab and supportive treatment.

2. Case Presentation

A 32-year-old Caucasian male with a past medical history of GPA presented with fatigue, dry cough, myalgia, and arthralgia since 2 weeks. Three days prior to presentation, he developed progressive shortness of breath. The patient did not have any hemoptysis on presentation. Previous medications included cyclophosphamide and prednisone. However, cyclophosphamide was held about a week before admission when the patient was noted to have significant hematuria, proteinuria, and possible hemorrhagic cystitis. The patient was continued on prednisone. The patient at admission was initially placed on noninvasive ventilation Bipap for acute hypoxemic respiratory failure. Vital signs at admission were as following: temperature 99.2F, heart rate 120–130 beats/min normal sinus rhythm, blood pressure 109/70 mmHg, and respiratory rate 28–34/min. Oxygen saturation was 90% on bipap (IPAP-14, EPAP-6). Chest X-ray showed bilateral diffuse patchy infiltrates (see Figure 1).

The patient's shortness of breath and mentation progressively worsened on noninvasive ventilation, and he was intubated. The patient was hypotensive after intubation and was started on norepinephrine.

Initial laboratory test was significant for acute rise in creatinine to 1.5 (baseline 0.9). Other relevant labs were as follows: hemoglobin is 10.0 gram/dL, hematocrit is 28.8, lactate 3.0 mmol/white blood cell count was 10.8 (10^3/uL),

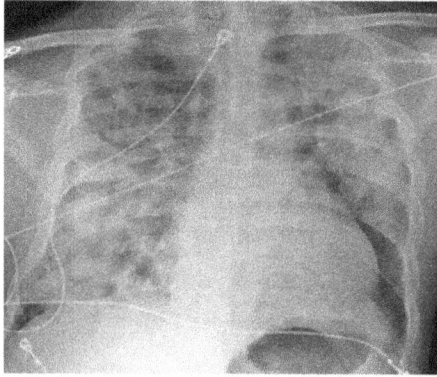

Figure 1: Chest X-ray showing diffuse bilateral patchy infiltrates at admission.

INR is 1.3, and PTT is 26.4 seconds. Immunological workup showed a normal myeloperoxidase (MPO) <9.0 U/mL (reference level 0.0–9.0 U/mL), increased antiproteinase antibodies (PR3) 17.6 units/mL (reference level—0.0–3.5 U/mL), c-ANCA titer of 1:640, and p-ANCA <1:20. CRP was also elevated at 15.7 mg/dL. The patient was started on piperacillin and tazobactam, levofloxacin, vancomycin, bactrim, and micafungin. The patient had a flexible bronchoscopy that showed progressive hemorrhagic bronchoalveolar lavage in serial samples consistent with diffuse alveolar hemorrhage (see Figure 2).

The patient was then started on methylprednisolone 1 gram daily for 3 days followed by solumedrol at 1 mg/Kg in divided doses. Plasmapheresis was also started on day 1 following the diagnosis of DAH and was continued daily for 5 days. On day 2, inspite of being on a 100% FiO_2, PEEP-18, sedated and paralyzed with cisatracurium, the patient's hypoxemia worsened and was unable to maintain PaO_2 > 55 mmHg or SaO_2 > 88%. Echocardiogram showed moderate pulmonary hypertension and no intra- or extracardiac shunt. The mode of ventilation was changed to APRV, and inhaled nitric oxide was also started. The patient was evaluated for extracorporeal life support (ECLS). As the patient's oxygenation started improving on APRV and nitric oxide, and the patient had bloody secretions from endotracheal tube, the patient was continued on current supportive care. He was not started on ECLS on day 4 although patient's oxygenation marginally improved with $SaO_2 \geq$ 88–90%; the patient persisted to have blood secretions in the endotracheal tube with a drop in hematocrit. With all the cultures for infectious workup being negative, the patient was started on 4 doses rituximab 375 mg/m^2 weekly. The patient was initially unstable to be moved for CT scan. However, with patient's improvement after 7 days of admission, a CT scan was obtained which showed extensive ground glass opacities, alveolar infiltrates areas of lobular consolidation, and patchy nodular foci with interstitial wall thickening compatible with GPA.

The patient clinically improved after 2 doses of rituximab and was able to be weaned off a ventilator. Hemoglobin was stable. His repeat antineutrophil cytoplasmic antibodies

(c-ANCA) titer decreased to 1:80, antiproteinase antibodies (PR3) decreased to 8.7 U/mL, and CRP decreased to 4.0 mg/dL after therapy. The patient was able to be soon transferred out of the ICU in a stable condition. The patient received the third dose in the hospital and completed his last dose as an outpatient. The patient's repeat of PR3 further decreased to 4.0 U/mL.

3. Discussion

GPA is an organ and a life-threatening autoimmune disease. It was previously named after Dr. Friedrich Wegener as Wegener's granulomatosis. However, in a recent effort to have vasculitis nomenclature free of eponyms it was changed to the current name of GPA [2]. It is typically characterized by necrotizing granulomatous inflammation of the upper and lower respiratory tract, necrotizing glomerulonephritis, and an autoimmune necrotizing systemic vasculitis affecting predominantly small vessels. The American College of Rheumatology (ACR) classified GPA based on fulfilling at least 2 of 4 criteria. These criteria include the following:

  (a) nasal or oral inflammation with development of painful or painless oral ulcers or purulent or bloody nasal discharge;

  (b) abnormal chest radiograph showing the presence of nodules, fixed infiltrates, or cavities;

  (c) urinary sediment characterized by microhematuria (>5 red blood cells per high-power field) or red cell casts in urine sediment;

  (d) Granulomatous inflammation within the wall of an artery or in the perivascular or extravascular area (artery or arteriole) on biopsy [3].

The Chapel Hill Consensus (CHC) Conference defines GPA as associated with cytoplasmic pattern ANCA (c-ANCA). Both c-ANCA and PR3 antibodies are closely associated with GPA with 85–90% sensitivity and 95% specificity for generalized active disease [4].

The cause of GPA is not exactly known. GPA can occur at any age, but most often between the ages of 40 and 65. It is rare in children. The most common radiographic and CT abnormalities seen at presentation in up to 90% of patients are pulmonary nodules or consolidation with cavitation. Diffuse alveolar hemorrhage (DAH) is a less common presentation of GPA and is associated with a higher mortality [5].

DAH is a clinical-pathologic syndrome characterized by disseminated injury of the pulmonary capillaries leading to accumulation of intra-alveolar RBCs originating from the alveolar capillaries. The clinical syndrome includes hemoptysis, anemia, diffuse radiographic pulmonary infiltrates, and hypoxemic respiratory failure. Hemoptysis, however, may be initially absent in up to 33% of cases. The diagnosis is established after flexible bronchoscopy shows progressively hemorrhagic BAL in serial samples [6]. In subacute or recurrent episodes, hemosiderin-laden macrophages may be useful for diagnosis. More than or equal to 20% of siderophages are considered an easier determinant of the

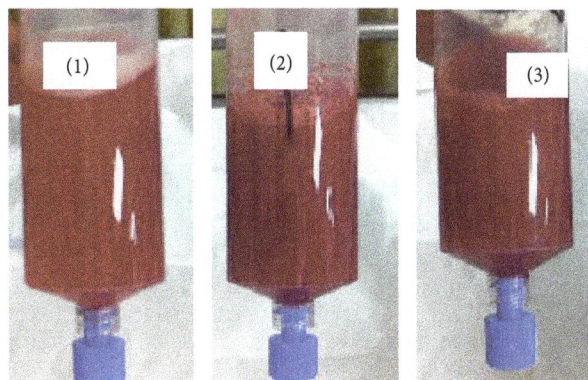

FIGURE 2: Bronchoscopy, bronchoalveolar lavage: The images show serial samples returned from bronchoalveolar lavage demonstrating progressive, hemorrhagic samples. These findings were consistent with diffuse alveolar hemorrhage.

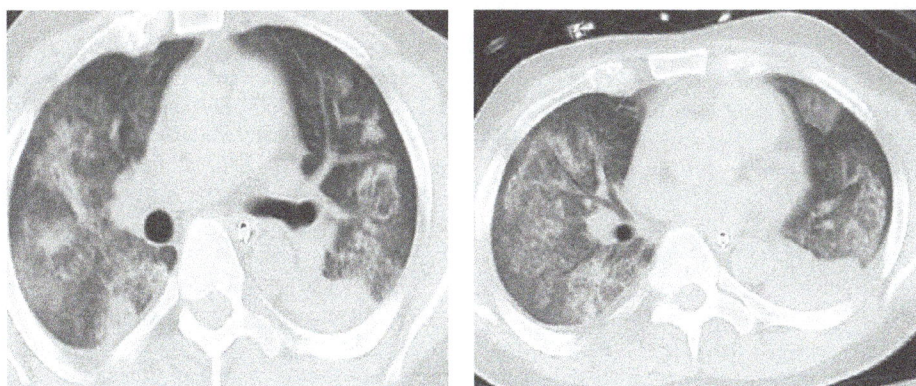

FIGURE 3

diagnosis of DAH [7]. The chest radiograph findings are nonspecific and consist of an alveolar filling process that can be a patchy, focal, or diffuse alveolar filling process (see Figure 3).

20–40% of GPA patients appear to be cured by conventional therapy. Immunosuppressive agents are the mainstay of therapy for DAH. Cyclophosphamide and corticosteroids with subsequent tapering, according to disease activity are the mainstay for the induction treatment in patients with severe organ and life-threatening disease manifestation. Maintenance therapy after remission is achieved either with methotrexate or azathioprine. However, disease flares are common. Treatment-induced side effects are a major cause of morbidity and mortality with conventional therapy. In patients with DAH and side effects from immunosuppressive drugs, there is a limited data for supportive management. Methotrexate should not be used in the acute setting of DAH [8].

Plasma exchange has also shown usefulness if instituted early in the disease course [9]. Recently, rituximab, a chimeric anti-CD20 monoclonal antibody, has been shown to induce remission in patients with refractory ANCA-associated granulomatous vasculitis. B-lymphocytes play a predominant role in autoimmune diseases. Rituximab is a chimeric monoclonal antibody directed against CD20 that leads to selective B-lymphocyte depletion. Rituximab may be considered for refractory GPA in patients not tolerating cyclophosphamide [10, 11].

In patients with persistent hypoxemic respiratory failure, the patients can be managed as per ARDS net protocol. However, as our patient was persistently hypoxemic his mode of ventilator was changed to airway pressure release ventilation (APRV). APRV has shown to improve oxygenation and decreased dead space ventilation in patients with refractory ARDS and can be used as an alternative mode in patients with refractory hypoxemia on traditional volume control [12, 13]. Steroids are routinely used as a part of induction remission for GPA and also recommended for moderate and severe ARDS [14]. Based on case reports, extracorporeal life support (ECLS) can also be considered in selected patients with pulmonary hemorrhage [15–17]. The cautious use of anticoagulation should be balanced with the risk of bleeding.

Our case illustrates a successful use of rituximab in addition to the supportive treatment as an effective remission induction agent for severe GPA with DAH and refractory hypoxemic respiratory failure.

Acknowledgment

The authors would like to thank Dr. Ashok Kirumaki, M.D., and Dr. Katherine Temprano, M.D.

References

[1] J. H. Stone, "Limited versus severe Wegener's granulomatosis: baseline data on patients in the Wegener's granulomatosis etanercept trial," *Arthritis and Rheumatism*, vol. 48, no. 8, pp. 2299–2309, 2003.

[2] R. J. Falk, W. L. Gross, L. Guillevin et al., "Granulomatosis with polyangiitis (wegener's): an alternative name for wegener's granulomatosis," *Arthritis and Rheumatism*, vol. 63, no. 4, pp. 863–864, 2011.

[3] R. Y. Leavitt, A. S. Fauci, D. A. Bloch et al., "The American College of Rheumatology 1990 criteria for the classification of Wegener's granulomatosis," *Arthritis and Rheumatism*, vol. 33, no. 8, pp. 1101–1107, 1990.

[4] K. Stephen Frankel, "The pulmonary vasculitides," *American Journal of Respiratory and Critical Care Medicine*, vol. 186, pp. 212–224, 2012.

[5] M. P. Chung, C. A. Yi, H. Y. Lee, J. Han, and K. S. Lee, "Imaging of pulmonary vasculitis," *Radiology*, vol. 255, no. 2, pp. 322–341, 2010.

[6] O. C. Ioachimescu and J. K. Stoller, "Diffuse alveolar hemorrhage: diagnosing it and finding the cause," *Cleveland Clinic Journal of Medicine*, vol. 75, no. 4, pp. 258–280, 2008.

[7] A. D. Lassence, J. Fleury-Feith, E. Escudier, J. Beaune, J. F. Bernaudin, and C. Cordonnier, "Alveolar hemorrhage: diagnostic criteria and results in 194 immunocompromised hosts," *American Journal of Respiratory and Critical Care Medicine*, vol. 151, no. 1, pp. 157–163, 1995.

[8] K. de Groot, N. Rasmussen, P. A. Bacon et al., "Randomized trial of cyclophosphamide versus methotrexate for induction of remission in early systemic antineutrophil cytoplasmic antibody-associated vasculitis," *Arthritis and Rheumatism*, vol. 52, no. 8, pp. 2461–2469, 2005.

[9] M. L. Krause, R. Cartin-Ceba, U. Specks, and T. Peikert, "Update on diffuse alveolar hemorrhage and pulmonary vasculitis," *Immunology and Allergy Clinics of North America*, vol. 32, pp. 587–600, 2012.

[10] R. Cartin-Ceba, F. C. Fervenza, and U. Specks, "Treatment of anti-neutrophil cytoplasmic antibody-associated vasculitis with rituximab," *Current Opinion in Rheumatology*, vol. 24, no. 1, pp. 15–23, 2012.

[11] K. A. Keogh, S. R. Ytterberg, F. C. Fervenza, K. A. Carlson, D. R. Schroeder, and U. Specks, "Rituximab for refractory Wegener's granulomatosis: report of a prospective, open-label pilot trial," *American Journal of Respiratory and Critical Care Medicine*, vol. 173, no. 2, pp. 180–187, 2006.

[12] E. M. Delgado, R. Cavallazzi, M. Baram, G. Gradwell, B. Dutill, and P. E. Marik, "Airway pressure release ventilation improves oxygenation and dead space ratio in medically critically ill patients with ards refractory to standard assist control mechanical ventilation," *Chest*, vol. 134, no. 4, p. 91002, 2008.

[13] N. Macintyre, "Guidelines for alternative modes of ventilation used in the management of patients with ARDS," http://www.thoracic.org/clinical/critical-care/salvage-therapies-h1n1/pages/alternative-modes.php.

[14] P. E. Marik, S. M. Pastores, D. Annane et al., "Recommendations for the diagnosis and management of corticosteroid insufficiency in critically ill adult patients: consensus statements from an international task force by the American College of Critical Care Medicine," *Critical Care Medicine*, vol. 36, no. 6, pp. 1937–1949, 2008.

[15] S. L. Barnes, M. Naughton, J. Douglass, and D. Murphy, "Extracorporeal membrane oxygenation with plasma exchange in a patient with alveolar hemorrhage secondary to Wegener's granulomatosis," *Internal Medicine Journal*, vol. 42, no. 3, pp. 341–342, 2012.

[16] S. H. Ahmed, T. Aziz, J. Cochran, and K. Highland, "Use of extracorporeal membrane oxygenation in a patient with diffuse alveolar hemorrhage," *Chest*, vol. 126, no. 1, pp. 305–309, 2004.

[17] M. Joseph and A. G. Charles, "Early extracorporeal life support as rescue for Wegener granulomatosis with diffuse alveolar hemorrhage and acute respiratory distress syndrome: a case report and literature review," *Pediatric Emergency Care*, vol. 27, no. 12, pp. 1163–1166, 2011.

The Wide and Unpredictable Scope of Synthetic Cannabinoids Toxicity

Jose Orsini, Christa Blaak, Eric Tam, Salil Rajayer, Joaquin Morante, Angela Yeh, and Ashvin Butala

Department of Medicine, New York University School of Medicine, Woodhull Medical and Mental Health Center, 760 Broadway, Brooklyn, NY 11206, USA

Correspondence should be addressed to Jose Orsini; jose.orsini@woodhullhc.nychhc.org

Academic Editor: Chiara Lazzeri

Drug use and abuse continue to be a large public health concern worldwide. Over the past decade, novel or atypical drugs have emerged and become increasingly popular. In the recent past, compounds similar to tetrahydrocannabinoid (THC), the active ingredient of marijuana, have been synthetically produced and offered commercially as legal substances. Since the initial communications of their abuse in 2008, few case reports have been published illustrating the misuse of these substances with signs and symptoms of intoxication. Even though synthetic cannabinoids have been restricted, they are still readily available across USA and their use has been dramatically increasing, with a concomitant increment in reports to poison control centers and emergency department (ED) visits. We describe a case of acute hypoxemic/hypercapnic respiratory failure as a consequence of acute congestive heart failure (CHF) developed from myocardial stunning resulting from a non-ST-segment elevation myocardial infarction (MI) following the consumption of synthetic cannabinoids.

1. Introduction

Synthetic cannabinoids are a heterogeneous group of compounds developed to investigate possible therapeutic effects and to study endocannabinoid receptor systems. Clandestine laboratories subsequently utilized published data to developed synthetic cannabinoids variations marketed as designer drugs, which have been emerging as popular recreational drugs due to their easy accessibility and undetectability on standard toxicology screens. First sold under the name "Spice," the drug has evolved into many different names (e.g., Black Diamond, Mojo, Spice Gold, Aroma, Dream, Genie, and Silver). K2 or "Spice" is made of a C8 homolog of the nonclassical cannabinoid CP-47, 497, 497-C8 (cannabicyclohexanol) and a cannabimimetic aminoalkylindole called JWH-018 [1]. They were distributed and sold legally in local smoke shops and gas stations in the USA until November 2010, when they were classified by the USA Drug Enforcement Agency (DEA) as Schedule-I controlled substances. Unlike partial agonist THC molecules, synthetic cannabinoids act as full nonselective agonists of the CB-1 and CB-2 receptors, making the substance 2–100 times more potent and longer lasting than THC [2]. They achieve euphoric effects by inhibiting glutamate synthesis and neurotransmission in the hippocampus [3].

Case reports of synthetic cannabinoids abuse have described patients presenting with alterations in mood and perception [4], xerostomia [5], and tachycardia [6]. Less common signs of intoxication included hypertension, agitation, paranoia, and hypokalemia [6]. There have been few cases describing more drastic features of intoxication such as ST-segment elevation MI [7], recurrent seizures [8], acute kidney injury [9], self-mutilation [10], serotonin syndrome [11], and cardiac arrest [12]. It has been estimated that more than 11,000 patients per year consult ED services in USA because of the side effects of synthetic cannabinoids [13]. As of May 2015, more than 40 deaths related to the use and abuse of synthetic cannabinoids have been reported in USA [14].

We describe a patient with acute hypoxemic/hypercapnic respiratory failure resulting from acute CHF developed from myocardial stunning as a consequence of a non-ST-segment elevation MI after consumption of synthetic cannabinoids.

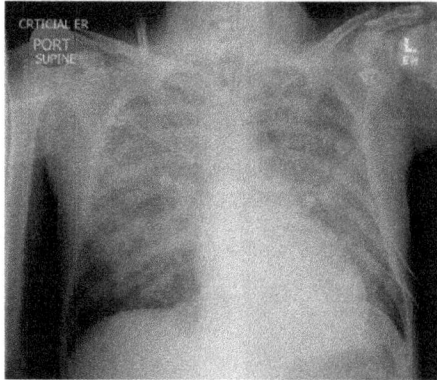

Figure 1: Initial CXR showing extensive bilateral infiltrates.

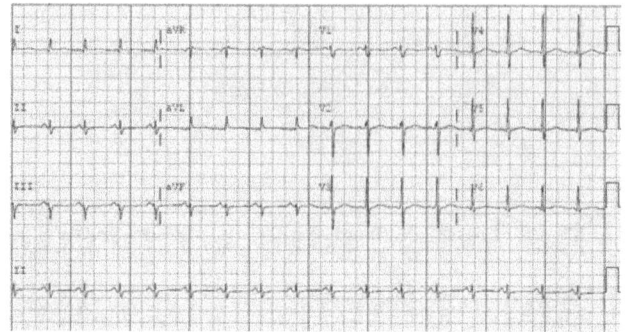

Figure 2: ECG showing sinus tachycardia without ST-segment or T-wave abnormalities.

2. Case Report

A 41-year-old Hispanic male was brought to our hospital ED after having a witnessed tonic-clonic seizure on the street. His past medical history was significant for polysubstance abuse (heroin, cocaine, benzodiazepines, and methadone) and chronic liver disease (hepatitis C). He had history of multiple admissions to our institution for opiates detoxification. On arrival to ED his vital signs were as follows: blood pressure of 98/63 mmHg, heart rate of 118 beats/minute, respiratory rate of 48 breaths/minute, temperature of 37.5°C, and an oxygen saturation of 90% while receiving oxygen by a non-rebreather mask. Emergency Medical Services (EMS) staffing reported finding a bag of K2 at the scene. Physical examination was remarkable for bilateral rales on lung auscultation. Old needle puncture areas were found over his arms and legs, without erythema. Pupils were equal with positive light reflex. While in ED, he was combative and developed another tonic-clonic seizure episode. Endotracheal intubation was performed and he was placed on mechanical ventilation. Remarkable laboratory findings included a white blood cell (WBC) count of 29.5 K/mm^3 (4.8–10.8), a bicarbonate level of 15 mmol/L (24–31), a lactic acid level of 4.4 mmol/L (0.5–2.2), and a urine toxicology screen positive for opiates, benzodiazepines, and methadone. Creatine kinase (CK) level was 5,590 U/L (25–215), and troponins were mildly elevated at 1.45 ng/mL (<0.1). Creatinine, coagulation, and liver function profiles were within normal limits. Arterial blood gas (ABG) while on mechanical ventilation and receiving FIO$_2$ of 100% showed a pH of 7.14 (7.35–7.45), a pCO$_2$ level of 79 mmHg (34–45), and a paO$_2$ level of 77 mmHg (80–100). Initial chest X-ray (CXR) showed bilateral infiltrates (Figure 1). Electrocardiogram (ECG) showed sinus tachycardia without ST-segment or T-wave abnormalities (Figure 2).

He was admitted to the intensive care unit (ICU) with the diagnosis of acute hypoxemic/hypercapnic respiratory failure presumptively secondary to drug overdose. He required propofol, fentanyl, and midazolam to achieve adequate sedation and ventilatory synchrony. Empiric intravenous antimicrobial therapy consisting of piperacillin/tazobactam (3.375 grams every 6 hours) was initiated for the possibility of aspiration pneumonitis. While in ICU, CK and troponin levels continued to increase to 18,589 U/L and 8.76 ng/mL,

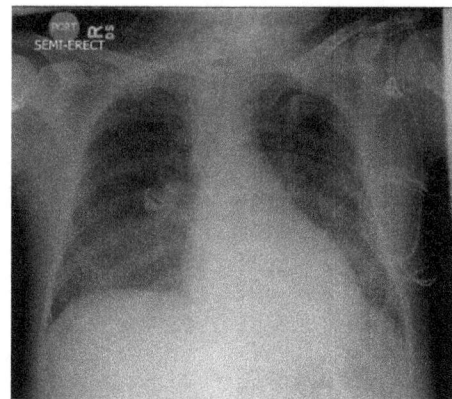

Figure 3: Follow-up CXR showing near resolution of bilateral infiltrates.

respectively. A new transthoracic echocardiogram (TTE) showed markedly decreased left ventricular ejection fraction of 30% (55–65), with severe global and segmental hypokinesis and no vegetations or valvular dysfunction. Given the echocardiographic and CXR findings as well as the elevated troponin levels, therapy for acute congestive heart failure probably secondary to a non-ST-segment elevation MI was initiated with low-molecular weight heparin, β-blockers, aspirin, clopidogrel, diuretics, statins, and angiotensin-converting enzyme (ACE) inhibitors. Repeated CXR after 24 hours showed near resolution of bilateral infiltrates (Figure 3). Blood, urine, and respiratory cultures were negative and antimicrobials were discontinued. He was extubated on day 4 of ICU admission but required reintubation because of severe agitation and hypoxemia, which were thought to be a clinical component of a possible withdrawal syndrome. His ICU course was further complicated by fevers, new bilateral infiltrates on CXR, and persistently elevated FIO$_2$ requirements. TTE was repeated, showing a remarkable improvement of left ventricular ejection fraction (63%), with a complete resolution of wall motion abnormalities. He was successfully extubated on day 11 of ICU admission, after being treated for acute respiratory distress syndrome (ARDS) secondary to ventilator-associated pneumonia.

3. Discussion

It is known that marijuana has pathophysiological effects on the cardiovascular system, which are mediated by stimulation of the sympathetic nervous system through release of nore-pinephrine and by parasympathetic blockade [15]. Marijuana consumption increases oxygen demands on the myocardium and also leads to an increase in carboxyhemoglobin levels, which results in decreased oxygen-carrying capacity [16, 17]. Interference with the integrity of peripheral vascular response has been postulated to be one of the mechanisms for cardiac events during cannabis smoking [14]. THC may also be associated with vascular inflammation and increased platelet activation, which is a potential mechanism of plaque rupture [18]. Few cases of MI associated with marijuana use have been reported in the literature [19–22]. Myocardial ischemia has also been reported with the use of synthetic cannabinoids [7, 23, 24]. In a large epidemiological study, THC and derivatives were reported to increase the risk of MI by 4.8 times in the first hour after use [25]. Given the presence of other substances in the urine toxicology screen which have been linked to acute coronary events, it was challenging to categorize the etiology of our patient's cardiovascular findings. Information about heroin-related MI is limited and its mechanisms are not well established. It has been postulated that heroin might have a direct toxic effect on the coronary arteries leading to coronary occlusion, either by provoking a local coronary spasm or inflammation [26]. The hypothesis of heroin-related myocardial injury might include rhabdomyolysis with cardiac involvement, hypoxia, acidosis, and vasoconstrictive substances released by muscle necrosis [27]. This hypothesis may explain the findings of rhabdomyolysis, hypoxia, and acidosis on the patient described in this report. However, the fact that our patient's pupils were not constricted and a bag of K2 was found at the scene makes heroin a less likely etiology for this patient's cardiac abnormalities. Although cases of myocardial ischemia possibly related to methadone use have been reported [28, 29], it has been proposed that methadone possesses cardioprotective properties that include reduction in infarct size in patients with myocardial infarction [30]. Cocaine was not found in the urine toxicology screen in our patient, which makes that substance an extremely unlikely cause for this patient's cardiovascular derangements.

To the best of our knowledge, this is the first report of synthetic cannabinoid-induced non-ST-segment elevation MI resulting in myocardial stunning and acute CHF in a patient without proven history of coronary artery disease. We hypothesized that our patient likely had transient myocardial ischemia resulting in ventricular stunning that might had led to acute CHF. This hypothesis is supported by the fact that subsequent troponin levels normalized within 48 hours and repeated TTE showed complete resolution of wall motion abnormalities with normal left ventricular ejection fraction. Patients with non-ST-segment elevation MI may present with heterogeneous conditions and, therefore, they may have varying degrees of reduction of coronary blood flow but without complete coronary occlusion in combination with distal embolization of thrombotic material and accompanying coronary spasm. In addition, myocardial necrosis (expressed by troponin elevation) may occur in the absence of coronary thrombosis but in the presence of stable but diffuse coronary artery disease and clinical conditions that increase myocardial demands (type-2 MI). Although the most common ECG findings in patients with non-ST-segment elevation MI are ST-segment depression and T-wave inversion, the presence of a normal ECG does not exclude the diagnosis of non-ST-segment elevation MI. Some studies have shown that approximately 1%–6% of patients with normal ECGs are found to have either an acute MI or unstable angina [31, 32].

Even though the main limitation of this report is the lack of biological testing of the patient's blood specimen, our subject's toxidrome fits perfectly with K2 overdose. Agitation and tachycardia are known side effects of synthetic cannabinoids [6]. Seizures have been reported in patients with synthetic cannabinoids intoxication [8, 33]. Rhabdomyolysis has been described in individuals abusing synthetic cannabinoids [9, 34]. Surely, the tonic-clonic seizures our patient developed contributed to the elevated CK levels. It is possible that myositis secondary to an autoimmune reaction to some of the inhaled antigens contained in synthetic cannabinoids may have played a role in the etiology of our patient's rhabdomyolysis. Another potential limitation of this paper is the lack of further follow-up studies such as coronary angiography and cardiac magnetic resonance imaging.

Our patient displayed other interesting clinical findings not commonly described in the literature. Based on a MED-LINE search and using the words "hypoxemia", "hypercapnea", "respiratory failure", and "synthetic cannabinoids", hypoxemic and/or hypercapnic respiratory failure has been infrequently reported in association with the consumption of synthetic cannabinoids. Berkowitz et al. reported a case series of patients with hypoxemic respiratory failure following the inhalation of synthetic cannabinoids [35]. Similarly, Alhadi et al. described another case of hypoxemia after the use of cannabinoids [36]. Hypoxemia related to synthetic cannabinoids use has also been outlined by Aksel et al. [37]. Diffuse miliary-micronodular infiltrates and centrilobular nodules with tree-in-bud pattern are the most common radiologic findings in patients with respiratory failure resulting from the use of synthetic cannabinoids [35]. The effects of synthetic cannabinoids on respiratory function have not been extensively detailed in humans and likely involve multiple mechanisms. Studies in rats demonstrated a marked respiratory depression, characterized by a decrease in respiratory rate, hypoxia, hypercapnea, and acidosis. Synthetic cannabinoids effect on peripheral receptors, such as chemo- and baroreceptors, increased airway resistance in bronchi, making CB-1 receptors stimulation a possible hypothesis for synthetic cannabinoid-induced respiratory depression [38]. Chemical gases released after inhalation of these substances may also cause damage to the bronchiolar epithelium, leading to acute respiratory distress that may progress to respiratory failure. We hypothesized that the etiology of respiratory failure in our patient was most likely acute congestive heart failure triggered by synthetic cannabinoids overdose.

4. Conclusion

This case illustrates to health care workers the possible life-threatening adverse effects of synthetic cannabinoids abuse. Although there is no specific toxidrome associated with synthetic cannabinoids intoxication, clinicians should suspect their involvement in patients presenting with signs and symptoms of drug overdose. Health care providers, especially those working in ED and critical care settings, should be on alert for drug-induced toxicities. Further research is needed to identify which contaminants are usually found in synthetic cannabinoids and to understand the interaction between different types of these substances to better predict adverse outcomes.

References

[1] S. Dresen, N. Ferreirós, M. Pütz, F. Westphal, R. Zimmermann, and V. Auwärter, "Monitoring of herbal mixtures potentially containing synthetic cannabinoids as psychoactive compounds," *Journal of Mass Spectrometry*, vol. 45, no. 10, pp. 1186–1194, 2010.

[2] M. S. Castaneto, D. A. Gorelick, N. A. Desrosiers, R. L. Hartman, S. Pirard, and M. A. Huestis, "Synthetic cannabinoids: epidemiology, pharmacodynamics, and clinical implications," *Drug and Alcohol Dependence*, vol. 144, pp. 12–41, 2014.

[3] A. F. Hoffman, A. C. Riegel, and C. R. Lupica, "Functional localization of cannabinoid receptors and endogenous cannabinoid production in distinct neuron populations of the hippocampus," *The European Journal of Neuroscience*, vol. 18, no. 3, pp. 524–534, 2003.

[4] D. Koethe, C. W. Gerth, M. A. Neatby et al., "Disturbances of visual information processing in early states of psychosis and experimental delta-9-tetrahydrocannabinol altered states of consciousness," *Schizophrenia Research*, vol. 88, no. 1–3, pp. 142–150, 2006.

[5] D. M. Berlach, Y. Shir, and M. A. Ware, "Experience with the synthetic cannabinoid nabilone in chronic noncancer pain," *Pain Medicine*, vol. 7, no. 1, pp. 25–29, 2006.

[6] M. Hermanns-Clausen, S. Kneisel, B. Szabo, and V. Auwärter, "Acute toxicity due to the confirmed consumption of synthetic cannabinoids: clinical and laboratory findings," *Addiction*, vol. 108, no. 3, pp. 534–544, 2013.

[7] A. Mir, A. Obafemi, A. Young, and C. Kane, "Myocardial infarction associated with use of the synthetic cannabinoid K2," *Pediatrics*, vol. 128, no. 6, pp. e1622–e1627, 2011.

[8] M. E. Bernson-Leung, L. Y. Leung, and S. Kumar, "Synthetic cannabis and acute ischemic stroke," *Journal of Stroke and Cerebrovascular Diseases*, vol. 23, no. 5, pp. 1239–1241, 2014.

[9] G. K. Bhanushali, G. Jain, H. Fatima, L. J. Leisch, and D. Thornley-Brown, "AKI associated with synthetic cannabinoids: a case series," *Clinical Journal of the American Society of Nephrology*, vol. 8, no. 4, pp. 523–526, 2013.

[10] K. A. Meijer, R. R. Russo, and D. V. Adhvaryu, "Smoking synthetic marijuana leads to self-mutilation requiring bilateral amputations," *Orthopedics*, vol. 37, no. 4, pp. e391–e394, 2014.

[11] C. D. Rosenbaum, S. P. Carreiro, and K. M. Babu, "Here today, gone tomorrow...and back again? A review of herbal marijuana alternatives (K2, Spice), synthetic cathinones (bath salts), kratom, *Salvia divinorum*, methoxetamine, and piperazines," *Journal of Medical Toxicology*, vol. 8, no. 1, pp. 15–32, 2012.

[12] S. Ibrahim, F. Al-Saffar, and T. Wannenburg, "A unique case of cardiac arrest following K2 abuse," *Case Reports in Cardiology*, vol. 2014, Article ID 120607, 3 pages, 2014.

[13] L. Fattore and W. Fratta, "Beyond THC: the new generation of cannabinoid designer drugs," *Frontiers in Behavioral Neuroscience*, vol. 5, article 60, 2011.

[14] J. Trecki, R. R. Gerona, and M. D. Schwartz, "Synthetic cannabinoid-related illnesses and deaths," *The New England Journal of Medicine*, vol. 373, no. 2, pp. 103–107, 2015.

[15] A. Gash, J. S. Karliner, D. Janowsky, and C. R. Lake, "Effects of smoking marihuana on left ventricular performance and plasma norepinephrine: studies in normal men," *Annals of Internal Medicine*, vol. 89, no. 4, pp. 448–452, 1978.

[16] J. L. Weiss, A. M. Watanabe, L. Lemberger, N. R. Tamarkin, and P. V. Cardon, "Cardiovascular effects of delta-9-tetrahydrocannabinol in man," *Clinical Pharmacology & Therapeutics*, vol. 13, no. 5, pp. 671–684, 1972.

[17] P. F. Renault, C. R. Schuster, R. Heinrich, and D. X. Freeman, "Marihuana: standardized smoke administration and dose effect curves on heart rate in humans," *Science*, vol. 174, no. 4009, pp. 589–591, 1971.

[18] M. A. Mittleman, M. Maclure, J. B. Sherwood et al., "Triggering of acute myocardial infarction onset by episodes of anger. Determinants of myocardial infarction onset study investigators," *Circulation*, vol. 92, no. 7, pp. 1720–1725, 1995.

[19] G. Kocabay, M. Yildiz, N. E. Duran, and M. Ozkan, "Acute inferior myocardial infarction due to cannabis smoking in a young man," *Journal of Cardiovascular Medicine*, vol. 10, no. 9, pp. 669–670, 2009.

[20] L. Bachs and H. Morland, "Acute cardiovascular fatalities following cannabis use," *Forensic Science International*, vol. 124, no. 2-3, pp. 200–203, 2001.

[21] Y. Velibey, S. Sahin, O. Tanik, M. Keskin, O. Bolca, and M. Eren, "Acute myocardial infarction due to marijuana smoking in a young man: guilty should not be underestimated," *American Journal of Emergency Medicine*, vol. 33, no. 8, pp. 1114.e1–1114.e3, 2015.

[22] C. J. Hodcroft, M. C. Rossiter, and A. N. Buch, "Cannabis-associated myocardial infarction in a young man with normal coronary arteries," *Journal of Emergency Medicine*, vol. 47, no. 3, pp. 277–281, 2014.

[23] R. G. McKeever, D. Vearrier, D. Jacobs, G. LaSala, J. Okaneku, and M. I. Greenberg, "K2-not the spice of life; synthetic cannabinoids and ST elevation myocardial infarction: a case report," *Journal of Medical Toxicology*, vol. 11, no. 1, pp. 129–131, 2015.

[24] B. C. Clark, J. Georgekutty, and C. I. Berul, "Myocardial ischemia secondary to synthetic cannabinoid (K2) use in pediatric patients," *The Journal of Pediatrics*, vol. 167, no. 3, pp. 757.e1–761.e1, 2015.

[25] M. A. Mittleman, R. A. Lewis, M. Maclure, J. B. Sherwood, and J. E. Muller, "Triggering myocardial infarction by marijuana," *Circulation*, vol. 103, no. 23, pp. 2805–2809, 2001.

[26] J. Sztajzel, H. Karpuz, and W. Rutishauser, "Heroin abuse and myocardial infarction," *International Journal of Cardiology*, vol. 47, no. 2, pp. 180–182, 1994.

[27] R. Melandri, I. De Tommaso, I. Zele et al., "Myocardial involvement in rhabdomyolysis caused by acute heroin intoxication," *Recenti Progressi in Medicina*, vol. 82, no. 6, pp. 324–327, 1991.

[28] D. G. Ioseliani, S. P. Semitko, D. G. Gromov et al., "Development of transmural myocardial infarction in young persons with intact coronary arteries during methadone use for the treatment of heroine addiction," *Kardiologiia*, vol. 44, no. 10, pp. 107–112, 2004.

[29] M. Backmund, K. Meyer, W. Zwehl, O. Nagengast, and D. Eichenlaub, "Myocardial infarction associated with methadone and/or dihydrocodeine," *European Addiction Research*, vol. 7, no. 1, pp. 37–39, 2001.

[30] E. R. Gross, A. K. Hsu, and G. J. Gross, "Acute methadone treatment reduces myocardial infarct size via the δ-opioid receptor in rats during reperfusion," *Anesthesia and Analgesia*, vol. 109, no. 5, pp. 1395–1402, 2009.

[31] G. W. Rouan, T. H. Lee, E. F. Cook, D. A. Brand, M. C. Weisberg, and L. Goldman, "Clinical characteristics and outcome of acute myocardial infarction in patients with initially normal or nonspecific electrocardiograms (a report from the Multicenter Chest Pain Study)," *The American Journal of Cardiology*, vol. 64, no. 18, pp. 1087–1092, 1989.

[32] B. D. McCarthy, J. B. Wong, and H. P. Selker, "Detecting acute cardiac ischemia in the emergency department: a review of the literature," *Journal of General Internal Medicine*, vol. 5, no. 4, pp. 365–373, 1990.

[33] C. R. Harris and A. Brown, "Synthetic cannabinoid intoxication: a case series and review," *Journal of Emergency Medicine*, vol. 44, no. 2, pp. 360–366, 2013.

[34] B. Sweeney, S. Talebi, D. Toro et al., "Hyperthermia and severe rhabdomyolysis from synthetic cannabinoids," *American Journal of Emergency Medicine*, 2015.

[35] E. A. Berkowitz, T. S. Henry, S. Veeraraghavan, G. W. Staton, and A. A. Gal, "Pulmonary effects of synthetic marijuana: chest radiography and CT findings," *American Journal of Roentgenology*, vol. 204, no. 4, pp. 750–757, 2015.

[36] S. Alhadi, A. Tiwari, R. Vohra, R. Gerona, J. Acharya, and K. Bilello, "High times, low sats: diffuse pulmonary infiltrates associated with chronic synthetic cannabinoid use," *Journal of Medical Toxicology*, vol. 9, no. 2, pp. 199–206, 2013.

[37] G. Aksel, Ö. Güneysel, T. Taşyürek, E. Kozan, and Ş. E. Çevik, "Intravenous lipid emulsion therapy for acute synthetic cannabinoid intoxication: clinical experience in four cases," *Case Reports in Emergency Medicine*, vol. 2015, Article ID 180921, 5 pages, 2015.

[38] K. Schmid, N. Niederhoffer, and B. Szabo, "Analysis of the respiratory effects of cannabinoids in rats," *Naunyn-Schmiedeberg's Archives of Pharmacology*, vol. 368, no. 4, pp. 301–308, 2003.

3

Internal Maxillary Artery Pseudoaneurysm: A Near Fatal Complication of Seemingly Innocuous Pharyngeal Trauma

M. P. Hennus[1] and L. Speleman[2]

[1] Department of Pediatric Intensive Care, Wilhelmina Children's Hospital, University Medical Center Utrecht, P.O. Box 85090, 3508 AB Utrecht, The Netherlands
[2] Department of Pediatric Otorhinolaryngology, Wilhelmina Children's Hospital, University Medical Center Utrecht, P.O. Box 85090, 3508 AB Utrecht, The Netherlands

Correspondence should be addressed to M. P. Hennus, m.p.hennus@umcutrecht.nl

Academic Editors: C. Mammina and A. J. Reddy

A 2-year-old boy presented with persistent pain and oral blood loss after falling with a toothbrush in his mouth. Initial routine inspection of the oropharynx showed no abnormalities. Recurrent blood loss instigated a reinspection under general anesthesia revealing the head of the toothbrush embedded in the nasopharynx. The toothbrush was removed without problems but several hours later a near fatal rebleeding occurred, requiring aggressive fluid resuscitation. Subsequently, the patient was transferred to our pediatric intensive care unit for further evaluation and treatment. CT angiography (CTA) showed a pseudoaneurysm of the internal maxillary artery which was successfully coiled, and further recovery was uneventful. Pediatric pharyngeal trauma is a common entity with rare, but potentially life-threatening, complications. In case of pharynx lesions, bleeding, and persistent pain, flexible endoscopy by an otolaryngologist is mandatory. In case of persistent bleeding vascular imaging is essential with CTA being a reliable alternative for the more invasive angiography.

1. Introduction

Pediatric pharyngeal trauma is relatively common in young children and usually caused by stick-like objects. Fortunately, most injuries are confined to mucosal and/or dermal surfaces and recovery is often uneventful without need for interventions. However rare, potentially devastating complications do occur, even in seemingly innocuous injuries. The first and most common complication is development of free air in the neck (subcutaneous emphysema) and/or chest (pneumomediastinum), which can lead to acute airway obstruction [1–4]. Furthermore, infections like retropharyngeal abscesses or mediastinitis may occur [1–4]. Vascular damage however, poses the greatest risk and is potentially life threatening [3, 5–9]. This paper not only illustrates how a common and seemingly innocuous injury can prove to be nearly fatal, it also emphasizes the need for vascular imaging in case of persistent blood loss after pharyngeal trauma.

2. Case Presentation

A previously healthy 2-year-old boy presented at the emergency department of a local hospital with persistent pain and oral blood loss after an unwitnessed fall. Immediately afterwards, he was found crying with only the base of a toothbrush in his hand. The head of the previously intact toothbrush was missing. During initial inspection of the oral cavity, the bleeding had stopped and no abnormalities were seen by the otolaryngologist. Although the parents repeatedly expressed their concern about their son's persisting abnormal behavior and the still missing head of the toothbrush, the patient was discharged with instructions to return to the hospital in case of a fever and/or recurrent blood loss. That same night, the boy started vomiting fresh blood and was taken to the hospital by ambulance. Again the bleeding had stopped spontaneously but the persistent character of the blood loss initiated a reinspection of the oronasopharynx under general anesthesia by an otolaryngologist. This revealed the missing

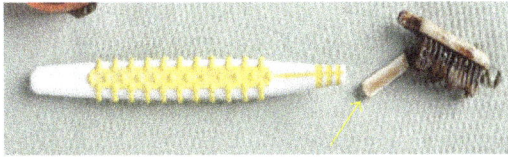

FIGURE 1: On the right, pieces of the head of the toothbrush (yellow arrow) immediately after removal from the patients oronasopharyngeal junction. On the left, the base of the toothbrush which the patient was found holding after his fall.

head of the toothbrush (Figure 1) lodged horizontally in the lateral walls of the nasopharynx with its sharp end embedded in the left lateral pharyngeal wall. It was removed without problems, making a small lesion visible in the left pharyngeal wall. The patient was successfully extubated and transferred to the pediatric ward.

Several hours afterwards however, he started vomiting large amounts of blood again, rapidly leading to progressive lethargy, tachycardia, and severe hypotension. Because of life-threatening hypovolemic shock with a hemoglobin level of 2.9 mmol/L, large amounts of intravenous saline and an unmatched blood transfusion were given. Crash reintubation followed, and during a second reinspection of the oro- and nasopharynx the bleeding again had stopped spontaneously. The site of the previous blood loss could not be identified. A Bellocq tampon was left in place and given the hemodynamic instability, and the still unknown origin of the massive bleeding the patient was transferred to our pediatric intensive care unit.

On admission, the patient was hemodynamically stable without signs of persisting blood loss, and invasive interventions were withheld. Mechanical ventilation was continued, antimicrobial therapy was started, and the Bellocq tampon was to be removed 48 hours later. That night however, during routine endotracheal suctioning, the patient started to cough inducing pulsatile oral blood loss suspect for an arterial vascular injury. The bleeding was successfully controlled, and subsequently a CT angiography (CTA) of the head and neck was performed. This showed a long, hypodense region in the right nasopharynx suspect for a hematoma as well as an aneurysmatic dilatation of the origin of the right internal maxillary artery (Figure 2). The subsequently performed conventional angiography confirmed the presence of an internal maxillary artery pseudoaneurysm, approximately 2 cm after the bifurcation of the arteria carotis communis which was successfully coiled (Figure 3). Two days later the Bellocq tampon was removed without problems, and a week after the initial fall, the patient could be extubated. He was discharged just 4 days after extubation. Clinical followup shortly after discharge and 1 year after the incident revealed no sequelae.

3. Discussion

Our patient survived a near fatal bleeding from an internal maxillary artery pseudoaneurysm resulting from a seemingly innocuous injury after a fall with a toothbrush in his mouth.

The incidence of pharyngeal trauma in young children is probably underreported. The initial trauma is usually unwitnessed and patients only present in case of persistent pain, dysphagia, or blood loss. Although the injuries are mostly confined to mucosal and/or dermal surfaces, seemingly innocuous injuries can result in severe blood loss and/or neurological deficits.

A careful medical history, including the time and cause of the incident as well as the initial and presenting complaints, is essential. Furthermore, persisting parental concern, especially when based on persisting complaints or abnormal behavior of their child as in this case, should always alert the physician. Routine inspection of the oral cavity and pharynx, even when meticulously performed, is not sufficient in pharyngeal trauma with persistent complaints. Here endoscopic inspection of the whole oro-, naso-, and hypopharynx is warranted. Unfortunately, vascular lesions can develop, even in the absence of a visible pharyngeal lesion: our patients' pseudoaneurysm was located on the right side of the pharynx and not on the left where the sharp, broken end of the toothbrush had left a small mucosal lesion. Compression of the carotid artery between the foreign body and the transverse process of a cervical vertebrae, namely, can result in an intimal tear in the vessel. This so-called "shearing effect" can lead to a pseudoaneurysm, dissection, and/or thrombosis of the vessel itself with the subsequent risk of migration of (a part of) the thrombus to the cerebral vessels [5].

Neurological complications develop in the first 3 to 60 hours after the initial trauma. This lucid period is believed to correlate with the time needed for formation and propagation of the thrombus [1]. Anticoagulants are recommended in the presence of a pseudoaneurysm and/or thrombus but only when the risk of an ischemic infarct outweighs the risk of a hemorrhagic infarct [1, 3, 4, 6]. Blood loss due to dissection of a vessel or pseudoaneurysm, as seen in our patient, also occurs within these first 60 hours. When refraining from admitting a patient, it is mandatory to provide parents or caregivers with necessary information concerning this lucid period, possible complications, and instructions how to act when problems occur.

Although the incidence of vascular injuries following pharyngeal trauma is less than 1% [2, 3], the sequelae can be disastrous [7–9]. Unfortunately, prognostic (risk) factors enabling early detection of vascular injuries before the onset of neurological signs and symptoms are still lacking [2]. Imaging studies are warranted in recurrent or persistent blood loss. The "gold standard" in diagnosing internal carotid artery damage is angiography, an invasive and rather time-consuming procedure with a small, but not neglectable, risk of neurological complications. A CTA offers a quick and effective alternative, which can be followed by an (intervention) angiography when a vascular injury is suspected [2, 10].

In conclusion, pediatric pharyngeal trauma is a common entity with rare, but potentially severe, complications. Vascular injuries can develop even in the absence of visible pharyngeal lesions. A thorough history and physical examination including inspection of the oro-naso-hypopharynx

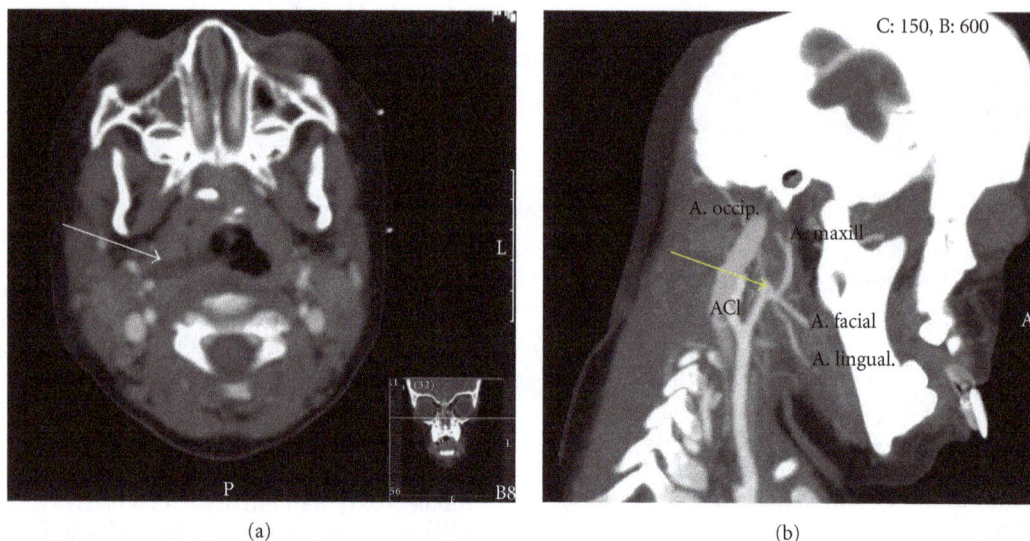

FIGURE 2: CT angiography of the head and neck showing a hematoma shaped like the head of the toothbrush in the right nasopharynx (white arrow) and the aneurysmatic dilatation of the origin of the internal maxillary artery (yellow arrow).

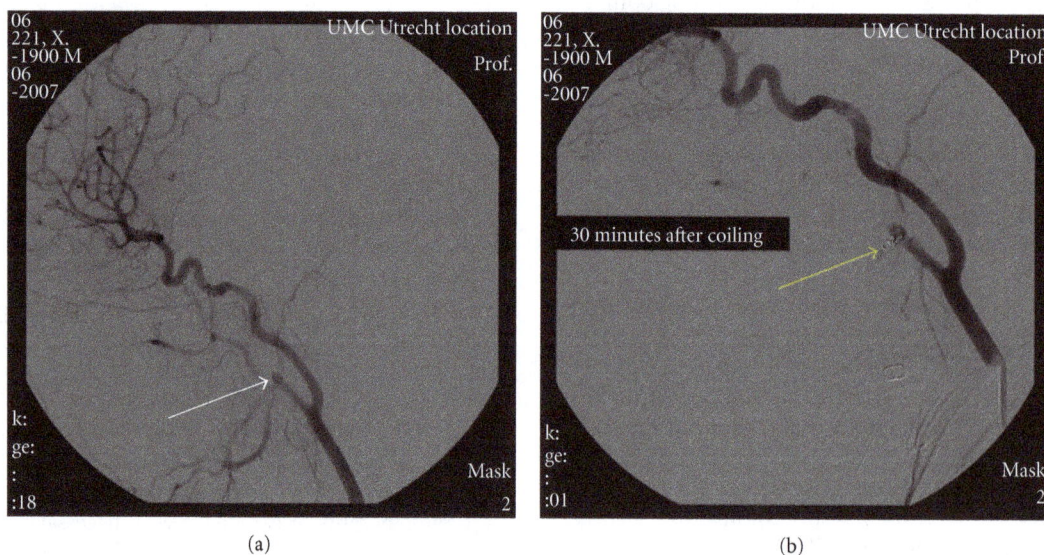

FIGURE 3: Conventional angiography of the head and neck showing the pseudoaneurysm at the base of the internal maxillary artery (white arrow) and the coil (yellow arrow) closing the pseudoaneurysm successfully.

are warranted. Flexible endoscopy by an otolaryngologist is mandatory in case of pharynx lesions, bleeding, and persistent pain. Vascular imaging is essential in persistent blood loss, with CTA offering a reliable alternative to the more invasive angiography. Given the possible lucid period in a vascular injury between the initial trauma and the development of sequelae, it is essential, when refraining from hospital admission, to provide parents or caregivers with the necessary information concerning these complications and with instructions how to act when problems do occur.

Acknowledgments

The authors would like to thank N. J. G. Jansen M.D., Ph.D., A. M. Schilder, M.D., Ph.D., both Wilhelmina Children's Hospital, and Professor Dr. W. P. Mali, University Medical Center Utrecht, for their critical appraisal of this paper.

References

[1] J. R. Hellmann, S. R. Shott, and M. J. Gootee, "Impalement injuries of the palate in children: review of 131 cases," *International Journal of Pediatric Otorhinolaryngology*, vol. 26, no. 2, pp. 157–163, 1993.

[2] R. J. Soose, J. P. Simons, and D. L. Mandell, "Evaluation and management of pediatric oropharyngeal trauma," *Archives of Otolaryngology—Head and Neck Surgery*, vol. 132, no. 4, pp. 446–451, 2006.

[3] D. A. Randall and D. R. Kang, "Current management of penetrating injuries of the soft palate," *Otolaryngology—Head and Neck Surgery*, vol. 135, no. 3, pp. 356–360, 2006.

Internal Maxillary Artery Pseudoaneurysm: A Near Fatal Complication of Seemingly...

13

[4] S. R. Schoem, S. S. Choi, G. H. Zalzal, and K. M. Grundfast, "Management of oropharyngeal trauma in children," *Archives of Otolaryngology—Head and Neck Surgery*, vol. 123, no. 12, pp. 1267–1270, 1997.

[5] S. Pitner, "Carotid thrombosis due to intraoral trauma. An unusual complication of a common childhood accident," *The New England Journal of Medicine*, vol. 274, no. 14, pp. 764–767, 1966.

[6] D. L. Suskind, M. A. Tavill, J. L. Keller, and M. B. Austin, "Management of the carotid artery following penetrating injuries of the soft palate," *International Journal of Pediatric Otorhinolaryngology*, vol. 39, no. 1, pp. 41–49, 1997.

[7] J. Caldwell, "Posttraumatig thrombosis of internal carotid artery," *The American Journal of Surgery*, vol. 32, no. 3, pp. 522–523, 1956.

[8] G. Higgins and J. Meredith, "Internal carotid artery thrombosis following penetrating trauma of the soft palate: an injury of youth," *Journal of Family Practice*, vol. 32, no. 3, pp. 316–322, 1991.

[9] C. Graham, J. Schwartz, and T. Stacy, "Stroke following oral trauma in children," *Annals of Emergency Medicine*, vol. 20, no. 9, pp. 1029–1031, 1991.

[10] S. E. Brietzke and D. T. Jones, "Pediatric oropharyngeal trauma: what is the role of CT scan?" *International Journal of Pediatric Otorhinolaryngology*, vol. 69, no. 5, pp. 669–679, 2005.

4

Alveolar Capillary Dysplasia with Misalignment of Pulmonary Veins (ACD/MPV)

Joana Miranda,[1] **Gustavo Rocha,**[1,2] **Henrique Soares,**[1] **Ana Vilan,**[1] **Otília Brandão,**[3] and **Hercília Guimarães**[1]

[1] *Division of Neonatology, Hospital of São João, Faculty of Medicine, University of Porto, Porto, Portugal*
[2] *Division of Neonatology, Hospital of São João, Piso 2, Alameda Professor Hernâni Monteiro, 4200-319 Porto, Portugal*
[3] *Department of Pathology, Hospital of São João, Faculty of Medicine, University of Porto, Porto, Portugal*

Correspondence should be addressed to Gustavo Rocha; gusrocha@oninet.pt

Academic Editors: R. Abouqal, M. Egi, and C. Zauner

Alveolar capillary dysplasia with misalignment of pulmonary veins (ACD/MPV) is a rare, fatal, developmental lung disorder, which usually presents as persistent pulmonary hypertension of the newborn (PPHN) unresponsive to treatment. The authors present their own experience with three cases admitted during the last 15 years.

1. Introduction

Alveolar capillary dysplasia with misalignment of pulmonary veins (ACD/MPV; OMIM number 265380) is a rare, fatal, developmental lung disorder, which usually presents as persistent pulmonary hypertension of the newborn (PPHN) unresponsive to treatment [1, 2]. The majority of the reported cases have been associated with other multiple congenital nonlethal anomalies, most frequently involving the cardiovascular, gastrointestinal, urogenital, and musculoskeletal systems [1]. Increasing awareness of this clinical entity may prevent the use of more invasive and futile treatments, including extracorporeal membrane oxygenation (ECMO).

We present three cases of ACD/MPV associated with gastrointestinal and urological malformations. All the newborns had an overwhelming course, with PPHN and hypoxemia refractory to treatment. The diagnosis of ACD/MPV was established by autopsy.

2. Cases Report

2.1. Case Report 1. Full-term female newborn admitted to our NICU (Neonatal Intensive Care Unit) in 1997 was diagnosed with severe bilateral hydronephrosis. She was the second daughter of a young healthy, unrelated couple. On prenatal ultrasounds severe bilateral hydronephrosis and oligoamnios were detected. Delivery occurred by C section at 38-week gestational age. The Apgar score was 5/8 and birth weight 3170 g. During the first hours of life patient developed increasing respiratory distress, with hypoxemia and bradycardia, and was intubated and ventilated. Chest radiograph showed a mild haziness pattern and echocardiogram excluded structural heart disease and demonstrated signs of PPHN. At hour 30 of life a rapid clinical deterioration was observed, with refractory hypoxemia and persistent severe metabolic acidosis, despite ventilatory optimization. Antibiotic therapy with ampicillin and gentamicin was administered since admission to NICU and was later adjusted to ampicillin, cefotaxime, and amicacin. Septic workup was negative, including blood, urine, and cerebrospinal fluid cultures.

The planned renal ultrasound and voiding cystourethrography (VCUG) were not preformed since the patient's clinical condition deteriorated rapidly and newborn died on the second day of life.

On autopsy severe bilateral hydronephrosis was confirmed and signs of severe renal corticomedullary parenchyma atrophy were observed. Histologic evaluation of

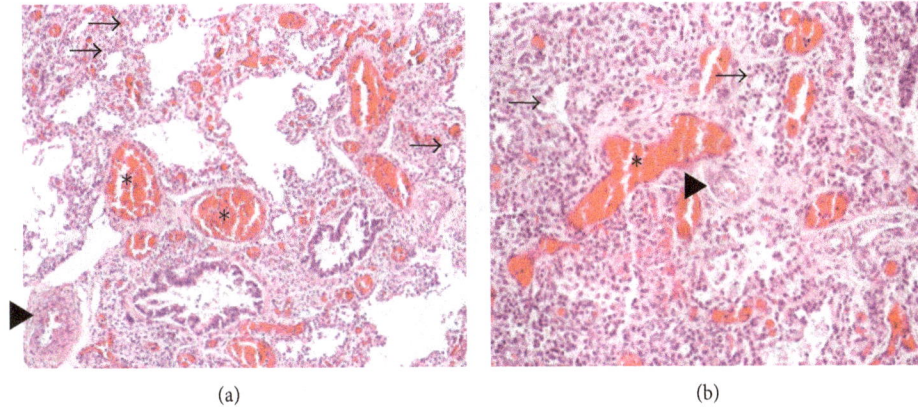

(a)   (b)

FIGURE 1: Case report 2: necropsy lung histology (hematoxylin and eosin staining) demonstrates the characteristic histologic features of ACD/MPV: thickened alveolar septae with scarce dilated pulmonary capillaries located away from the alveolar epithelium, with absence of the usual alveolar-capillary barrier (→); medial hypertrophy of small pulmonary arteries and muscularization of distal arterioles (▶); congested pulmonary veins malpositioned, adjacent to pulmonary arteries in the same adventitial sheath (∗); lymphangiectasis not present.

lung tissue showed the characteristic histological features of ACD/MPV.

2.2. Case Report 2.

A neonate was admitted to our NICU during 2011 for surgical correction of duodenal atresia. She was a 36-week gestational age female newborn, of birth weight of 3800 g, and of a healthy 15-year-old primigravida. After an uneventful pregnancy, the delivery occurred by vacuum extraction and the newborn required resuscitation with oxygen mask. The Apgar score was 5/9/9. The newborn was submitted to an exploratory laparotomy which detected a duodenal stenosis secondary to annular pancreas. A surgical correction with duodenoduodenostomy was performed.

By hour 9 of life, a rapidly increasing respiratory distress syndrome developed and she was started on mechanical ventilation with FiO_2 1.0. After surgery, a clinical picture of PPHN with increasing oxygenation index became obvious, corroborated by echocardiographic findings. The patient's condition progressively deteriorated despite aggressive treatment for severe pulmonary hypertension, including inotropic support with dopamine, dobutamine and noradrenalin, inhaled nitric oxide (up to 40 ppm), oral sildenafil (maximum 2 mg/kg/day), and nebulized iloprost (maximum 3 μg/kg/dose, 4/4 h). A diffuse reticulogranular pattern on chest radiographs became evident. Five doses of surfactant were administered. Infectious workup, metabolic screening, thyroid function, and cranial and abdominal ultrasounds were normal. Karyotype was 46,XX. The neonate presented an overwhelming course, with hypoxemia refractory to treatment, and died on day 15 of life.

Autopsy confirmed the annular pancreas and revealed an associated intestinal malrotation. The lung histology was diagnostic of ACD/MPV (Figure 1).

DNA sequence analysis was performed, applying the protocol described by Sen and colleagues [3]. DNA sequence analysis revealed a heterozygous nonsense mutation c.539C>A, p.S180X, in the first exon of *FOXF1*. The mutation was not present in the mother. The father, an unrelated, healthy 21-year-old, refused testing.

2.3. Case Report 3.

A male preterm newborn, of 34-week gestational age, with prenatal diagnosis of severe bilateral hydronephrosis associated with hydramnios, right pleural effusion, and ascites, was admitted to our NICU in 2012. Amniocentesis showed a normal karyotype (46, XY) and maternal serologic screening was negative. He was the first baby of a healthy young couple.

After a C-section delivery due to fetal distress, he presented with anasarca and respiratory distress, which improved temporarily with positive end-expiratory pressure during initial ventilation. The Apgar score was 2/8/8 and birth weight 2465 g.

During the first hour of life he was started on nasal CPAP, due to an increasing respiratory distress syndrome. Although, at hour 6 of life patient required intubation and mechanical ventilation owing to a persistent pulmonary hypertension, with increasing oxygenation index. Echocardiographic evaluation revealed a severe PPHN with a normal cardiac anatomy and chest radiographs showed ground glass opacities and right pleural effusion (Figure 2(a)). A rapidly increasing FiO_2 to 1.0 was required and at hour 22 of life inhaled nitric oxide with 20 ppm was initiated, which was later increased to 40 ppm. Surfactant was administered twice. Nevertheless a severe hypoxemia refractory to treatment was settled. Cardiorespiratory arrest occurred on the second day of life, requiring respiratory and cardiac resuscitation with chest compressions and adrenaline. Pneumomediastinum with spontaneous resolution was observed, (Figure 2(b)). On the third day of life the newborn died after an unsuccessful trial of high-frequency oscillatory ventilation.

To investigate prenatal diagnosis of hydronephrosis a postnatal renal ultrasound and a VCUG were performed. The postnatal ultrasound revealed bilateral renal dilatation, with loss of corticomedullary differentiation, marked calyceal dilatation (renal pelvis anteroposterior diameter in the right kidney 35 mm and in the left kidney 25 mm), and ureteral dilatation. VCUG showed a bladder with an atypical morphology, elongated and irregular in its upper portion, but it was not suggestive of posterior urethral valves. To

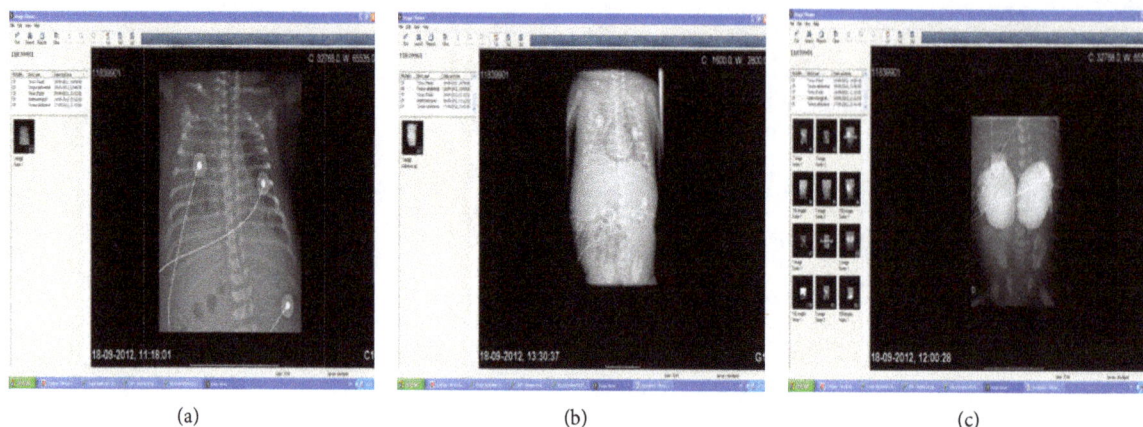

(a)   (b)   (c)

FIGURE 2: Case report 3: (a) chest radiograph with pulmonary ground glass opacities and right pleural effusion. (b) Chest radiograph showing pneumomediastinum. (c) Percutaneous nephrostomy using water-soluble contrast revealing very severe bilateral hydronephrosis.

complement the study, an ultrasound-guided percutaneous nephrostomy using water-soluble contrast was preformed, revealing a very severe bilateral hydronephrosis with obstruction to contrast flow from the renal pelvis to the proximal ureter, suggestive of ureteropelvic junction obstruction, (Figure 2(c)). Bilateral percutaneous nephrostomies kept functioning until newborn's death.

Treatment with ampicillin and cefotaxime was initiated on admission to NICU. Blood and urine cultures were negative. The morphological study, including cranial and abdominal ultrasounds, was normal.

On autopsy the lungs were both heavy and globoid on gross appearance and the histopathologic study showed the characteristic features of ACD/MPV. Giant hydronephrosis secondary to ureteropelvic junction obstruction was evident. Renal corticomedullary parenchyma was normally developed, however with secondary atrophy and rare cortical tubules with cystic dilatation.

Due to the fulminate course of the disease, DNA was not extracted to further analysis and metabolic screening was not preformed.

3. Discussion

Newborns affected with ACD/MPV develop respiratory distress and severe PPHN within the first 48 hours of life and die of respiratory failure within the first month of life, although longer survivals and later presentations have been reported [2, 4–6]. PPHN secondary to ACD/MPV may be difficult to distinguish from idiopathic PPHN. ACD/MPV should be suspected in patients with severe hypoxemia and PPHN who fail to improve with ventilatory support and pulmonary vasodilator therapy [2]. The clinical approach to infants with ACD/MPV is similar to other neonates presenting with PPHN, including inhaled nitric oxide, oral sildenafil, nebulized iloprost, and inotropic support with noradrenalin and milrinone. However, the response to this therapy is often minimal and not sustained, which may serve as an initial diagnostic clue. In some centres, ECMO is offered while awaiting definitive diagnosis. ACD/MPV should always

be considered in infants with idiopathic PPHN without sustained response to ECMO [2].

Histological examination of lung remains the gold standard for ACD/MPV diagnosis. Thus, approximately 90% of reported cases of ACD/MPV have been diagnosed on autopsy and 10% of diagnoses have been made from lung tissue obtained during *ante mortem* lung biopsy [2]. Histologically, ACD/ MPV is characterized by malpositioned (misaligned) pulmonary veins, paucity of capillaries close to the alveolar epithelium, anomalous distended pulmonary veins within the bronchovascular bundle instead of the interlobular septa, and immature alveolar development with medial thickening of small pulmonary arteries [1, 2]. ACD/MPV is a rare developmental disorder of the lung affecting both the parenchyma and the vasculature [7].

More than 80% of infants with ACD/MPV have multiple other congenital malformations [1]. All of our newborns presented with other congenital malformations; two of them presented with severe bilateral hydronephrosis and the other with annular pancreas, and intestinal malrotation, anomalies already reported in literature [2, 8–10].

DNA sequencing and comparative genomic hybridization have led to the identification of *FOXF1* as one of the genes responsible for ACD/MPV. Using array CGH analysis, Stankiewicz and colleagues identified six overlapping microdeletions encompassing the *FOX* transcription factor gene cluster in chromosome 16q24.1q24.2 in patients with ACD/MPV and multiple congenital anomalies. Subsequently, they identified four different heterozygous mutations in unrelated patients with sporadic ACD/MPV and multiple congenital anomalies [11].

Using DNA sequencing analysis we identify a new heterozygous nonsense mutation in the first exon of *FOXF1* gene, c.539C>A, p.S180X in the patient with ACD/MPV, annular pancreas, and intestinal malrotation.

Unfortunately, in the two patients with ACD/MPV and severe bilateral hydronephrosis we did not have the opportunity to perform DNA sequencing analysis. Patients with ACD/MPV and hydronephrosis had already been described with mutations in the *FOXF1* gene by Stankiewicz and colleagues [11], as well as with 16q24.1 microdeletion in a case reported by Zufferey and colleagues [10].

In conclusion, our experience with ACD/MPV is according to the rare nature of the disease. There is no pathognomonic laboratory or imaging criteria for the disease. Initial chest radiographs are often reported to be unremarkable or to show a mild haziness pattern. The deteriorating course is a challenging task for diagnosis and treatment. Management of infants with ACD/MPV is not different than management of other causes of PPHN. Histological examination of lung remains the gold standard for ACD/MPV diagnosis.

Abbreviations

ACD/MPV: Alveolar capillary dysplasia with misalignment of pulmonary veins
PPHN: Persistent pulmonary hypertension of the newborn
NICU: Neonatal intensive care unit
VCUG: Voiding cystourethrography
ECMO: Extracorporeal membrane oxygenation.

References

[1] J. M. Abu-Shaweesh, "Respiratory disorders in preterm and term infants," in *Fannaroff and Martin's Neonatal-Perinatal Medicine, Diseases of the Fetus and Infant*, R. J. Martin, A. A. Fanaroff, and M. C. Walsh, Eds., pp. 1141–1170, Elsevier Mosby, St Louis, Miss, USA, 9th edition, 2011.

[2] N. B. Bishop, P. Stankiewicz, and R. H. Steinhorn, "Alveolar Capillary dysplasia," *American Journal of Respiratory and Critical Care Medicine*, vol. 184, no. 2, pp. 172–179, 2011.

[3] P. Sen, R. Gerychova, P. Janku et al., "A familial case of alveolar capillary dysplasia with misalignment of pulmonary veins supports paternal imprinting of *FOXF1* in human," *European Journal of Human Genetics*. In press.

[4] H. I. Abdallah, N. Karmazin, and L. A. Marks, "Late presentation of misalignment of lung vessels with alveolar capillary dysplasia," *Critical Care Medicine*, vol. 21, no. 4, pp. 628–630, 1993.

[5] S. Ahmed, V. Ackerman, P. Faught, and C. Langston, "Profound hypoxemia and pulmonary hypertension in a 7-month-old infant: Late presentation of alveolar capillary dysplasia," *Pediatric Critical Care Medicine*, vol. 9, no. 6, pp. e43–e46, 2008.

[6] V. Shankar, A. Haque, J. Johnson, and J. Pietsch, "Late presentation of alveolar capillary dysplasia in an infant," *Pediatric Critical Care Medicine*, vol. 7, no. 2, pp. 177–179, 2006.

[7] P. Sen, T. Choudhury, E. O. Smith, and C. Langston, "Expression of angiogenic and vasculogenic proteins in the lung in alveolar capillary dysplasia/misalignment of pulmonary veins: An immunohistochemical study," *Pediatric and Developmental Pathology*, vol. 13, no. 5, pp. 354–361, 2010.

[8] P. Sen, N. Thakur, D. W. Stockton, C. Langston, and B. A. Bejjani, "Expanding the phenotype of alveolar capillary dysplasia (ACD)," *Journal of Pediatrics*, vol. 145, no. 5, pp. 646–651, 2004.

[9] B. Antao, M. Samuel, E. Kiely, L. Spitz, and M. Malone, "Congenital alveolar capillary dysplasia and associated gastrointestinal anomalies," *Fetal and Pediatric Pathology*, vol. 25, no. 3, pp. 137–145, 2006.

[10] F. Zufferey, D. Martinet, M. C. Osterheld et al., "16q24. 1 microdeletion in a premature newborn: usefulness of array-based comparative genomic hybridization in persistent pulmonary hypertension of the newborn," *Pediatric Critical Care Medicine*, vol. 12, no. 6, pp. e427–e432, 2011.

[11] P. Stankiewicz, P. Sen, S. S. Bhatt et al., "Genomic and genic deletions of the *FOX* gene cluster on 16q24.1 and inactivating mutations of *FOXF1* cause alveolar capillary dysplasia and other malformations," *American Journal of Human Genetics*, vol. 84, no. 6, pp. 780–791, 2009.

5

Contained Left Ventricular Free Wall Rupture following Myocardial Infarction

Arthur Shiyovich[1] and Lior Nesher[1, 2]

[1] Internal Medicine E, Soroka University Medical Center, P.O. Box 151, 84101 Beer Sheva, Israel
[2] Department of Emergency Medicine, Rekanati School for Community Health Professions, Faculty of Health Sciences,
  Ben-Gurion University of the Negev, 84105 Beer Sheva, Israel

Correspondence should be addressed to Arthur Shiyovich, arthur.shiyovich@gmail.com

Academic Editors: Y. D. Durandy, Z. Molnar, and S. Natoli

Rupture of the free wall of the left ventricle occurs in approximately 4% of patients with infarcts and accounts for approximately 20% of the total mortality of patients with myocardial infractions. Relatively few cases are diagnosed before death. Several distinct clinical forms of ventricular free wall rupture have been identified. Sudden rupture with massive hemorrhage into the pericardium is the most common form; in a third of the cases, the course is subacute with slow and sometimes repetitive hemorrhage into the pericardial cavity. Left ventricular pseudoaneurysms generally occur as a consequence of left ventricular free wall rupture covered by a portion of pericardium, in contrast to a true aneurysm, which is formed of myocardial tissue. Here, we report a case of contained left ventricular free wall rupture following myocardial infarction.

1. Introduction

Rupture of the free wall of the left ventricle occurs in approximately 4% of patients with myocardial infarction (MI) and accounts for approximately 20% of mortality of these patients [1, 2]. Premortem diagnosis of rupture is made in approximately 15% of in-hospital deaths from acute MI in a coronary care unit [3]. However, one series of autopsies claims that up to 31% of MI fatalities had cardiac rupture. Hence, relatively few cases of left ventricular free wall rupture (LVFWR) are diagnosed before death. Nevertheless, the increased availability of bedside echocardiography has contributed to a progressive rise in the number of cases of LVFWR being diagnosed and reported. Several distinct clinical forms of ventricular free wall rupture have been identified [4]. Sudden rupture with massive hemorrhage into the pericardium is the most common form; in a third of the cases, the course is subacute with slow and sometimes repetitive hemorrhage into the pericardial cavity [5]. Left ventricular pseudoaneurysm is a variant of left ventricular rupture that generally occurs as a consequence of LVFWR covered by a portion of pericardium. Here, we report a case of contained left ventricular free wall rupture following myocardial infarction.

2. Patient Description

An 80-year-old retired female resident of a home for the aged was admitted with recent complaints of dyspnea, dizziness, and a falling episode with a possible loss of consciousness. Her personal history revealed mild dementia, Parkinson's disease treated with carbidopa and levodopa, hypertension treated by nifedipine, and dyslipidemia treated by statins. Additional medications included acetylsalicylic acid (100 mg qd), calcium supplements, and brotizolam as a sleep inducer. The patient did not take any other medication or vitamin supplements. At admission to the Emergency Department, the patient's respiratory rate was 16 breaths/min, blood pressure was 96/60 mm Hg, heart rate was regular at 100/min, room-air oxygen saturation was 92% and temperature was 36.7°C. Physical examination revealed no apparent distress, pale 80-year-old Caucasian female, good breath sounds bilaterally, heart sounds were regular

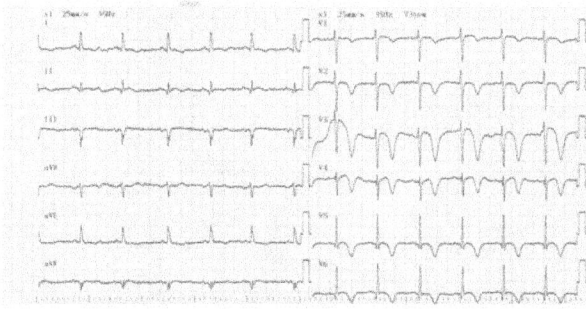

FIGURE 1: Twelve-lead ECG of the patient: sinus rhythm 73 p/minute, axis of 5 degrees with pathological Q waves in leads V4–V6, ST-segment elevations in leads V1–V3, and T wave inversions in V1–V6 and in leads I and AVL.

and distant, abdomen was nontender, no organomegaly was observed, and pulses were palpated as normal in the radial and femoral points of examination. A 12-lead electrocardiogram obtained in supine posture showed an axis of 5 degrees with pathological Q waves in leads V4–V6, ST-segment elevation in leads V1–V3, and T wave inversion in V1–V6 and in leads I and AVL (Figure 1). Cardiac enzymes were indicative of myocardial injury; troponin T levels were 1.93 ng/mL (normal 0–0.014); creatine kinase was 9684 U/L (normal 20–180 U/L); lactate dehydrogenase was 1443 U/L (normal 230–480); myoglobin was 1865 ng/mL (normal 19–51 ng/mL). Creatinine levels were 0.71 mg/dL (normal 0.51–0.95 mg/dL); urea was 57 mg/dL (normal 17–43 mg/dL). Liver function tests were mildly elevated. Aspartate aminotransferase was 217 U/L (normal 0–31 U/L); alanine transaminase was 84 (normal 0–34). Sodium was 129 mEq/L (normal 125–135), otherwise the complete blood count and electrolytes were all within normal limits. Chest X-ray image (Figure 2(a)) revealed a space-occupying lesion with clearly defined borders. The lesion was of single consistency without calcification. The lesion merged with the lower border of the heart situated at a wide angle to the shadow of the heart, appearing as a mass in the anterior middle mediastinum. Cranial computerized tomography (CT) scan, performed to rule out intracranial hemorrhage related to the falling episode, was interpreted as normal. The patient was admitted to a monitored bed. A chest CT scan with contrast material was performed. Frame 143 of the scan revealed a cystic process in the anterior middle mediastinal region with a double layer of fluid lucency, one of which is consistent with blood. The process merged with the left ventricle. CT Frame 205 of the same exam revealed thinning of the posterior lateral wall of the left ventricle with an aneurysm of approximately 50 millimeters, expanding from the left ventricle (Figure 2(b)). A transthoracic echocardiogram was performed that demonstrated severe left ventricular dysfunction, severe mitral regurgitation, moderate-to-severe pulmonary hypertension, and a huge left ventricular lateral wall aneurysm.

At this point, it was evident that the patient had a contained left ventricular free wall rupture following myocardial infarction. Following a detailed explantation of the

treatment options to the patient and her family, a noninvasive/nonsurgical treatment modality was chosen. Combined pharmacological therapy including acetylsalicylic acid (aspirin 100 mg), ACE inhibitor (ramipril 5 mg), diuretic (lasix 40 mg), and beta blocker (carvedilol 6.25 mg × 2) improved the patient's hemodynamic status and reduced the symptoms of heart failure (mostly dyspnea), additional treatment included a statin (simvastatin 20 mg), and a benzodiazepine for sleeping (britazolam 0.25 mg). After six days of hospitalization, the patient was discharged for ambulatory followup. Approximately two months following discharge, the patient was admitted with exacerbation of the heart failure complaints. Echocardiography demonstrated no change in the aneurysm or the ventricular function. Following an increase in the dose of the diuretics and stabilization of the symptoms, home oxygen was arranged and the patient was discharged.

3. Comment

Ventricular free wall rupture occurs up to ten times more frequently than septal or papillary muscle rupture [6]. It progresses from the endocardium to the pericardium and occurs through an area of necrosis. Risk factors for rupture include hypertension, older age, female sex, first infarction, anterior infarction, and large transmural infarction of at least 20% [7]. In the case considered here most of the risk factors were present.

Most ventricular ruptures occur within the first week after MI, approximately 50% within the initial four days; however, some cases have been reported as late as one month or even later. Acute LVFWR may present by chest pain, or by the classic features of cardiac tamponade, namely, shock with hypotension, pulsus paradoxus, elevated venous pressure, quiet heart sounds, sinus bradycardia, or frank electromechanical dissociation. Death usually ensues in a matter of minutes to hours. Cardiopulmonary resuscitation maneuvers are uniformly unsuccessful in these cases.

In the subacute form, the presentation may evolve over hours, days, or even longer. This form usually presents mainly with pericardial effusion signs and symptoms and may present with dysrhythmias, syncope, prolonged or recurrent chest pain (sometimes of the pericardial type), and heart failure [8]. In this form, the rupture is often sealed by the epicardium or alternatively by a haematoma in the epicardial surface of the heart, forming a contained myocardial rupture. Pathologically, this situation stands somewhere between free rupture into the pericardial cavity and formation of pseudoaneurysm [7].

Opinions differ as to the most common site of the left ventricular rupture. It was suggested that a lateral wall infarction is more likely to rupture than an anterior or inferior infarction. However, anterior MIs are more frequent than lateral MIs and thus the anterior wall is the most common site. Another possible explanation for the greater prevalence of posterior subacute ruptures is that ruptures of the anterior wall cannot be tolerated, as they are rarely compressed by an adherent pericardium. The inflammatory

(a) Chest X-ray

(b) Computerized tomography scan

(c) Computerized tomography scan

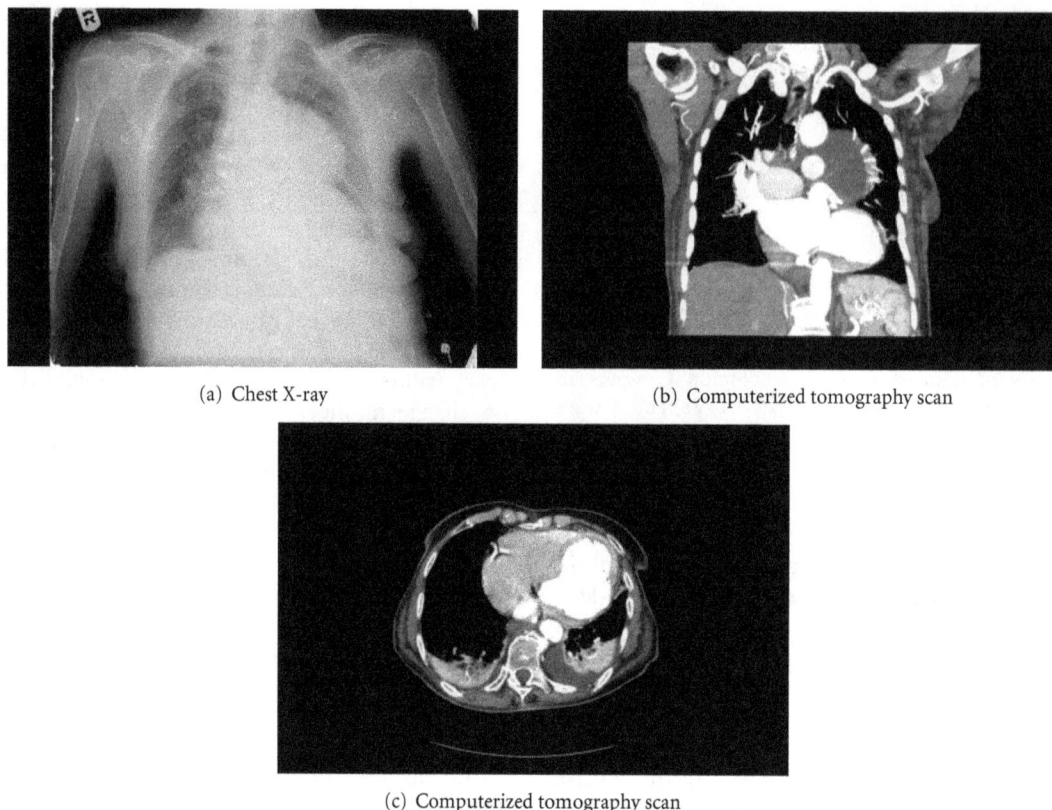

FIGURE 2: (a) A posterior-anterior X-ray of the chest which reveals a space-occupying lesion with clearly defined borders. The lesion is of single consistency without calcification and merges with the lower border of the heart situated at a wide angle to the shadow of the heart, appearing as a mass in the anterior middle mediastinum. (b) Computerized tomography scan reveals a cystic process in the anterior middle mediastinale region with a double layer of fluid, one of which is consistent with blood. The process merges with the left ventricle. (c) CT Frame 205 of the same exam revealed thinning of the posterior lateral wall of the left ventricle with an aneurysm of approximately 50 millimeters, expanding from the left ventricle.

reaction of the posterior pericardium might result in pericardial adhesions and formation of a posterior left ventricular pseudoaneurysm.

Electrocardiographic findings in LV rupture patients may be related to its type and severity. Electromechanical dissociation and bradycardia are features of the acute variety, while new ST elevation ("saddle shaped") in the affected leads or persistent noninversion of T waves may suggest the less noisy "stuttering" type of rupture.

Echocardiography (transthoracic or transesophageal) is usually the preferred imaging test when LVFWR is suspected and is considered highly accurate. Color flow imaging and pulsed Doppler may be useful in the assessment of flow characteristics at the presumed rupture site, and an intravenous echocardiographic contrast agent may be useful in identifying intrapericardial hemorrhage caused by myocardial rupture or the development of ventricular pseudoaneurysm. The most common finding is pericardial effusion and its absence excludes the diagnosis of ventricular rupture.

Recent evidence indicates that cardiac magnetic resonance imaging (MRI), especially with contrast enhancement, is emerging as a valuable diagnostic tool providing visualization of the entire heart and clear differentiation of

structures such as the pericardium, myocardium, thrombus, and epicardial fat [9, 10]. Clearly MRI is not the investigation of choice in acute patients with hemodynamic instability; however, in subacute cases, timely contrast-enhanced MRI may help to delineate the anatomical location of FWR and aneurismal change, thereby enabling planned surgical intervention. Additionally, it may identify areas of ischemic myocardium even in the absence of definite ECG findings and myocardium at risk of impending rupture.

Multidetector computed tomography has also been shown to be effective in detecting LVFWR and may assist in the diagnosis [11, 12], especially when MRI is not available or when time is imperative.

Early diagnosis is imperative in these cases as many ventricular ruptures may be surgically corrected with a good long-term outcome. Although it is a generally acceptable that surgery provides the only definitive treatment of subacute LVFWR [13], cases of patients with long-term survival following medical management have been reported. Medical management usually includes avoidance of obstipation, prolonged bed rest, strict blood pressure control (preferably with beta blockers), and pericardiocentesis as needed. The goals of surgery should be to stop bleeding, to relieve cardiac tamponade, and to prevent a second rupture. Multiple surgical techniques have been described but all involve extensive debridement into normal muscle, thrombectomy of the ventricle, and closure with or without a patch, with preservation of left ventricular geometry. Coronary angiography is also warranted in cases of ventricular rupture, in order to determine whether coronary artery bypass grafting is needed in addition to the repair of the rupture [13].

The overall hospital mortality in patients with and without surgery was reported to be approximately 60% [14]. Surgery-related mortality is up to 33% but in those who survive the complicated operation, the long-term outcome is good.

In conclusion, it remains clear that despite the significant risk, surgery is the cornerstone treatment of subacute LVFWR. Nevertheless, nonsurgical management may be considered for carefully selected patients, especially for those at high surgical risk. We believe it is imperative for physicians in various specialties to be well acquainted with this entity to be able to consider it in the differential diagnosis while there is still time to save these patients' lives.

References

[1] E. Eren, N. Bozbuga, M. E. Toker et al., "Surgical treatment of post-infarction left ventricular pseudoaneurysm: a two-decade experience," *Texas Heart Institute Journal*, vol. 34, no. 1, pp. 47–51, 2007.

[2] R. C. Becker, J. M. Gore, C. Lambrew et al., "A composite view of cardiac rupture in the United States National Registry of Myocardial Infarction," *Journal of the American College of Cardiology*, vol. 27, no. 6, pp. 1321–1326, 1996.

[3] S. G. Reddy and W. C. Roberts, "Frequency of rupture of the left ventricular free wall or ventricular septum among necropsy cases of fatal acute myocardial infarction since introduction of coronary care units," *American Journal of Cardiology*, vol. 63, no. 13, pp. 906–911, 1989.

[4] K. Balakumaran, C. J. Verbaan, C. E. Essed et al., "Ventricular free wall rupture: sudden, subacute, slow, sealed and stabilized varieties," *European Heart Journal*, vol. 5, no. 4, pp. 282–288, 1984.

[5] J. Lopez-Sendon, A. Gonzalez, E. Lopez de Sa et al., "Diagnosis of subacute ventricular wall rupture after acute myocardial infarction: sensitivity and specificity of clinical, hemodynamic and echocardiographic criteria," *Journal of the American College of Cardiology*, vol. 19, no. 6, pp. 1145–1153, 1992.

[6] R. J. Bates, S. Beutler, L. Resnekov, and C. E. Anagnostopoulos, "Cardiac rupture-challenge in diagnosis and management," *American Journal of Cardiology*, vol. 40, pp. 429–437, 1977.

[7] S. S. Chen, P. Ruengsakulrach, R. J. Dick, and B. F. Buxton, "Post-infarct left ventricular free wall rupture—not always a lethal complication of acute myocardial infarction," *Heart Lung and Circulation*, vol. 13, no. 1, pp. 26–30, 2004.

[8] D. Dubreuil, G. Gosselin, Y. Hébert, and L. P. Perrault, "Contained rupture of left ventricular false aneurysm after acute myocardial infarction secondary to left anterior descending artery embolism," *Canadian Journal of Cardiology*, vol. 24, no. 12, pp. e94–e95, 2008.

[9] A. A. Shiozaki, R. A. Filho, L. A. Dallan, S. A. de Oliveira, J. C. Nicolau, and C. E. Rochitte, "Left ventricular free-wall rupture after acute myocardial infarction imaged by cardiovascular magnetic resonance," *Journal of Cardiovascular Magnetic Resonance*, vol. 9, no. 4, pp. 719–721, 2007.

[10] U. Krishnan, G. P. McCann, M. Hickey, and M. Schmitt, "Role of contrast-enhanced magnetic resonance imaging in detecting early adverse remodeling and subacute ventricular wall rupture complicating myocardial infarction," *Heart and Vessels*, vol. 23, no. 6, pp. 430–432, 2008.

[11] R. Suzuki, A. Mikamo, H. Kurazumi, and K. Hamano, "Left ventricular free wall rupture detected by multidetector computed tomography after mitral valve replacement," *Journal of Cardiac Surgery*, vol. 25, no. 6, p. 699, 2010.

[12] R. A. Crossley, G. J. Morgan-Hughes, and C. A. Roobottom, "Post myocardial infarction left ventricular free wall rupture diagnosed by multidetector computed tomography," *Heart*, vol. 93, no. 6, p. 653, 2007.

[13] L. Raposo, M. J. Andrade, J. Ferreira et al., "Subacute left ventricle free wall rupture after acute myocardial infarction: awareness of the clinical signs and early use of echocardiography may be life-saving," *Cardiovascular Ultrasound*, vol. 4, article 46, 2006.

[14] J. Slater, R. J. Brown, T. A. Antonelli et al., "Cardiogenic shock due to cardiac free-wall rupture or tamponade after acute myocardial infarction: a report from the SHOCK Trial Registry," *Journal of the American College of Cardiology*, vol. 36, no. 3, pp. 1117–1122, 2000.

6

Boerhaave's Syndrome: Still a Diagnostic and Therapeutic Challenge in the 21st Century

J. Spapen,[1] J. De Regt,[2] K. Nieboer,[3] G. Verfaillie,[4] P. M. Honoré,[2] and H. Spapen[2]

[1] Department of Internal Medicine, University Hospital, Vrije Universiteit Brussel, Laarbeeklaan 101, 1090 Brussels, Belgium
[2] Department of Intensive Care, University Hospital, Vrije Universiteit Brussel, Laarbeeklaan 101, 1090 Brussels, Belgium
[3] Department of Radiology, University Hospital, Vrije Universiteit Brussel, Laarbeeklaan 101, 1090 Brussels, Belgium
[4] Department of Thoracic Surgery, University Hospital, Vrije Universiteit Brussel, Laarbeeklaan 101, 1090 Brussels, Belgium

Correspondence should be addressed to H. Spapen; herbert.spapen@uzbrussel.be

Academic Editors: M. Egi, P. Kopterides, C. Lazzeri, and C. Mammina

Boerhaave's syndrome is a rare but potentially fatal condition characterised by a transmural tear of the distal oesophagus induced by a sudden increase in pressure. Diagnosis is challenging as the classic triad of vomiting, abdominal or chest pain, and subcutaneous emphysema is absent in many patients. Management is multidisciplinary and relies on rapid, distinct, and repeated imaging. Treatment has not been standardised and may be conservative, endoscopic, or surgical. We present a typical case which illustrates possible diagnostic pitfalls and the therapeutic conundrum surrounding management of the syndrome. Based on time of presentation and eventual presence of sepsis, a therapeutic algorithm is proposed.

1. Introduction

Boerhaave's syndrome, first described in the 18th century by the Dutch physician Herman Boerhaave, refers to an oesophageal tear caused by an abrupt rise of intraluminal pressure [1]. It is a rare but life-threatening condition that requires urgent diagnosis and treatment. If treatment is delayed, severe and potentially lethal complications such as mediastinitis, pleural empyema, septic shock, and multiple organ failure may develop. A high index of suspicion is imperative for timely diagnosis and to assure well-selected radiological and endoscopic investigations. Prompt and adequate therapy reduces mortality. Some centers advocate early and extensive surgery as the cornerstone of treatment, yet others prefer a more conservative, endoscopic, or less invasive surgical approach. Such experience-based difference in attitude likely explains the lack of well-established treatment guidelines.

2. Case Report

A 41-year-old man with an extensive medical history, including Child-Pugh B liver cirrhosis and chronic pancreatitis, consulted his family doctor with progressive dyspnea, retrosternal pain radiating to the back, repeated vomiting, and fever for 3 days. On admission at the emergency ward, the patient appeared confused and agitated. Core temperature was 38.5°C, heart rate was regular at 150 beats/min, and respiratory rate was 40 breaths/min. Physical examination revealed a supple but tender abdomen, normal peristalsis, and muffled breath sounds over the right lung. Blood analysis showed macrocytic anemia, 18500 leukocytes/mm^3, normal enzymes, a C-reactive protein (CRP) of 303 mg/L, and a lactate level of 7.4 mmol/L. Chest X-ray showed a silhouette sign over the right heart border and small mediastinal radiolucent streaks of air (Figure 1). A contrast-enhanced computed tomography (CT) scan of the thorax confirmed the pneumomediastinum (Figure 2(a)) and showed a dilated oesophagus with a distal tear, bilateral pleural effusions, and heterogeneous retro- and paracardiac collections (Figure 2(b)). The diagnosis of Boerhaave's syndrome was made. Blood cultures were taken; intravenous antibiotic therapy (β-lactam + aminoglycoside) and ample fluid resuscitation were initiated. The patient was transferred to the ICU. Two hours after ICU admission, the patient became increasingly oxygen- and vasopressor-dependent. A

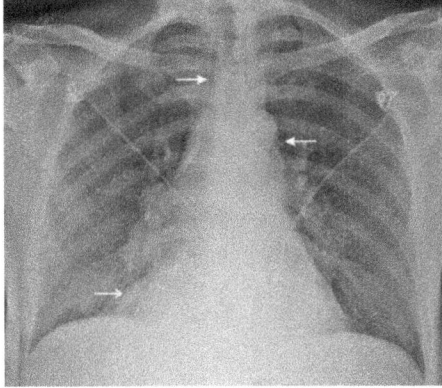

FIGURE 1: Chest X-ray at admission at the emergency ward showing a pneumomediastinum (closed arrows) and silhouette sign over the right heart border (open arrow). No pleural effusions were observed in the costolateral sinuses.

new chest X-ray revealed a rapidly evolving right pleural effusion (Figure 3). Subsequently, the patient was intubated and mechanically ventilated. A chest tube was inserted in the right pleural space. A brown, foul-smelling fluid was evacuated. The pleural fluid did not contain food particles, pH was 7, and amylase was 685 U/L. Gastroscopy confirmed an oesophageal tear in the lower one-third of the oesophagus. At that time, a severe concomitant mucosal inflammation precluded further endoscopic treatment because of a too high risk of oesophageal rupture. A control CT scan demonstrated a left-sided paravertebral encapsulated air-fluid collection and a left pleural effusion that had substantially increased in size. A pigtail catheter was inserted into the left pleural space. CT guided drainage of encapsulated pleural collections was performed. Four days after ICU admission, a self-expandable oesophageal stent was endoscopically placed. Despite stenting, continuous bilateral pleural drainage, and broad antimicrobial covering, the patient remained septic with hectic fever and persistently high leukocyte counts and CRP levels. Video-assisted thoracoscopic surgery was performed with drainage and rinsing of the mediastinum and pleural cavities. Thereafter, fever subsided and clinical and biological parameters progressively normalised. After an ICU stay of 33 days, the patient was discharged.

3. Discussion

Boerhaave's syndrome is a barogenic tear of the oesophagus caused by a sudden rise of intraluminal pressure in its distal end. It accounts for approximately 15% of all cases of oesophageal rupture and has a mortality rate up to 40%. In the majority of cases, the rupture is located in the left posterolateral wall of the distal third of the oesophagus [2].

Boerhaave's syndrome is readily suspected in a patient with a history of overindulgence in food or drinks who, after severe or repeated vomiting, experiences excruciating chest pain and develops subcutaneous emphysema [3]. However, up to one-third of patients have atypical symptoms or are admitted with severe respiratory distress and/or shock. The

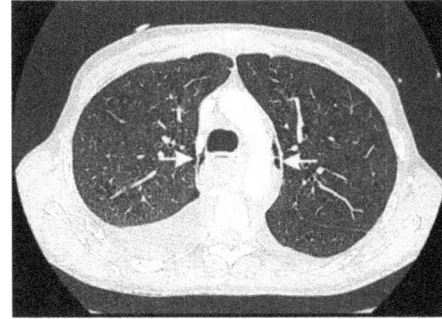

(a)

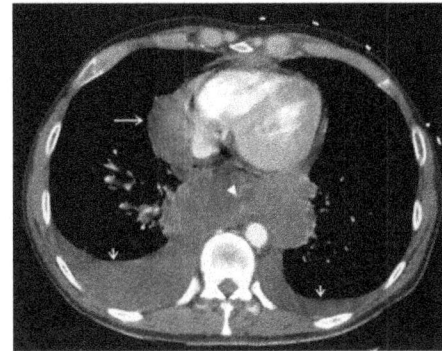

(b)

FIGURE 2: Contrast-enhanced CT scan of the thorax: (a) lung window, confirming pneumomediastinum (closed arrows), and (b) mediastinal window showing a tear in the right posterolateral wall of the distal oesophagus (arrowhead), bilateral pleural effusions (short arrows), massive retrocardiac collections, and a paracardial collection (open arrow) corresponding with the silhouette sign on chest X-ray.

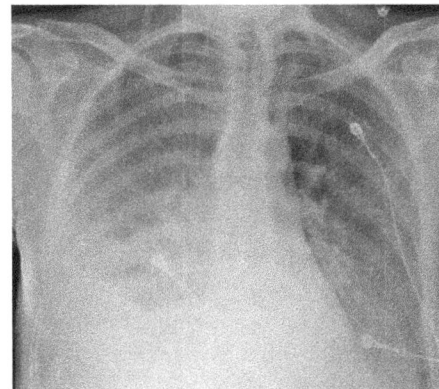

FIGURE 3: Chest X-ray, 2 h after admission, revealing a rapidly evolving right pleural effusion.

differential diagnosis of Boerhaave's syndrome includes a variety of acute thoracic and abdominal conditions including myocardial infarction, pulmonary embolus, dissecting aorta, ruptured aortic aneurysm, perforated peptic ulcer, Mallory-Weiss syndrome, pancreatitis, pneumonia, and spontaneous pneumothorax [4].

Standard treatment
• Cessation of oral intake
• Administration of fluids and parenteral nutrition
• Broad-spectrum antibiotics (consider antifungal prophylaxis)
• H_2-blockers

Sepsis

Yes   No

Diagnosis within 24 h   Diagnosis after 24 h

Patient's clinical condition   Yes   Widespread mediastinal and/or   Conservative
allows surgery   pleural contamination   Standard treatment
                                                                                              ± mediastinal and/or
                                                                                              pleural drainage

Yes   No   No

Surgery   Endoscopy   Clinical improvement without
(open thoracotomy or VATS)   If failure   ± pleural and/or   mediastinal and/or pleural
                                                   mediastinal drainage   contamination
Debridement and drainage of mediastinum
and/or pleural cavities
± resection of thoracic oesophagus with
reconstruction if large tear and extensive   No   Yes
necrosis

                                                                                        Continue conservative
                                                                                        treatment

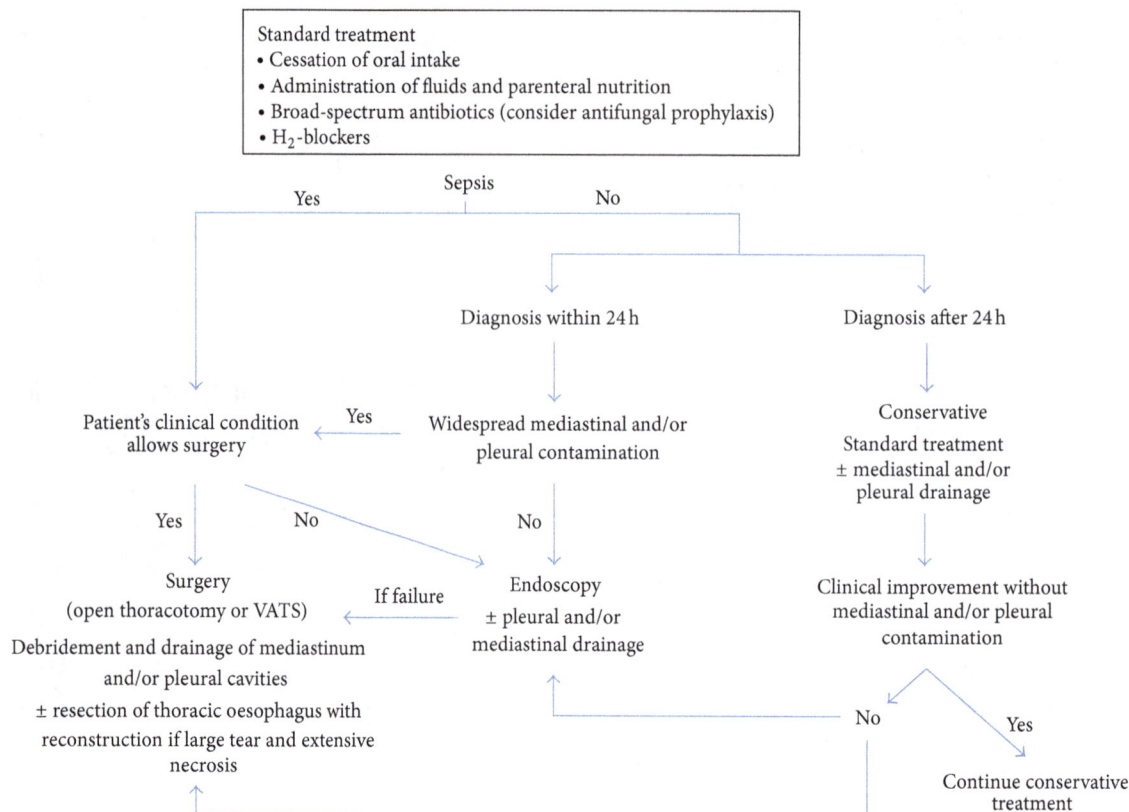

FIGURE 4: Boerhaave's syndrome treatment algorithm.

On physical examination, patients generally appear acutely ill with tachycardia and tachypnea. Fever may be present or not. Auscultation occasionally reveals decreased breath sounds on the perforation side. When mediastinal emphysema is present, Hamman's sign (i.e., a mediastinal "crackling" accompanying every heart beat) may be heard in left lateral decubitus position [2].

Blood laboratory tests are of little help to support the diagnosis, except for excluding other pathologies (e.g., myocardial infarction, pancreatitis). Presence of food particles, a high amylase content, and a low pH in pleural fluid are either highly confirmatory or very suggestive of oesophageal perforation [2, 3].

Imaging is of key importance for diagnosis. Plain chest X-rays may reveal subcutaneous and/or mediastinal emphysema, mediastinal widening, pleural effusion(s), pneumothorax, hydrothorax, and intrathoracic air-fluid levels or masses [5]. In 20% of cases, a "V sign" is noticed which appears as a radiolucent streak of air dissecting the retrocardiac fascial planes [6]. A rapidly developing or evolving effusion requires urgent investigation. Importantly, up to 15% of patients have normal chest roentgenograms. CT scanning of thorax and mediastinum has largely replaced the former gastrografin swallow tests. CT indeed allows a more detailed assessment of the lungs, mediastinum, pleura, and aorta. CT also is more sensitive than plain radiography for detection of small amounts of paraspinal or pleural air-fluid collections [7]. Finally, endoscopy enables direct visualisation of the location

and extent of the perforation but must be performed with caution since it may potentially aggravate the oesophageal tear.

Management of Boerhaave's syndrome remains a controversial issue. Basically, three levels of treatment are distinguished: a conservative, an endoscopic, and a surgical approach [8, 9]. Conservative treatment consists of cessation of oral intake, administration of fluids and parenteral nutrition, broad-spectrum antibiotics, H_2-blockers, and eventual mediastinal, pleural, or abscess drainage. It can be offered to selected, nonseptic patients with a small or well-contained perforation [10]. Endoscopic therapy is increasingly used in patients whose perforation is diagnosed early without widespread contamination and sepsis. Endoluminal placement of a self-expandable metallic stent to bridge an oesophageal tear has shown encouraging results. Yet, endoscopic stenting in Boerhaave's syndrome has a rather undetermined and center-dependent success rate and may not be devoid of side effects such as enhanced mediastinal or pleural contamination and accidental stent migration [11]. Finally, surgical treatment ranges from a less invasive approach consisting of debridement and drainage of mediastinum and pleural cavities to extensive resection of the thoracic oesophagus [8, 9, 12]. Factors determining surgical intervention are the extent of the perforation, eventual concomitant pathologies that require synchronous management, the degree of mediastinal or pleural contamination, and the presence of sepsis. Abbas et al. advocate primary surgical repair when patients present with sepsis, large uncontained leaks, and extensive contamination [13]. Based on a literature review, de Schipper et al. propose to perform surgery (i.e., open thoracotomy with resection, hemifundoplication, and pleural/mediastinal drainage) in patients diagnosed early (<48 h), regardless sepsis is present or not, and in patients diagnosed beyond 48 h who remain or become septic under conservative treatment [14]. Experience with less invasive surgical procedures is scarce. Haveman et al. compared open thoracotomy with video-assisted thoracoscopic surgery (VATS) and found similar success rates [15]. More prospective studies are warranted to establish the potential advantage of VATS in treating patients with Boerhaave's syndrome. To deal with single incident cases, a treatment algorithm is composed and presented in Figure 4. According to this algorithm, it could be argued that early surgical intervention might have been the preferred optimal first-line treatment in our patient.

4. Conclusion

Boerhaave's syndrome still represents a diagnostic and therapeutic challenge. Timely recognition shouldered by repeated radiological imaging is an important prognostic determinant. The choice of treatment depends upon critical and continuous assessment of the patient's clinical status, the extent and duration of the leak, and the presence of sepsis. Minimally or less invasive treatment options have been applied successfully, but their impact must be evaluated in prospective trials.

References

[1] V. J. Derbes and R. E. Mitchell Jr., "Hermann Boerhaave's (1) *Atrocis, nec Descripti Prius, Morbi Historia* (2) the first translation of the classic case report of rupture of the esophagus, with annotations," *Bulletin of the Medical Library Association*, vol. 43, no. 2, pp. 217–240, 1955.

[2] J. J. Curci and M. J. Horman, "Boerhaave's syndrome: the importance of early diagnosis and treatment," *Annals of Surgery*, vol. 183, no. 4, pp. 401–408, 1976.

[3] J. A. M. Henderson and A. J. M. Peloquin, "Boerhaave revisited: spontaneous esophageal perforation as a diagnostic masquerader," *The American Journal of Medicine*, vol. 86, no. 5, pp. 559–567, 1989.

[4] R. B. Brauer, D. Liebermann-Meffert, H. J. Stein, H. Bartels, and J. R. Siewert, "Boerhaave's syndrome: analysis of the literature and report of 18 new cases," *Diseases of the Esophagus*, vol. 10, no. 1, pp. 64–68, 1997.

[5] N. Ghanem, C. Altehoefer, O. Springer et al., "Radiological findings in Boerhaave's syndrome," *Emergency Radiology*, vol. 10, no. 1, pp. 8–13, 2003.

[6] E. A. Naclerio, "The "v sign" in the diagnosis of spontaneous rupture of the esophagus (an early roentgen clue)," *The American Journal of Surgery*, vol. 93, no. 2, pp. 291–298, 1957.

[7] F. Fadoo, D. E. Ruiz, S. K. Dawn, W. R. Webb, and M. B. Gotway, "Helical CT esophagography for the evaluation of suspected esophageal perforation or rupture," *The American Journal of Roentgenology*, vol. 182, no. 5, pp. 1177–1179, 2004.

[8] D. Wolfson and J. S. Barkin, "Treatment of Boerhaave's syndrome," *Current Treatment Options in Gastroenterology*, vol. 10, no. 1, pp. 71–77, 2007.

[9] P. W. Carrott Jr. and D. E. Low, "Advances in the management of esophageal perforation," *Thoracic Surgery Clinics*, vol. 21, no. 4, pp. 541–555, 2011.

[10] J. P. Platel, P. Thomas, R. Giudicelli, J. Lecuyer, A. Giacoia, and P. Fuentes, "Oesophageal perforation and rupture: a plea for conservative management," *Annales de Chirurgie*, vol. 51, no. 6, pp. 611–616, 1997.

[11] E. Johnsson, L. Lundell, and B. Liedman, "Sealing of esophageal perforation or ruptures with expandable metallic stents: a prospective controlled study on treatment efficacy and limitations," *Diseases of the Esophagus*, vol. 18, no. 4, pp. 262–266, 2005.

[12] J. Jougon, T. Mc Bride, F. Delcambre, A. Minniti, and J. F. Velly, "Primary esophageal repair for Boerhaave's syndrome whatever the free interval between perforation and treatment," *European Journal of Cardiothoracic Surgery*, vol. 25, no. 4, pp. 475–479, 2004.

[13] G. Abbas, M. J. Schuchert, B. L. Pettiford et al., "Contemporaneous management of esophageal perforation," *Surgery*, vol. 146, no. 4, pp. 749–756, 2009.

[14] J. P. de Schipper, A. F. Pull ter Gunne, H. J. M. Oostvogel, and C. J. H. M. van Laarhoven, "Spontaneous rupture of the oesophagus: Boerhaave's syndrome in 2008—literature review and treatment algorithm," *Digestive Surgery*, vol. 26, no. 1, pp. 1–6, 2009.

[15] J. W. Haveman, V. B. Nieuwenhuijs, J. P. M. Kobold, G. M. van Dam, J. T. Plukker, and H. S. Hofker, "Adequate debridement and drainage of the mediastinum using open thoracotomy or video-assisted thoracoscopic surgery for Boerhaave's syndrome," *Surgical Endoscopy and Other Interventional Techniques*, vol. 25, no. 8, pp. 2492–2497, 2011.

7

Rare Strain of *Vibrio cholerae* Septicemia in a Patient with Multiple Myeloma

Deepu Daniel[1] and Sunil Kumar[2]

[1]*Broward Health Medical Center, Fort Lauderdale, FL 33316, USA*
[2]*Pulmonary/Critical Care Medicine, Broward Health Medical Center, Fort Lauderdale, FL 33316, USA*

Correspondence should be addressed to Deepu Daniel; deepudaniel17@yahoo.com

Academic Editor: Mehmet Doganay

Introduction. Non-O1/non-O139 is a rare strain of *Vibrio cholera* that has been documented to cause significant morbidity and mortality in the immunosuppressed population. *Case Presentation.* A patient with multiple myeloma develops non-O1/non-O139 *Vibrio cholera* septicemia, leading to multiorgan failure and ultimately death. *Discussion.* An exceedingly rare strain of *Vibrio cholera*, non-O1/non-O139, may be an important factor of morbidity and mortality in certain immunosuppressed populations, such as patients with multiple myeloma and malignancies. *Conclusion.* Bacteremia involving generally noninvasive microbes, such as non-O1/non-O139 *Vibrio cholerae*, can have significant deleterious effects in the immunosuppressed patients as shown by this case report. Physicians need to be more diligent when treating these patients.

1. Introduction

Reported cases of non-O1/non-O139 *Vibrio cholerae* bacteremia are extremely uncommon in the literature [1]. This strain has, on rare occasions, been shown to cause invasive and systemic manifestations beyond the commonly associated gastrointestinal symptoms of diarrhea, nausea, and emesis [2–4]. Bacterial infections, including such rare instances of non-O1/non-O139 *Vibrio cholerae*, are more prone to occur in the immunosuppressed and may carry worse prognoses in this population [5]. One such population of patients is those with multiple myeloma. This case study presents a peculiar incidence of severe sepsis induced by non-O1/non-O139 *Vibrio cholerae* bacteremia in a multiple myeloma patient leading to severe sepsis, pulmonary hemorrhage, and ventilator dependent respiratory failure.

2. Case Presentation

A 54-year-old Haitian male with a past medical history of multiple myeloma diagnosed one year prior was admitted to Broward Health Medical Center due to septic shock and acute renal injury. He had his last chemotherapy session for the multiple myeloma over 3 months ago and was lost to follow-up since that time period. Symptomatically, he was complaining of diffuse abdominal pain, nausea, vomiting, and diarrhea for 3 days after returning from a trip to Haiti.

Initial vital signs included temperature of 102 degrees Fahrenheit, heart rate 90 beats per minute, blood pressure 86/40 mmHg, and oxygen saturation 100% on 2 L/min of oxygen via nasal cannula. Labs showed a white blood cell count of $2.85 \times 10^3/\mu L$, hemoglobin 8.7 g/dL, hematocrit 25.5%, platelets $43 \times 10^3/\mu L$, segmented neutrophils 76%, bands 8%, and lymphocytes 12%. Comprehensive metabolic panel showed sodium 144 mmol/L, potassium 3.9 mmol/L, chloride 119 mmol/L, bicarbonate 12 mmol/L, BUN 31 mg/dL, creatinine 3.5 mg/dL, alkaline phosphatase 39 units/L, aspartate aminotransferase 55 units/L, alanine aminotransferase 65 units/L, and albumin 2 g/dL. Initial X-ray and CT of the chest did not indicate any acute infiltrates. A CT of the abdomen showed mild circumferential wall thickening of the colon extending from the cecum to the rectum indicative of colitis. Aggressive IV fluid hydration was initiated and he was empirically started on piperacillin-tazobactam. Initial blood cultures preliminarily grew gram negative rods, at which time levofloxacin was added to his regimen.

Within 48 hours of admission he began to experience worsening respiratory distress and severe tachypnea, with ABG indices showing a pH of 7.26, pCO_2 of 43, pO_2 of 64, base excess of (-8), and O_2 saturation of 91%. Patient was switched to a nonrebreather. He was found to be fluid overloaded with a significant positive fluid balance. The patient had to be placed on BiPap and diuresed with bumetanide. Repeat chest X-ray indicated new right upper lobe infiltrates. After being stabilized he was weaned back to 4 L of O_2 via nasal cannula.

Blood culture identification showed growth of *Vibrio cholerae* non-O1/non-O139. Based on identification and susceptibility studies, antibiotic treatment was deescalated to intravenous levofloxacin. The bacterial strain was isolated and identified by the Florida Department of Health in Jacksonville, FL.

However, the patient's clinical status once again deteriorated. He began to develop episodes of copious hemoptysis and worsening thrombocytopenia. Intermittent platelet transfusions and a trial of desmopressin were started; however no significant increase in platelet count was seen. Patient's respiratory status continued to worsen through his course progressing to respiratory failure requiring emergent intubation. He continued to have bloody secretions suctioned from the endotracheal tube. Chest X-rays indicated worsening bilateral fluffy infiltrates. In the setting of continued bloody secretions it was felt that the radiological findings may correlate with pulmonary hemorrhage.

Patient was sent to the operating room for tracheostomy placement and oral packing by the otolaryngologist. Secondary to the extensive amount of oropharyngeal bleeding, vaginal pads were required. The patient was also started on aminocaproic acid, a fibrinolytic inhibitor without any significant improvement. He continued to require full ventilator support and was too hemodynamically unstable to attempt weaning from the ventilator. As his clinical status deteriorated further, he became less responsive and comatose. A CT of the brain revealed a 2 cm hemorrhage in the left cerebellum with mild surrounding edema. He later underwent cardiac arrest and was unable to be revived, ultimately succumbing to his illness.

3. Discussion

As mentioned earlier, immunosuppressive states such as multiple myeloma and other hematologic malignancies do place patients at an overall increased risk of bacteremia [7–12]. Hypogammaglobulinemia and a decrease in the production of IgA and IgG may lead to an overall increased risk of infection specifically among those with multiple myeloma. These patients are functionally asplenic and are thus susceptible to bacterial infections, particularly encapsulated microbes [13, 14]. However, a non-O1/non-O139 *Vibrio cholerae* infection has rarely been documented. This case showed the deleterious effects of an exceedingly rare bacterium on an immunosuppressed host.

Shelton et al. described a case report of recurrent non-O1 *Vibrio cholerae* bacteremia in a patient with multiple myeloma [15]. The patient had been admitted both instances, approximately one year apart, with symptoms of fever, malaise, and cough. During both instances, patient did not have any gastrointestinal complaints of diarrhea, nausea, or vomiting. Patient had also denied consumption of raw seafood. The blood cultures drawn during both admissions revealed infection with non-O1 *Vibrio cholerae*. Comparison of the two strains of non-O1 *Vibrio cholerae* showed minor differences to each other. Patient was discharged home both instances on oral antibiotic therapy.

Majority of pathogenic *Vibrio cholerae* strains express two "O antigens," O1 and O139. Those that do not express these antigens are classified as non-O1/non-O139 *Vibrio cholerae*. The majority of these latter strains are for the most part nonpathogenic. However there has been a minority that has caused significant pandemics and outbreaks [16–20]. Two main virulence factors that are found in O1 and O139 *Vibrio cholerae* are the cholera toxin (CT) and toxin coregulated pilus (TCP) [21]. CT is responsible for causing diarrhea whereas TCP functions in allowing the microbe to colonize the colon [22]. However the mechanism of pathogenicity in non-O1/non-O139 *Vibrio cholerae* is less well established.

Dziejman et al. performed genetic analyses on four strains of non-O1/non-O139 *Vibrio cholerae* (AM-19226, AM-15622, MZO-2, and MZO-3) which were isolated from stool studies from patients in Bangladesh in 2001 [23]. Genomic analyses of the AM-19226 strain showed similarities to genes found in *Vibrio parahaemolyticus* that encode for the Type III Secretion System (TTSS). TTSS produces virulence factors in *V. parahaemolyticus*, as well as in several gram negative organisms (i.e., *Salmonella*, *Shigella*, *Vibrio*, *E. coli*, *Pseudomonas*, *Aeromonas*). TTSS found in *Vibrio parahaemolyticus* functions in causing enterotoxicity. This study suggested the possibility that the TTSS gene cluster in AM-19226 would produce similar virulence factors and that similar TTSS clusters may lead to virulence factors in other non-O1/non-O139 strains.

The reported incidence of non-O1/non-O139 bacteremia is very rare in the United States. According to the CDC's 2011 COVIS (Cholera and Other *Vibrio* Illness Surveillance) annual summary, there were only 68 reported cases of bacteremia attributable to non-O1/non-O139 *Vibrio cholerae* in the United States (Table 1 and Figure 1) [6].

One of the most significant cholera outbreaks ever to occur in the western hemisphere occurred in Haiti in 2010. The patient in this case had confirmed to hospital staff that he has been living in Haiti for nearly 6 months prior to his admission. Chin et al., implementing third generation single molecule DNA sequencing, analyzed the genetic sequences of two prominent *Vibrio cholerae* strains isolated during the Haiti outbreak and compared them to strains seen during earlier outbreaks in South Asia and Latin America [24]. Studies indicated that the likely causative strain of the Haiti outbreak was *Vibrio cholerae* El Tor. This was the same strain isolated from Bangladesh in 2002 and 2008.

This patient passed away from severe sepsis, respiratory failure, pulmonary hemorrhage and copious retropharyngeal bleeding exacerbated by unrelenting thrombocytopenia.

TABLE 1: Reported *Vibrio* cases in the United States in 2011, taken directly from the 2011 COVIS annual report published in the CDC website [6].

| *Vibrio* species | Cases | | Demographic characteristics | | | | Outcomes | | | |
| | | | Age (years) | | Sex | | Hospitalizations | | Deaths | |
	N	%	Median	Range	Male (n/N)	%	n/N	%	n/N	%
V. alginolyticus	156	18	33	2–86	118/155	76	16/146	11	0/144	0
V. cholerae (excluding toxigenic O1 and O139)*	86	10	48	1–85	59/86	69	28/82	34	3/80	4
Photobacterium damselae subsp. *damselae* (formerly *V. damselae*)	7	1	55	6–77	4/7	57	3/6	50	0/1	0
V. fluvialis	37	4	65	20–108	18/37	49	18/34	53	0/33	0
Grimontia hollisae (formerly *V. hollisae*)	7	1	50	42–75	7/7	100	4/7	57	0/6	0
V. mimicus	15	2	45	4–87	11/14	79	6/15	47	0/15	0
V. parahaemolyticus	334	39	45	1–94	225/334	67	75/315	24	7/304	2
V. vulnificus	113	13	60	8–91	87/111	78	89/113	87	34/108	31
Species not identified	87	10	44	3–93	51/86	59	19/82	23	4/78	5
Multiple species†	11	1	52	23–80	7/11	64	4/11	36	0/10	0
Total	**853**	**100**	**47**	**1–108**	**587/848**	**69**	**272/811**	**34**	**48/785**	**6**

*Including 86 nontoxigenic *V. cholerae* (non-O1/non-O139 [68 cases], O1 [2 cases], O139 [1 case], and no serogroup specified [2 cases]) and 13 toxigenic *V. cholerae* (O75 [12 cases] and O141 [1 case]).

†The following combinations of *Vibrio* species were isolated from patients infected with multiple species: *V. alginolyticus, V. parahaemolyticus* (3 patients); *V. cholerae* O1, *V. parahaemolyticus* (1 patient); *V. fluvialis, V. parahaemolyticus* (1 patient); *P. damselae* subsp. *damselae, Vibrio* species not identified (1 patient); *V. fluvialis, V. furnissii* (1 patient); *V. parahaemolyticus, V. vulnificus* (1 patient); *V. cholerae* non-O1/non-O139, *Vibrio* species not identified (1 patient); *V. alginolyticus, Vibrio* species not identified (1 patient); *V. alginolyticus, P. damselae* subsp. *damselae* (1 patient). None of these are included in the rows for individual species.

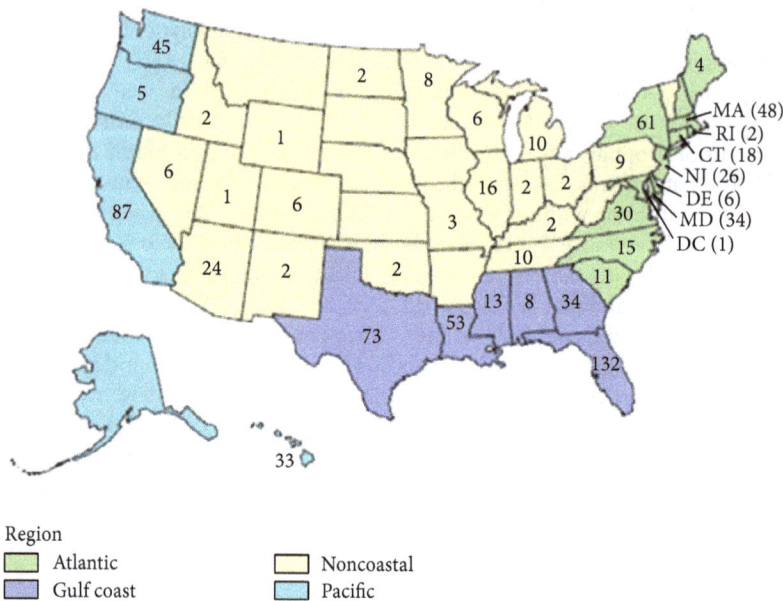

FIGURE 1: Geographic distribution of *Vibrio* infections in the United States in 2011, also taken directly from the 2011 COVIS report published on the CDC website [6].

Despite aggressive intravenous fluid hydration, appropriate antibiotic therapy, and multiple transfusions of packed red blood cells and platelets, his illness proved fatal. His underlying multiple myeloma was his most significant comorbidity contributing to his unfortunate outcome. Virulence factors produced by this rare strain of *Vibrio cholerae* may have further attributed to his prognosis; however we are unable to definitively make this conclusion at this time. Further studies will be required to identify and study the pathogenicity virulence factors associated with this microbe.

4. Conclusion

In our case report, we described a fatal case of severe sepsis in a patient with multiple myeloma. The patient's clinical course was complicated by his history of multiple myeloma. It is important to reemphasize the rarity of reported cases of bacteremia caused by these strains of bacteria and that the immunosuppressed population is more prone to bacterial infections, including such rare strains.

It is important for physicians to understand the deleterious effects that a generally nonpathogenic strain of bacteria can have on immunosuppressed patients. Physicians need to be vigilant on this particular population of patients to avoid these consequences. Our case was important in reiterating this fact.

References

[1] Centers for Disease Control and Prevention (CDC), *Non-O1 and Non-O139 Vibrio cholerae Infections*, US Department of Health and Human Services, CDC, Atlanta, Ga, USA, 2014.

[2] F. M. T. Ulloa, T. L. Porte, J. S. Braun et al., "Acute gastroenteritis caused by a *Vibrio cholerae* non-O1, non-O139 strain harboring a genetic region homologous to the VpaI-7 pathogenicity Island," *Revista Chilena de Infectologia*, vol. 28, no. 5, pp. 470–473, 2011.

[3] Y.-L. Lee, P.-P. Hung, C.-A. Tsai, Y.-H. Lin, C.-E. Liu, and Z.-Y. Shi, "Clinical characteristics of non-O1/non-O139 *Vibrio cholerae* isolates and polymerase chain reaction analysis of their virulence factors," *Journal of Microbiology, Immunology and Infection*, vol. 40, no. 6, pp. 474–480, 2007.

[4] K. K. Tan, K. S. Sin, A. J. Ng, H. Yahya, and P. Kaur, "Non-O1 *Vibrio cholerae* septicaemia: a case report," *Singapore Medical Journal*, vol. 35, no. 6, pp. 648–649, 1994.

[5] J. M. Fernández, M. Serrano, J. J. De Arriba, M. V. Sánchez, E. Escribano, and P. Ferreras, "Bacteremic cellulitis caused by Non-O1, Non-O139 Vibrio cholerae: Report of a case in a patient with hemochromatosis," *Diagnostic Microbiology and Infectious Disease*, vol. 37, no. 1, pp. 77–80, 2000.

[6] Centers for Disease Control and Prevention (CDC), *COVIS Annual Summary, 2011*, US Department of Health and Human Services, CDC, Atlanta, Ga, USA, 2011.

[7] J. M. Hughes, D. G. Hollis, E. J. Gangarosa, and R. E. Weaver, "Non-cholera Vibrio infections in the United States: clinical, epidemiologic, and laboratory features," *Annals of Internal Medicine*, vol. 88, no. 5, pp. 602–606, 1978.

[8] K. C. Klontz, "Fatalities associated with *Vibrio* parahaemolyticus and *Vibrio cholerae* non-O1 infections in Florida (1981 to 1988)," *Southern Medical Journal*, vol. 83, no. 5, pp. 500–502, 1990.

[9] S. Safrin, J. G. Morris Jr., M. Adams, V. Pons, R. Jacobs, and J. E. Conte Jr., "Non-O:1 *Vibrio cholerae* bacteremia: case report and review," *Reviews of Infectious Diseases*, vol. 10, no. 5, pp. 1012–1017, 1988.

[10] M. I. Siegel and A. I. Rogers, "Fatal non-O1 *Vibrio cholerae* septicemia in chronic lymphocytic leukemia," *Gastroenterology*, vol. 83, no. 5, pp. 1130–1131, 1982.

[11] E. Platia and K. L. Vosti, "Noncholera *Vibrio* septicemia," *Western Journal of Medicine*, vol. 132, no. 4, pp. 354–357, 1980.

[12] C. C. Young, Y. C. Chuang, and C. D. Young, "Non-0:1 *Vibrio cholerae* bacteremia: report of two cases," *Kansenshogaku Zasshi*, vol. 65, no. 11, pp. 1479–1483, 1991.

[13] L. Cone and J. W. Uhr, "Immunological deficiency disorders associated with chronic lymphocytic leukemia and multiple myeloma," *The Journal of Clinical Investigation*, vol. 43, pp. 2241–2248, 1964.

[14] D. R. Jacobson and S. Zolla-Pazner, "Immunosuppression and infection in multiple myeloma," *Seminars in Oncology*, vol. 13, no. 3, pp. 282–290, 1986.

[15] C. H. Shelton III, R. L. Martino, and K. M. Ramsey, "Recurrent non-0:1 *Vibrio cholerae* bacteremia in a patient with multiple myeloma," *Cancer*, vol. 72, no. 1, pp. 105–107, 1993.

[16] J. G. Morris Jr., "Non-O group 1 Vibrio cholerae: a look at the epidemiology of an occasional pathogen," *Epidemiologic Reviews*, vol. 12, pp. 179–191, 1990.

[17] A. Dalsgaard, O. Serichantalergs, A. Forslund et al., "Clinical and environmental isolates of *Vibrio cholerae* serogroup O141 carry the CTX phage and the genes encoding the toxin-coregulated pili," *Journal of Clinical Microbiology*, vol. 39, no. 11, pp. 4086–4092, 2001.

[18] S. Rudra, R. Mahajan, M. Mathur, K. Kathuria, and V. Talwar, "Cluster of cases of clinical cholera due to *Vibrio* cholerae 010 in east Delhi," *Indian Journal of Medical Research*, vol. 103, pp. 71–73, 1996.

[19] K. Bagchi, P. Echeverria, J. D. Arthur, O. Sethabutr, O. Serichantalergs, and C. W. Hoge, "Epidemic of diarrhea caused by *Vibrio cholerae* non-O1 that produced heat-stable toxin among Khmers in a camp in Thailand," *Journal of Clinical Microbiology*, vol. 31, no. 5, pp. 1315–1317, 1993.

[20] T.-Y. Ou, J.-W. Liu, and H.-S. Leu, "Independent prognostic factors for fatality in patients with invasive Vibrio cholerae non-O1 infections," *Journal of Microbiology, Immunology and Infection*, vol. 36, no. 2, pp. 117–122, 2003.

[21] S. M. Faruque, M. J. Albert, and J. J. Mekalanos, "Epidemiology, genetics, and ecology of toxigenic *Vibrio cholerae*," *Microbiology and Molecular Biology Reviews*, vol. 62, no. 4, pp. 1301–1314, 1998.

[22] D. A. Herrington, R. H. Hall, G. Losonsky, J. J. Mekalanos, R. K. Taylor, and M. M. Levine, "Toxin, toxin-coregulated pili, and the toxR regulon are essential for Vibrio cholerae pathogenesis in humans," *Journal of Experimental Medicine*, vol. 168, no. 4, pp. 1487–1492, 1988.

[23] M. Dziejman, D. Serruto, V. C. Tam et al., "Genomic characterization of non-O1, non-O139 *Vibrio cholerae* reveals genes for a type III secretion system," *Proceedings of the National Academy of Sciences of the United States of America*, vol. 102, no. 9, pp. 3465–3470, 2005.

[24] C.-S. Chin, J. Sorenson, J. B. Harris et al., "The origin of the Haitian cholera outbreak strain," *The New England Journal of Medicine*, vol. 364, no. 1, pp. 33–42, 2011.

8

Neurogenic Stunned Myocardium Associated with Acute Spinal Cord Infarction

Gillian A. Beauchamp,[1] **Jason T. McMullan,**[1] **and Jordan B. Bonomo**[1,2]

[1] *Department of Emergency Medicine, University of Cincinnati, Cincinnati, OH 45267, USA*
[2] *Division of Neurocritical Care, Department of Neurosurgery, University of Cincinnati, 231 Albert Sabin Way, ML 0769, MSB 1654, Cincinnati, OH 45267, USA*

Correspondence should be addressed to Gillian A. Beauchamp, beauchgn@ucmail.uc.edu

Academic Editors: K. Chergui, Y. Kluger, and C. D. Roosens

Introduction. Neurogenic stunned myocardium (NSM) is a reversible cardiomyopathy resulting in transient left ventricular apical ballooning presumed to result from catecholamine surge occurring under physiologic stress. Acute spinal cord ischemia is a rare ischemic vascular lesion. We report a case of neurogenic stunned myocardium occurring in the setting of acute spinal cord infarction. *Methods.* Singe case report was used. *Results.* We present the case of a 63-year-old female with a history of prior lacunar stroke, hypertension, chronic back pain, and hypothyroidism who presented with a brief episode of diffuse abdominal and bilateral lower extremity pain which progressed within minutes to bilateral lower extremity flaccid paralysis. MRI of the spinal cord revealed central signal hyperintensity of T2-weighted imaging from conus to T8 region, concerning for acute spinal cord ischemia. Transthoracic echocardiogram was performed to determine if a cardiac embolic phenomenon may have precipitated this ischemic event and showed left ventricular apical hypokinesis and ballooning concerning for NSM. *Conclusion.* Neurogenic stunned myocardium is a reversible cardiomyopathy which has been described in patients with physiologic stress resulting in ventricular apical ballooning. Our case suggests that it is possible for neurogenic stunned myocardium to occur in the setting of acute spinal cord ischemia.

1. Introduction

Neurogenic stunned myocardium (NSM) is a reversible cardiomyopathy resulting in transient left ventricular apical ballooning which has been described to occur in the setting of catecholamine release [1, 2] during situations of physiologic stress such as subarachnoid hemorrhage [3–5], reversible posterior leukoencephalopathy [6], atrial fibrillation [7], hemorrhagic cerebral contusion [8], status epilepticus [9], ischemic cerebrovascular accident [10], limbic encephalitis [11], and severe emotional stress [12]. NSM has also been referred to as "broken heart syndrome" [12], "takotsubo cardiomyopathy," "apical ballooning syndrome," "neurogenic stress cardiomyopathy," [13] and "transient left ventricular dysfunction syndrome." [14] This condition typically presents with mildly elevated cardiac biomarkers [14] and reversible regional-wall motion abnormalities on echocardiogram [15]. Care for NSM involves treatment of the underlying cause and supportive care.

Acute spinal cord ischemia is a rare ischemic vascular lesion with high morbidity and mortality [16]. To the best of our knowledge, this is the first case report of the occurrence of neurogenic stunned myocardium in the context of acute spinal cord infarction.

2. Case Presentation

A 63-year-old female with a history of prior lacunar stroke, hypertension, chronic back pain, and hypothyroidism presented to a community emergency department one hour after the acute onset of severe bilateral lower extremity pain which progressed, within minutes, to bilateral lower extremity generalized weakness and then flaccid paralysis. In addition, within an hour of symptom onset, she developed dull, diffuse abdominal pain with radiation to the bilateral flanks, lasting one hour with subsequent resolution.

At presentation, she was found to have a blood pressure of 131/88 mmHg, tachycardia with a heart rate of 110 beats

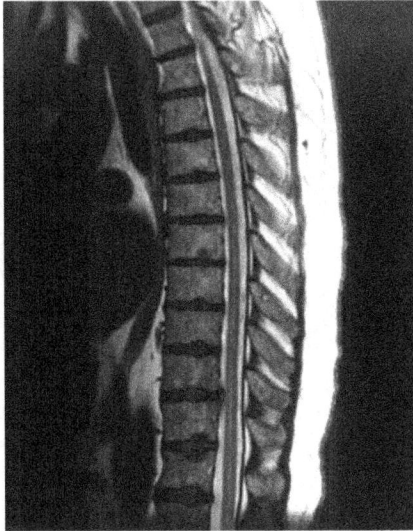

FIGURE 1: MRI thoracic spine showing acute spinal cord infarction. Sagittal T2-weighted MRI of the patient's thoracic spine demonstrating nonspecific central intrinsic signal hyperintensity of the spinal cord located in conus region with extension to T8 level. Multilevel thoracic disc disease at T1 and T10-T11 is also present.

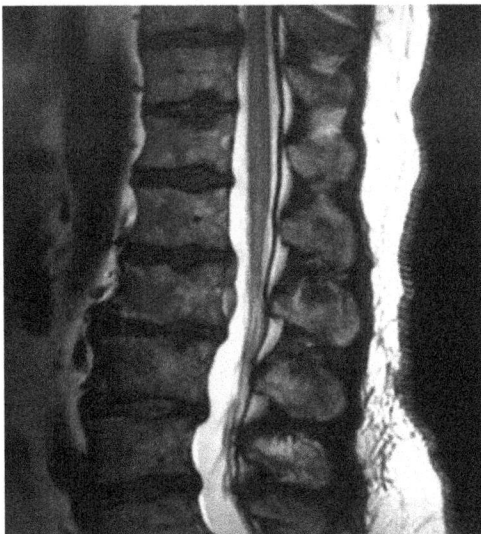

FIGURE 2: MRI of the lumbar spine showing acute spinal cord infarction. Sagittal T2-weighted MRI of the patient's lumbar spine showing a nonspecific central intrinsic signal hyperintensity of the spinal cord located in conus region with extension to T8 level. Image also shows multilevel degenerative disc disease with noncompressive disc herniation at L1-L2.

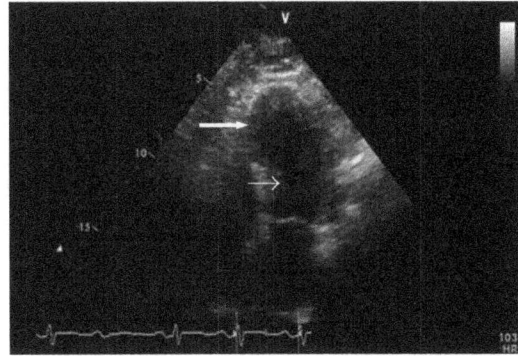

FIGURE 3: Transthoracic echocardiogram. The patient's apical four-chamber transthoracic echocardiogram at end systole showing left ventricle, left atrium, and mitral valve. There is left ventricular basilar contraction (small arrow), with near apposition of the endomyocardium, and severe apical hypokinesia (large arrow) with apical ballooning.

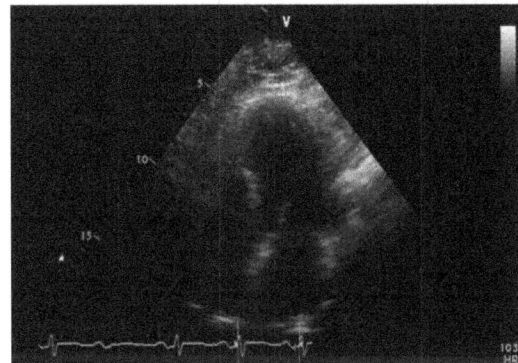

FIGURE 4: Transthoracic echocardiogram. The patient's transthoracic echocardiogram in diastole showing neurogenic stunned myocardium. Apical four-chamber view showing left ventricle, left atrium, and mitral valve during diastole. Note the uniformity of the endomyocardium resulting in a "bullet shape" of the left ventricle in which all three segments of the ventricle: base, mid, and apex relax equally.

per minute, oral temperature of 96.8 degrees, F and SpO$_2$ of 97% on room air. The patient presented with 0/5 strength and decreased sensation to light touch and areflexia of the bilateral lower extremities. Noncontrast computed tomography (CT) of the head showed a remote lacunar infarct. CT angiography of the abdomen and pelvis showed no evidence of pulmonary embolus, abdominal aortic aneurysm, or aortic dissection. Surface electrocardiogram showed sinus tachycardia without ischemia.

The patient was transferred to a tertiary care center for advanced imaging and care, where a T2-weighted magnetic resonance image (MRI) showed a nonspecific central intrinsic signal hyperintensity in the conus region extending to the level of T8, concerning for acute spinal cord ischemia (Figures 1 and 2). Transthoracic echocardiogram, performed to determine if there was a cardiac source of emboli, showed atypical dyskinesia with left ventricular apical ballooning and an ejection fraction of 35%, a characteristic of neurogenic stunned myocardium (Figures 3 and 4). Cardiology was consulted, and a diagnosis of takotsubo cardiomyopathy was made, with no further recommendation for heparinization or catheterization. Pertinent laboratory results are shown in Table 1.

The patient was admitted to the neurology inpatient service for supportive care including physical and

TABLE 1: Pertinent laboratory data. Values and normal reference range noted for each laboratory test. All reported data is from time of presentation to emergency department unless otherwise specified.

Laboratory test	Value	Normal reference range
White blood cell count	$9.2 \times 10^3/\mu L$	$3.8–10.8 \times 10^3/\mu L$
Blood urea nitrogen	21 mg/dL	7–25 mg/dL
Creatinine	1.32 mg/dL	0.5–1.2 mg/dL
Point of care troponin $T = 0$ h	2.04 ng/mL	0.00–0.05 ng/mL
Point of care troponin at $T = 3$ h	1.72 ng/mL	0.00–0.05 ng/mL
Troponin I at $T = 9$ h	0.47 ng/mL	0.00–0.05 ng/mL
Point of care CKMB at $T = 0$ h	16.4 ng/mL	0.00–3.5 ng/mL
Point of care CKMB at $T = 3$ h	15.8 ng/mL	0.00–3.5 ng/mL
CKMB at $T = 9$ h	4.6 ng/mL	0.00–2.4 ng/mL
Lactate	1.9 mmol/L	0.5–2.2 mmol/L
International normalized ratio	1.1	0.9–1.1
Prothrombin time	14.1 seconds	11.6–14
Total cholesterol	255 mg/dL	0–200 mg/dL
High-density lipoprotein	48 mg/dL	30–60 mg/dL
Low-density lipoprotein	176 mg/dL	0–160 mg/dL
Triglycerides	154 mg/dL	10–150 mg/dL

occupational therapy. During admission, the patient was evaluated for stroke risk factors, and statin therapy was subsequently initiated for hyperlipidemia. No other specific underlying etiology of the spinal cord ischemia was found. Cerebrospinal fluid studies were performed to rule out other etiologies for paralysis and were unremarkable. The patient was started on low-dose beta-blocker and ACE-inhibitor therapy per cardiology recommendations, and the patient was discharged to a rehabilitation facility with the recommendation to have a transthoracic echocardiogram six months after discharge. The patient was subsequently lost to followup.

3. Discussion

Neurogenic stunned myocardium (NSM) has most recently been explained by the "catecholamine hypothesis," which describes the underlying activation of sympathetic nervous system activity as the cause of reversible apical ballooning and left ventricular dysfunction [1, 2]. Specifically, catecholamine release from sympathetic nerves innervating the myocardium leads to the development of reversible wall motion abnormalities, typically presenting as apical ballooning on echocardiogram and occurring with mild troponin elevations [3, 5, 17]. Although not performed in this patient, coronary artery disease is ideally ruled out with coronary angiography and resolution of cardiac stun confirmed with a repeated echocardiogram performed two to four weeks after the onset of NSM [2].

The occurrence of NSM in the face of acute spinal cord ischemia suggests underlying physiologic or emotional stress as a possible etiology for this myocardial regional wall motion abnormality. Additionally, it is also possible that an underlying cardiomyopathy might have actually precipitated the spinal cord ischemia—although it is our hypothesis that

the spinal stroke led to the development of NSM, we are limited to supposition and without definitive proof. It is likely that this phenomenon of myocardial stunning is underrecognized in patients who present with acute neurological disease and that the identification of this co-occurrence by echocardiography may inform the approach to supportive care during the patient's recovery period. Awareness of this phenomenon may encourage vigilant observation for rare but serious sequelae of NSM. Although not seen in this patient, these sequelae may include arrhythmias, hypotension, and cardiogenic shock, as well as dyskinesia of the left ventricle and the attendant risk of thrombus formation.

References

[1] A. Kothavale, N. M. Banki, A. Kopelnik et al., "Predictors of left ventricular regional wall motion abnormalities after subarachnoid hemorrhage," Neurocritical Care, vol. 4, no. 3, pp. 199–205, 2006.

[2] I. S. Wittstein, D. R. Thiemann, J. A. C. Lima et al., "Neurohumoral features of myocardial stunning due to sudden emotional stress," New England Journal of Medicine, vol. 352, no. 6, pp. 539–548, 2005.

[3] J. M. Levine, "Critical care management of subarachnoid hemorrhage," Current Treatment Options in Neurology, vol. 11, no. 2, pp. 126–136, 2009.

[4] R. Jain, J. Deveikis, and B. G. Thompson, "Management of patients with stunned myocardium associated with subarachnoid hemorrhage," American Journal of Neuroradiology, vol. 25, no. 1, pp. 126–129, 2004.

[5] T. Kono, H. Morita, T. Kuroiwa, H. Onaka, H. Takatsuka, and A. Fujiwara, "Left ventricular wall motion abnormalities in patients with subarachnoid hemorrhage: neurogenic stunned myocardium," Journal of the American College of Cardiology, vol. 24, no. 3, pp. 636–640, 1994.

[6] P. A. Banuelos, R. Temes, and V. H. Lee, "Neurogenic stunned myocardium associated with reversible posterior

leukoencephalopathy syndrome," *Neurocritical Care*, vol. 9, no. 1, pp. 108–111, 2008.

[7] E. L. Leung Ki, A. Delabays, X. Lyon, and E. Pruvot, "A case of recurrent transient left ventricular apical ballooning associated with atrial fibrillation," *International Journal of Cardiology*, vol. 118, no. 2, pp. e35–e38, 2007.

[8] D. Deleu, M. A. Kettern, Y. Hanssens, S. Kumar, K. Salim, and F. Miyares, "Neurogenic stunned myocardium following hemorrhagic cerebral contusion," *Saudi Medical Journal*, vol. 28, no. 2, pp. 283–285, 2007.

[9] M. Shimizu, A. Kagawa, T. Takano, H. Masai, and Y. Miwa, "Neurogenic stunned myocardium associated with status epileptics and postictal catecholamine surge," *Internal Medicine*, vol. 47, no. 4, pp. 269–273, 2008.

[10] A. S. Dande, A. S. Pandit, and I. D. Galin, "Takotsubo cardiomyopathy followed by neurogenic stunned myocardium in the same patient: gradations of the same disease?" *Cardiology*, vol. 118, no. 3, pp. 175–178, 2011.

[11] J. Gelow, M. Kruer, V. Yadav, and S. Kaul, "Apical ballooning resulting from limbic encephalitis," *American Journal of Medicine*, vol. 122, no. 6, pp. 583–586, 2009.

[12] H. Khallafi, V. Chacko, N. Varveralis, and F. Elmi, "'Broken heart syndrome': catecholamine surge or aborted myocardial infarction?" *Journal of Invasive Cardiology*, vol. 20, no. 1, pp. E9–E13, 2008.

[13] V. H. Lee, J. K. Oh, S. L. Mulvagh, and E. F. M. Wijdicks, "Mechanisms in neurogenic stress cardiomyopathy after aneurysmal subarachnoid hemorrhage," *Neurocritical Care*, vol. 5, no. 3, pp. 243–249, 2006.

[14] S. Cimarelli, F. Sauer, O. Morel, P. Ohlmann, A. Constantinesco, and A. Imperiale, "Transient left ventricular dysfunction syndrome: patho-physiological bases through nuclear medicine imaging," *International Journal of Cardiology*, vol. 144, no. 2, pp. 212–218, 2010.

[15] H. Nguyen and J. G. Zaroff, "Neurogenic stunned myocardium," *Current Neurology and Neuroscience Reports*, vol. 9, no. 6, pp. 486–491, 2009.

[16] D. S. Geldmacher and B. C. Bowen, "Vascular disease of the nervous system," in *Neurology in Clinical Practice*, W. G. Bradley, R. B. Daroff, G. M. Fenichel, and J. Jankovic, Eds., p. 1313, Butterworth Heinemann, Philadelphia, Pa, USA, 4th edition, 2004.

[17] Y. Abe, M. Kondo, R. Matsuoka, M. Araki, K. Dohyama, and H. Tanio, "Assessment of clinical features in transient left ventricular apical ballooning," *Journal of the American College of Cardiology*, vol. 41, no. 5, pp. 737–742, 2003.

9

Myasthenic Crisis in an Elderly Patient with Positive Antibodies against Acetylcholine and Anti-MuSK, Successfully Treated with Noninvasive Mechanical Ventilation

José A. Fernández, Antonio Fernández-Valiñas, Daniel Hernández, Joel Orozco, and Antonio Lugo

Hospital Ángeles Clínica Londres, Durango No. 50, Roma Norte, Cuauhtémoc, 06700 Ciudad de México, DF, Mexico

Correspondence should be addressed to José A. Fernández; ariagv988@yahoo.com.mx

Academic Editor: Nicolas Nin

Myasthenia gravis is an autoimmune disease characterized by muscle weakness. Subjects with antibodies against acetylcholine usually have greater ocular symptoms, lower bulbar weakness, and fewer respiratory complications, compared to individuals with anti-MuSK antibodies. The presence of positivity to both types of antibodies in the same patient is uncommon, and the clinical behavior of these individuals is uncertain. A myasthenic crisis is characterized by respiratory and bulbar muscle weakness, causing acute respiratory failure which requires mechanical ventilatory support. We present the case of a 73-year-old man with a medical history of myasthenia gravis and positive antibody titers against acetylcholine and anti-MuSK, who sought for medical assessment because of respiratory tract infection symptoms, dysphagia, and generalized weakness. Initially, no respiratory distress was found. After 24 hours the patient showed respiratory deterioration and neurological impairment. Endotracheal intubation was rejected, so ventilatory support with noninvasive ventilation was started. The patient was supported by intense respiratory therapy, and infusion of immunoglobulin was initiated. The individual responded favorably, improving his general condition. Weaning from noninvasive mechanical ventilation was possible after six days. Our case illustrates that noninvasive ventilation, properly supported by intense respiratory therapy, can be a great option to avoid intubation in the myasthenic patient.

1. Introduction

Myasthenia gravis is an autoimmune disease characterized by the formation of autoantibodies against nicotinic acetylcholine receptors at the neuromuscular junction or by the presence of antibodies directed against other postsynaptic muscle fiber components like muscle specific tyrosine kinase (MuSK). Clinically it is manifested as muscle weakness of varying intensity [1]. It is recognized that the type of present antibodies determines the clinical behavior of the disease. Antibodies against acetylcholine can be found in young or elderly patients. These subjects usually have more weakness of the limbs in comparison to the bulbar muscles and marked ptosis, and thymoma or thymic hyperplasia is present in 80% of cases. Recurrent crisis is not usual in these patients. Individuals with anti-MuSK antibodies have a more complex clinical course. This group of patients are usually female and under 40 years. They show predominance of the bulbar symptoms, less ocular disturbances, and often lack of thymoma. In addition, they may show poor response to conventional therapy and recurrent myasthenic crisis. The presence of both kinds of antibodies in an individual is very rare, and therefore, the clinical behavior of these patients is extremely uncertain [2].

Myasthenic crisis should be considered a neurological emergency. It is characterized by weakness of the bulbar and respiratory muscles, severe enough to compromise ventilation and airway permeability, causing acute respiratory failure which requires mechanical ventilatory support [3]. Currently, the prognosis of these patients has improved dramatically thanks to the immunomodulatory therapy with plasmapheresis, immunoadsorption, or immunoglobulin.

The development and appropriate use of noninvasive ventilation have helped to avoid the complications involved in endotracheal intubation, which has further improved the prognosis of these patients. With proper treatment, mortality from this condition is less than 5% [4].

We report the case of an elderly patient with positive antibodies against acetylcholine and anti-MuSK, who, despite generalized muscular weakness and bulbar muscles involvement, showed an adequate response to noninvasive ventilation.

2. Case Presentation

The patient is a 73-year-old male with medical history of diabetes mellitus, hypertension, chronic obstructive pulmonary disease, and obesity grade 2, plus myasthenia gravis of two years of diagnosis, with positive antibody titers against acetylcholine (normal value by immunoradiometric assay <0.25 nmol/L; patient value 6.5 nmol/L) and anti-MuSK (normal value by enzymatic immunoassay <0.4 U/mL; patient value 4.2 U/mL), treated with pyridostigmine (60 mg every 4 hours), azathioprine (50 mg twice a day), and prednisone (5 mg once a day). He is not bearer of thymoma. He had a myasthenic crisis a year ago, which required invasive mechanical ventilation and admission to the intensive care unit for a week. After this event, with established medical treatment, he was wearing an acceptable quality of life.

The individual began his current condition three days before his hospitalization with productive cough, pleuritic pain, and fever. Later he presented difficulty swallowing, nasal voice, ptosis, and generalized weakness. After first medical evaluation in our hospital unit, bulbar symptoms reported by the patient were corroborated along with the weakness of upper and lower extremities, with no observed data of respiratory distress. Clinically, a pulmonary condensation syndrome was integrated in the right hemithorax, so both diagnostics of exacerbation of myasthenia gravis in stage IIa of the Osserman and Genkins classification, and community-acquired pneumonia, were established. The patient entry arterial gases showed no disturbances.

During the first 24 hours of hospitalization, the subject presented respiratory deterioration, referring to dyspnea and showing bradypnea, thoracoabdominal dissociation, and employment of auxiliary breathing muscles. An aggravation in the Osserman and Genkins classification was declared, setting the patient status in stage IVb. Neurologically he was observed to be stuporous, with a Glasgow coma scale of 10 points. Blood gases demonstrated hypoxemia and hypercapnia. Patient was assessed by the critical care service, who indicated need for admission to their unit to start invasive mechanical ventilation and immunomodulatory therapy; however, the responsible relative of the individual did not accept advanced management of the airway and signed a nonintubation order. Therefore keeping the patient in the intermediate care unit and initiating treatment with immunoglobulin (2 grams per kilo of body weight, for 4 days) and noninvasive mechanical ventilation in bilevel continuous positive airway pressure mode, with initial parameters of positive inspiratory airway pressure of 12, positive expiratory

airway pressure of 5, inspired oxygen fraction of 60%, and respiratory rate of 20 breaths per minute, were decided. A CareFusion *VELA* ventilator in noninvasive mechanical ventilation mode was employed. Blood gases prior to the start of noninvasive mechanical ventilation showed pH of 7.34, pO_2 of 54.1 mmHg, pCO_2 of 44 mmHg (normal values for Mexico City 28–32 mmHg), and HCO_3 of 28.3 mmol/L (normal values for Mexico City 18 to 22 mmol/L). Initially the use a nasal mask was decided, but the patient was not able to keep his mouth closed due facial muscle weakness, which generated a big leak of air. For this reason, changing to an orofacial mask was necessary. After one hour of noninvasive respiratory therapy, the patient showed gasometric improvement with a pH of 7.36, pO_2 of 64 mmHg, pCO_2 of 36.4 mmHg, and HCO_3 of 29.1 mmol/L. He also presented significant neurological amelioration, recovering alertness, but at times he showed restlessness and uncooperativeness, so an infusion of dexmedetomidine was started at a dose of 0.5 μg/kg/hr. With this measure a better coupling to the noninvasive ventilatory therapy was achieved. Clinically the patient kept an adequate respiratory frequency, with no use of the accessory muscles of respiration and no thoracoabdominal dissociation. Due to the significant bulbar weakness presented by the individual, the face mask was recurrently removed to allow coughing, suctioning of secretions, and pulmonary percussion therapy. Micronebulization treatment with ipratropium bromide was initiated to prevent bronchospasm. After six hours, the patient showed a complete recovery of neurological status. Dexmedetomidine infusion was no longer necessary. The gas analysis reflected total remission of hypoxemia and hypercapnia, with pH of 7.45, pO_2 of 84 mmHg, pCO_2 of 28 mmHg, and HCO_3 of 24.3 mmol/L. Oxygen saturation was 97%.

After 48 hours of continuous therapy with noninvasive ventilation and immunoglobulin treatment, the patient was able to restart the oral route. Besides removing of noninvasive mechanical ventilation mask to allow the elimination of secretions, patient was put on pap diet with assisted technique and was allowed to rest for the ventilatory support during two hours after every meal. During resting times, the patient was maintained with a venturi mask with an inspired oxygen fraction of 60%. Blood gases kept in acid-base balance and hypoxemia did not recur.

As part of the support management, starting prophylactic anticoagulation with low molecular weight heparin, protection of the gastric mucosa with proton pump inhibitor, and glycemic control by insulin scheme every six hours and basal insulin was decided. Hemodynamic monitoring with telemetry was established. Treating the respiratory tract infection with third-generation cephalosporin and clarithromycin was decided. The treatment with azathioprine was maintained and pyridostigmine was put off until the patient was able to completely retake the oral route. The chronic steroid treatment was kept intravenously until the patient was able to take it orally.

After completing four days of immunoglobulin therapy and noninvasive mechanical ventilation, the patient evolved favorably, leaving the bilevel positive airway pressure therapy during the day and keeping it only overnight. Patient status was set in stage IIa of Osserman and Genkins. Solid diet was initiated and adequately tolerated, and significant improvement in lung infection that triggered the myasthenic crisis was observed. On the sixth day, pulmonary rehabilitation was initiated with incentive spirometry, and noninvasive mechanical ventilation was withdrawn definitely. After seven days of treatment, the patient was discharged home with his usual treatment.

3. Discussion

Respiratory infections are one of the most common etiologies in the development of myasthenic crisis. Our patient, after starting with clinical data from respiratory infection three days before seeking medical attention, suddenly evolved from class IIa of the Osserman and Genkins score to class IVb, demonstrating how quickly the respiratory impairment in these diseases can be presented, demanding mechanical ventilatory support at any time.

The vast majority of patients with respiratory failure of neuromuscular origin initially develop CO_2 retention, and, particularly in patients with myasthenic crisis, hypoxemia is often seen late [4]. Our patient, however, quickly showed a mixed respiratory failure, probably triggered both by weakness of the respiratory muscles and by alveolar commitment caused by infection. Because of the clinical data of respiratory failure, bulbar weakness, gasometric evidence of hypoxemia and hypercapnia, and neurological deterioration observed in the patient, endotracheal intubation and the use of invasive mechanical ventilation was initially decided. Noninvasive mechanical ventilation appeared as a therapeutic resource of great value after the nonintubation order signed by the relative of the patient.

Because the noninvasive ventilatory support in continuous positive airway pressure mode (cPAP) does not actively assist during inspiration [5], the myasthenic patient usually responds more favorably to the bilevel positive airway pressure mode (BiPAP) that delivers adjustable degrees of continuous positive airway pressure, which is higher during inspiration and lower during expiration. Each cycle begins with the breathing efforts of the patient. The positive inspiratory airway pressure helps to decrease the resistance of the upper airway, reducing the work of breathing. The positive end-expiratory airway pressure prevents airway collapse before the end of the respiratory cycle, reducing the risk of atelectasis. This type of ventilatory support is particularly effective in patients with neuromuscular weakness, who are capable of starting the respiratory cycle but are unable to mobilize sufficient amounts of air to prevent the development of atelectasis [6].

The noninvasive ventilation is strongly contraindicated in patients who cannot protect their airway and in subjects who are unable to effectively manage secretions despite receiving support by aspiration and respiratory therapy [5]. In myasthenia gravis, the presence of anti-MuSK antibodies is associated with marked bulbar symptoms, which tend to cause problems in swallowing and difficulty in handling secretions. In the patient in myasthenic crisis, the exacerbation of these symptoms is an inconvenience for the use of

noninvasive mechanical ventilation [3]. Although there are various face masks, and most guidelines of noninvasive ventilatory support do not give superiority to any in particular [7], aspiration and secretions management is facilitated by using a nasal mask; however, this has the disadvantage of generating a large air leak if the patient keeps his mouth open. Our patient, due to muscle weakness, was unable to keep his mouth closed. For this reason it was preferred to place an orofacial mask, withdrawing it frequently for aspiration and to allow coughing. Despite this measure, noninvasive ventilation might have failed if it was not for the excellent response after the initiation of the treatment with immunoglobulin and the intense respiratory therapy given. In addition to continuous suctioning, the patient received lung physiotherapy very often, his position was changed up to six times per day, and he was treated with bronchodilators to prevent bronchospasm. These measures, often neglected, prevent pulmonary complications in patients with myasthenic crisis [8]. After starting the pap diet, delaying the placement of BiPAP up to two hours after meals was decided to avoid episodes of aspiration.

Some predictors of response to noninvasive mechanical ventilation in the myasthenic patient have been identified. Seneviratne et al. conducted a retrospective cohort study of 60 episodes of myasthenic crisis. They found that pCO_2 greater than 45 mmHg prior to initiation of treatment with BiPAP is a failure predictor in the use of this therapy. In this same study, the initiation of noninvasive mechanical ventilation prevented intubation in 14 of 24 patients, and the only variable that showed decrease in the duration of endotracheal intubation was the early use of BiPAP [6]. Another retrospective study by Wu et al. showed that an APACHE II score of less than 6 points and a serum bicarbonate below 30 mmol/L are predictors of BiPAP therapy success in myasthenic crisis [9]. Despite the limitations of both studies, these results are worth taking into account when making the decision about the mechanical ventilatory therapy to employ in the myasthenic patient.

It must be taken into consideration that the main causes of death in myasthenic crisis are lethal arrhythmias and pulmonary embolism [3]. Our patient was maintained with continuous hemodynamic monitoring and remained under prophylactic anticoagulation scheme his entire hospitalization. Weaning from noninvasive mechanical ventilation was conducted favoring the daily clinical evaluation, with the support of scores of assessment designed for myasthenic patient, using mainly the myasthenia gravis composite scale [10].

4. Conclusions

Myasthenic crisis is a neurological emergency. The presence of antibodies against acetylcholine and anti-MuSK in the same individual is an unusual form of presentation of the disease and confers increased therapeutic difficulty. Commonly, the presence of anti-MuSK antibodies is associated with bulbar symptoms, which tend to cause problems in swallowing and difficulty in handling secretions. The exacerbation of these symptoms is a strong inconvenience for the use of noninvasive mechanical ventilation. Our patient, however, by being supported by an intense respiratory therapy, and thanks to the timely start of immunomodulatory therapy, responded favorably to the treatment with noninvasive ventilation. We expect that the way the respiratory support and the immunomodulatory treatment were implemented in this case could serve other physicians who face a similar clinical situation.

References

[1] B. R. Thanvi and T. C. N. Lo, "Update on myasthenia gravis," *Postgraduate Medical Journal*, vol. 80, no. 950, pp. 690–700, 2004.

[2] A. Chaudhuri and P. Behan, "Myasthenic crisis," *QJM: An International Journal of Medicine*, vol. 102, no. 2, pp. 97–107, 2009.

[3] D. A. Godoy, L. J. V. de Mello, L. Masotti, and M. Di Napoli, "The myasthenic patient in crisis: an update of the management in Neurointensive Care Unit," *Arquivos de Neuro-Psiquiatria*, vol. 71, no. 9, pp. 627–639, 2013.

[4] D. Lacomis, "Myasthenic crisis," *Neurocritical Care*, vol. 3, no. 3, pp. 189–194, 2005.

[5] S. Nava and N. Hill, "Non-invasive ventilation in acute respiratory failure," *The Lancet*, vol. 374, no. 9685, pp. 250–259, 2009.

[6] J. Seneviratne, J. Mandrekar, E. F. M. Wijdicks, and A. A. Rabinstein, "Noninvasive ventilation in myasthenic crisis," *Archives of Neurology*, vol. 65, no. 1, pp. 54–58, 2008.

[7] S. P. Keenan, T. Sinuff, K. E. A. Burns et al., "Clinical practice guidelines for the use of noninvasive positive-pressure ventilation and noninvasive continuous positive airway pressure in the acute care setting," *Canadian Medical Association Journal*, vol. 183, no. 3, pp. E195–E214, 2011.

[8] P. N. Varelas, H. C. Chua, J. Natterman et al., "Ventilatory care in myasthenia gravis crisis: assessing the baseline adverse event rate," *Critical Care Medicine*, vol. 30, no. 12, pp. 2663–2668, 2002.

[9] J.-Y. Wu, P.-H. Kuo, P.-C. Fan, H.-D. Wu, F.-Y. Shih, and P.-C. Yang, "The role of non-invasive ventilation and factors predicting extubation outcome in myasthenic crisis," *Neurocritical Care*, vol. 10, no. 1, pp. 35–42, 2009.

[10] T. M. Burns, M. Conaway, and D. B. Sanders, "The MG composite. A valid and reliable outcome measure for myasthenia gravis," *Neurology*, vol. 74, no. 18, pp. 1434–1440, 2010.

10

Opiate Withdrawal Complicated by Tetany and Cardiac Arrest

Irfanali R. Kugasia and Nehad Shabarek

Department of Internal Medicine, Lincoln Medical and Mental Health Center, 234 East 149th Street, Bronx, NY 10451, USA

Correspondence should be addressed to Irfanali R. Kugasia; irfanali102@gmail.com

Academic Editor: Joel Starkopf

Patients with symptoms of opiate withdrawal, after the administration of opiate antagonist by paramedics, are a common presentation in the emergency department of hospitals. Though most of opiate withdrawal symptoms are benign, rarely they can become life threatening. This case highlights how a benign opiate withdrawal symptom of hyperventilation led to severe respiratory alkalosis that degenerated into tetany and cardiac arrest. Though this patient was successfully resuscitated, it is imperative that severe withdrawal symptoms are timely identified and immediate steps are taken to prevent catastrophes. An easier way to reverse the severe opiate withdrawal symptom would be with either low dose methadone or partial opiate agonists like buprenorphine. However, if severe acid-base disorder is identified, it would be safer to electively intubate these patients for better control of their respiratory and acid-base status.

1. Introductions

Withdrawal from opiates is considered to be generally benign with the common symptoms being diaphoresis, piloerection, lacrimation, diarrhea, anxiousness, nonspecific abdominal and bodily pain sensation, and hyperventilation. It is rarely associated with life threatening complications, unlike withdrawal from benzodiazepine and alcohol which are frequently associated with life threatening complications and need close monitoring in an inpatient setting [1–3]. As a result, opiate antagonist like naloxone has been extensively and successfully used in the field and the emergency departments for diagnosing altered mental status from opiate overdose and reversing their complication of respiratory depression which is considered to be more life threatening [3–5]. However, in rare cases serious complications and fatal outcomes have been reported during opiate withdrawals, particularly in patients who are undernourished or have underlying electrolyte or cardiorespiratory abnormalities [3, 5, 6]. These complications considered to be either from direct toxic effects of naloxone or from increased catecholamine surge due to severe opiate withdrawal [4–6]. This case emphasizes the need for a cautious approach towards severe manifestations of simple opiate withdrawal symptom, like hyperventilation.

2. Case

A 54-year-old female was brought to the hospital by EMT (emergency medical team) with suspicion of opiate overdose. EMT was called by a family member after the patient was found to be less responsive and difficult to arouse. The patient received 4 mg of naloxone subcutaneously in field by the EMT which improved patient's responsiveness but pushed her into severe opiate withdrawal. In the emergency department, the patient was found to be awake, alert, and anxious. She was not oriented but was able to follow simple commands. The patient was also diaphoretic, tachypneic with respiratory rate in 30 and tachycardic with heart rate in 150 s. Lungs were clear on auscultation with good bilateral air entry. Cardiovascualr exam was unremarkable with regular rhythm good pulses present in all four extremities. Abdominal exam was also unremarkable. Neuromuscular exam showed tremulousness and muscle fasciculation in different muscle groups of the face, upper limb, and lower extremities, exacerbated deep tendon reflex and normal motor strength with severe pain on movement of left hip. The patient had a past medical history of AIDS, hepatitis C, and bipolar disorder but as per her home medication list she was not on any treatment for them. At home, the patient was on 150 mg of methadone for maintenance and oral morphine sustained release and immediate

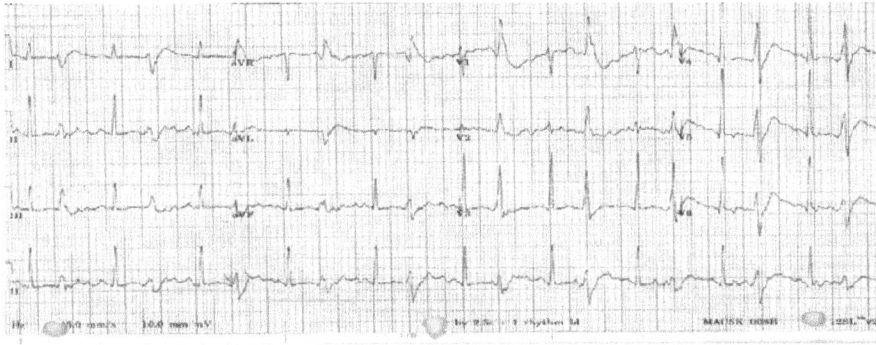

FIGURE 1: Initial EKG showing bigeminy—showing increased cardiac muscle excitability with origination of ventricular ectopics.

release for pain control for her recent hip fracture. The first ABG done at the time of patient's ED presentation was on a nonrebreather mask; it showed pH 7.694, PCO_2 19.6 mmHg, PO_2 224 mmHg, O_2 saturation of 100%, and lactate of 2.97 and her initial EKG showed bigeminy with the rest of the details obscured by artifacts as seen in Figure 1. In the next 30 minutes patient's respiratory rate had decreased to 18–25 breaths per minute at which time a repeat ABG was done on room air that showed pH of 7.641, PCO_2 20.3 mmHg, PO_2 of 86 mmHg, and O_2 saturation of 98% with lactate of 2.48. While being on telemetry, the patient had sinus tachycardia with PVCs and runs of bigeminy. The patient was subsequently deemed stable and taken for CT scan of heat and chest for further evaluation, while in CT room the patient went into generalized tetany and then into cardiac arrest with initial rhythm of ventricular tachycardia that degenerated to torsade de pointes and ventricular fibrillation. Code was run for 25 minutes, during which the patient was intubated and received 2 doses of epinephrine and 4 gm of magnesium and was shocked 3 times. She had a return of spontaneous circulation after the third shock. The patient was initially started on hypothermia protocol; however, it was abandoned as patient showed movement of extremities. The labs obtained prior to patient's cardiac arrest showed Na^+ 138, K^+ 3.4, Mg^+ 2.0, Ca^{2+} 8.9, HCO_3 18, and anion gap of 16; however, this sample was hemolyzed. Repeat labs obtained 30 minutes after intubation showed K^+ 3.5, Ca^{2+} 7.6, iCa^{2+} 3.92, Mg^+ 2.6, and HCO_3 16 with anion gap of 17. EKG obtained after cardiac arrest showed sinus tachycardia. Urine toxicology obtained for the patient was positive only for methadone and opiates. Patient's serum albumin level was 2.9. The patient was extubated on day 2 and was discharged from hospital on day 8 of hospitalization.

3. Discussion

The most important concern after giving naloxone to a patient with opiate overdose is reversal of naloxone antagonism and patient slipping back into respiratory depression from opiate overdose. This is because the half-life of naloxone action is only 20–80 minutes, much shorter than many of the opiates [2, 3]. The initial impression in this case was that patient had respiratory alkalosis from her tachypnea

due to acute opiate withdrawal and this was expected to reverse as quickly as the effect of naloxone wears off. However, repeat clinical evaluation and ABG after 30 minutes did not show any major change as the patient was still breathing at 25 breaths per minute and was tachycardic to 120–140 s. So other explanations for the clinical findings were sought. The consideration of pulmonary embolism was high on the differential as the patient had recent history of hip fracture and had an A-a gradient of almost 40 mmHg on the repeat arterial blood gas. As a result, decision was made to rule it out with a chest CT which came out to be negative for pulmonary embolism or any lung pathology. CT brain was also negative for any intracranial bleed.

The cardiac arrest observed in this case can be explained by three main reasons. Firstly, it could be from naloxone itself. Pulmonary edema and cardiac arrest from ventricular fibrillation have been reported with administration of naloxone. This was mostly seen in postoperative patient to whom naloxone was given to reverse the effect of opiates and in patient who was on high dose of opiate for pain relief who had some kind of cardiac comorbidity [6, 7]. These complications were considered to be from a sudden surge in catecholamine levels and have been mostly reported within minutes of IV naloxone administration [6, 7]. Since the cardiac arrest in this case occurred almost 1 hour after the naloxone which was given subcutaneously and negative chest CT for pulmonary edema, naloxone as the cause of cardiac arrest is less likely. Secondly, the cardiac arrhythmias observed in this patient like torsades de pointes and ventricular fibrillation are found in patient with prolonged QT interval. This is commonly seen with methadone overdose. The incidence of torsades de pointes with methadone is increased when methadone overdose is associated with electrolyte abnormality especially hypokalemia [8]. The cardiac arrest in this case could be easily attributed to methadone overdose associated with some electrolyte abnormalities. However, there was no conclusive evidence of prolonged QTc. The waves in initial EKG were obscured by artifacts and repeat EKG after successful resuscitation showed a QTc of 473. Also, none of this could explain the simultaneous occurrence of tetany and cardiac arrest observed in this case. Lastly, the cardiac arrhythmia and tetany could be explained by the severe alkalemia secondary to hypocapnia from patient's hyperventilation. As

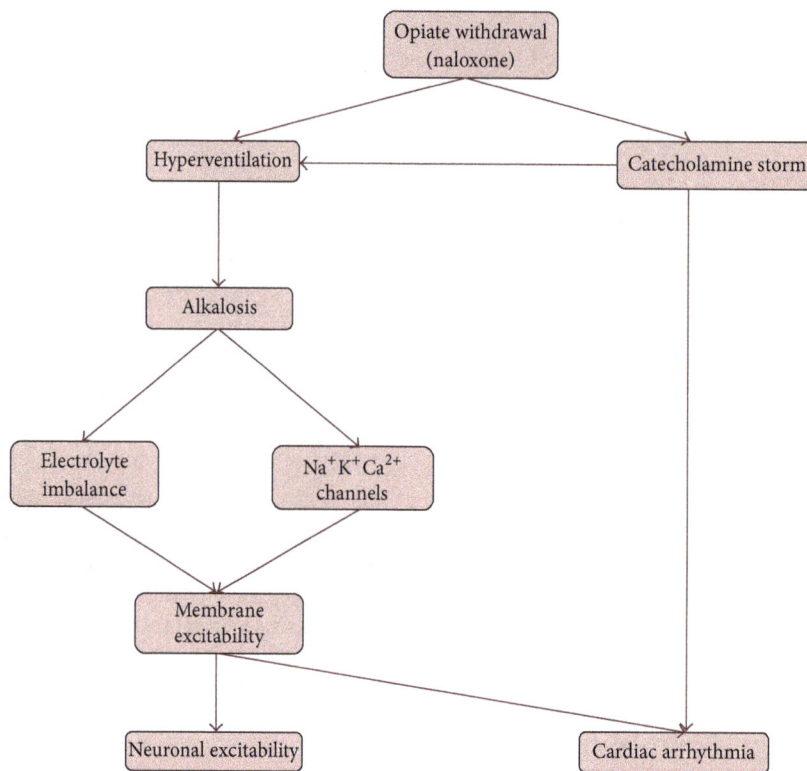

FIGURE 2: Mechanism explaining neuronal and cardiac excitability in opiate withdrawal.

per patient's initial lab and ABG, she had severe primary respiratory alkalosis with mild high anion gap metabolic acidosis which was considered to be from patient's elevated lactate level from her tachypnea. Voluntary hyperventilation in normal healthy patients has been found to be associated with severe respiratory alkalosis, increase in anion gap from lactic acidosis, and significant change in serum K^+ level [9, 10]. Severe alkalemia resulting from hyperventilation and hypocapnia has been shown to cause perioral numbness, cardiac arrhythmias, seizure, and tetany [11–13]. These complications can be either due to the direct effect of alkalemia on ion gated channels controlling membrane potential or secondary to its effect on serum potassium (K^+) and ionized calcium (iCa^{2+}) levels or from combination of both [14]. Putting together these pathophysiologic effects of severe alkalemia can result in neuronal and cardiac excitability. This can explain the initial findings of muscle fasciculation and bigeminy and later the tetany, polymorphic ventricular tachycardia, and ventricular fibrillation which were observed in this patient. A simplified schematic for this mechanism is depicted in Figure 2. Also notable was the rapid improvement in patient's clinical status and EKG finding after intubation with resolution of arrhythmia and overall good patient outcome.

To avoid severe opiate withdrawals and complications, a more conservative and cautious use of naloxone is advised. Intravenous route by well-trained personnel to better titrate the naloxone dose is recommended, as at low dose naloxone can reverse the respiratory depression from opiate overdose without causing overt withdrawal from opiates [3]. With

subcutaneous and intramuscular administration of naloxone, the time to peak effect and peak effect are less predictable than intravascular administration. However, once severe withdrawal symptoms are identified, immediate treatment with low dose of methadone or partial opiate agonists like buprenorphine could help in reversing some of these severe withdrawal symptoms [2, 3]. Nonetheless, with concerns of respiratory depression from opiate overdose and risk of severe alkalosis from hyperventilation, early elective intubation and sedation should be highly considered, as these would provide better control of patient's respiratory system and in turn their acid-base status.

References

[1] E. J. Khantzian and G. J. McKenna, "Acute toxic and withdrawal reactions associated with drug use and abuse," *Annals of Internal Medicine*, vol. 90, no. 3, pp. 361–372, 1979.

[2] T. R. Kosten and P. G. O'Connor, "Management of drug and alcohol withdrawal," *The New England Journal of Medicine*, vol. 348, no. 18, pp. 1786–1795, 2003.

[3] E. W. Boyer, "Management of opioid analgesic overdose," *The New England Journal of Medicine*, vol. 367, no. 2, pp. 146–155, 2012.

[4] D. M. Yealy, P. M. Paris, R. M. Kaplan, M. B. Heller, and S. E. Marini, "The safety of prehospital naloxone administration by paramedics," *Annals of Emergency Medicine*, vol. 19, no. 8, pp. 902–905, 1990.

[5] J. J. Osterwalder, "Naloxone-for intoxications with intravenous heroin and heroin mixtures-harmless or hazardous? A prospec-

tive clinical study," *Clinical Toxicology*, vol. 34, no. 4, pp. 409–416, 1996.

[6] F. M. Cuss, C. B. Colaco, and J. H. Baron, "Cardiac arrest after reversal of effects of opiates with naloxone," *British Medical Journal*, vol. 288, no. 6414, pp. 363–364, 1984.

[7] E. L. A. van Dorp, A. Yassen, and A. Dahan, "Naloxone treatment in opioid addiction: the risks and benefits," *Expert Opinion on Drug Safety*, vol. 6, no. 2, pp. 125–132, 2007.

[8] G. B. Ehret, C. Voide, M. Gex-Fabry et al., "Drug-induced long QT syndrome in injection drug users receiving methadone: high frequency in hospitalized patients and risk factors," *Archives of Internal Medicine*, vol. 166, no. 12, pp. 1280–1287, 2006.

[9] R. Krapf, P. Caduff, P. Wagdi, M. Staubli, and H. N. Hulter, "Plasma potassium response to acute respiratory alkalosis," *Kidney International*, vol. 47, no. 1, pp. 217–224, 1995.

[10] M. G. Sanchez and D. C. Finlayson, "Dynamics of serum potassium change during acute respiratory alkalosis," *Canadian Anaesthetists Society Journal*, vol. 25, no. 6, pp. 495–498, 1978.

[11] J. W. Edmondson, R. E. Brashear, and T. K. Li, "Tetany: quantitative interrelationships between calcium and alkalosis," *American Journal of Physiology*, vol. 228, no. 4, pp. 1082–1086, 1975.

[12] E. B. Brown Jr., "Physiological effects of hyperventilation," *Physiological Reviews*, vol. 33, no. 4, pp. 445–471, 1953.

[13] N. W. Lawson, G. H. Butler III, and C. T. Ray, "Alkalosis and cardiac arrhythmias," *Anesthesia and Analgesia*, vol. 52, no. 6, pp. 951–964, 1973.

[14] G. C. Tombaugh and G. G. Somjen, "Effects of extracellular pH on voltage-gated Na^+, K^+ and Ca^{2+} currents in isolated rat CA1 neurons," *Journal of Physiology*, vol. 493, no. 3, pp. 719–732, 1996.

11

Systemic Capillary Leak Syndrome: Is Methylene Blue the Silver Bullet?

Michele Umbrello,[1] **Marco Gardinali,**[2] **Davide Ottolina,**[1]
Giancarlo Zanforlin,[1] **and Gaetano Iapichino**[1,3]

[1]*Unità Operativa di Anestesia e Rianimazione, Azienda Ospedaliera San Paolo, Polo Universitario,*
Via A. Di Rudinì 8, 20142 Milano, Italy

[2]*Unità Operativa di Medicina IV, Azienda Ospedaliera San Paolo, Polo Universitario, Via A. Di Rudinì 8, 20142 Milano, Italy*

[3]*Dipartimento di Fisiopatologia Medico-Chirurgica e dei Trapianti, Università degli Studi di Milano,*
Via F. Sforza 35, 20122 Milano, Italy

Correspondence should be addressed to Michele Umbrello; michele.umbrello@ao-sanpaolo.it

Academic Editor: Zsolt Molnar

Background. Systemic capillary leak syndrome (SCLS) is a rare disorder characterized by unexplained, recurrent episodes of transient, abrupt increase in endothelial permeability, leading to severe hypotension, generalized edema, and hemoconcentration. *Case Report.* We report the case of a patient suffering from systemic capillary leak syndrome and present a possible interpretation of the pathophysiology of this condition. Besides the classical triad of hypotension, edema, and hemoconcentration, we recorded increased levels of methemoglobin, an index of NO overproduction. We present a possible interpretation of the pathophysiology of this condition based on the fast and complete reversal of symptoms after methylene blue administration (which opposes NO-induced effects) and speculate that increased NO levels could be implicated in the pathophysiology of the capillary leak phase. *Why should an emergency physician be aware of this?* The safety of this treatment and its fluid- and cathecolamine-sparing effect deserve consideration and further research.

1. Introduction

Systemic capillary leak syndrome (SCLS) is a rare disorder characterized by unexplained, recurrent episodes of transient, abrupt increase in endothelial permeability, leading to severe hypotension, generalized edema, and hemoconcentration [1]. Both etiology and pathogenesis are currently unknown, and systematic research is clearly limited by the rarity of the disease. Several hypotheses have been formulated, but clear evidence is lacking to support any.

We describe the improvement of one patient with SCLS in two occasions with acute IV administration of methylene blue after failure of the medications commonly used in this setting. We present a possible interpretation of the pathophysiology of this response to therapy.

2. Case Presentation

In March 2013, a 56-year-old man, otherwise healthy, suffered from a cold and low-grade fever and gradually developed oliguria and weight gain. The general practitioner prescribed some biochemical tests, which resulted normal except for serum albumin 3 g/dL and a monoclonal IgG/κ peak. An empirical course of broad-spectrum antibiotic and furosemide was started.

Ten days later, he developed massive peripheral edema, bilateral pleural and pericardial effusion, and ascites. Body temperature was normal, arterial blood pressure (ABP) was 90/60, and heart rate was (HR) 120/min. Blood tests showed albumin 2.3 g/dL, creatinine 1.4 mg/dL, sodium 129 mEq/L, hemoglobin (Hb) 22 g/dL, and hematocrit (Ht)

TABLE 1: Time course of hemodynamic and laboratory parameters at baseline and during the second acute episode.

Time (hours)	BL	0	+5	+13.5	+24.5*	+36.5	+39.5	+47.5	+54.5	+61.5	+65.5
ABP (mmHg)	125/75	80/50	90/60	65/30	135/80	110/60	100/70	110/50	129/61	110/50	115/60
HR (1/min)	73	140	134	120	105	100	97	112	98	102	101
CVP (mmHg)	—	—	—	2/−3 (−1)	—	2/−3 (−1)	—	16/7 (12)	—	7/0 (4)	8/4 (6)
Hb (g/dL)	12.5	22.0	22.4	22.7	17.5	15.2	13.4	12	10.9	10.5	10.2
Ht (%)	37.1	67.1	68.2	69	53.4	46.5	41.2	36.9	33.5	32.3	31.5
Albumin (g/dL)	3.9	3.7	3.3	—	2.7	—	2.4	—	—	—	—
Creatinine (mg/dL)	1	1.2	0.9	1.2	1.5		1.2				
pH	7.4	7.4	7.4	7.4	7.35	7.4	7.46	7.46	7.46	7.47	7.43
BE (mmol/L)	1.1	−2.8	−0.8	−4	−0.9	4.9	8.2	9.8	11.4	12.1	10.1
HCO$_3$ (mmol/L)	26.4	22.9	24.2	22.6	24	29.6	32.4	34.3	36.1	36.6	35
Lactate (mmol/L)	0.6	1.6	1.7	2.2	2	1.3	1.6	1.2	1	1.1	1.3
Na (mEq/L)	141	134	134	131	137	139	141	142	143	143	143
K (mEq/L)	3.7	4.3	4.6	5.6	4.2	3.7	3.8	3.4	3.3	3.5	4.1
MetHb (%)	—	0.5	0.6	0.4	1.3	1.4	1.5	1.4	1.5	1.3	1.7

BL: baseline (3 months before the acute episode). First line refers to hours after admission. *Denotes methylene blue administration.
ABP: arterial blood pressure; HR: heart rate; CVP: central venous pressure; Hb: haemoglobin; Ht: hematocrit; MetHb: methaemoglobin; BE: base excess; HCO$_3$: bicarbonate; Na: sodium; K: potassium.

62%. Crystalloid loading was started, but despite a positive balance of about 7000 mL over 12 hours, ABP kept falling down to 70/40 and the patient became anuric. Norepinephrine (NE) up to 0.2 mcg/kg/min was then added, with ABP only rising to 80/60. Despite the presence of only tachycardia as a SIRS sign (WBC 11780/mm^3, PaCO2 37 with RR 18/min, core body temperature 36.4°C, HR 120/min), the case was interpreted as refractory septic shock of unknown origin (cultures later resulted negative), and empirical treatment with methylene blue (1.5 mg/kg IV bolus over 1 hour) was given. Soon after the end of the infusion, ABP rose to 140/80, HR 75/min, diuresis restarted, and norepinephrine was suspended in 2 hours. Renal function improved and edema and effusions reduced. The patient was discharged home with no therapy, whilst awaiting more tests.

In the following months he experienced two less severe episodes, requiring admittance to a nephrology ward for fatigue, hypotension, peripheral swelling, oliguria, hypoalbuminemia, and hemoconcentration. During the course of these admissions, a series of tests were run, showing normal levels of complement and C1-esterase inhibitor, negative cancer markers, no autoantibodies; immunoglobulin levels, including IgE, were in the normal range. Absence of diarrhea excluded a protein losing enteropathy. Renal biopsy yielded no alterations, and brain MR excluded pituitary lesions. Thyroid and adrenal functions were normal. Bone marrow biopsy excluded malignancies. Subcutaneous fatty tissue biopsy excluded systemic amyloidosis. POEMS syndrome was excluded by the absence of any sign of polyneuropathy. Determination of vascular endothelial growth factor (VEGF) showed increased levels (1429 pg/mL—normal values <450 pg/mL). The recurrence of episodes of hypotension, hypoalbuminemia, and hemoconcentration and the presence of a monoclonal IgG/κ peak led to the diagnosis of systemic capillary leak syndrome: prophylactic treatment with theophylline 300 mg bid was started.

In October 2013, the patient again experienced symptoms of a cold similar to those before the first admission. On arrival to the hospital, he was hypotensive and tachycardic; blood tests (Table 1) showed severe hemoconcentration with normal albumin levels. He was oliguric and had peripheral edema. Again, SIRS was not present. Echocardiography showed a pericardial effusion 18 mm, with no sign of tamponade, normal valves, hypertrophic left ventricle with slightly reduced end-diastolic volume (70 mL), and 60% ejection fraction, normal diastolic pattern, TAPSE 20 mm. Inferior vena cava diameter was unmeasurable. Fluid loading with crystalloids was started, but despite a positive balance of 5500 mL/12 h, ABP kept falling (Figure 1) and urine output remained low. NE was started and rapidly increased up to 0.2 mcg/kg/min, with minimal response in terms of ABP. ABG showed increasing levels of lactic acid and methaemoglobin (Table 1). Organ failure was quantified, yielding a SOFA score of 8, only depending, however, from complete failure of cardiocirculatory and renal system (norepinephrine 0.2 mcg/kg/min, anuria) with no sign of compromise of any other organ (GCS 15, bilirubin 1.1, platelet count 180000, PaO2 81 mmHg at room air).

Given the lack of response to treatment, bearing in mind the previous anecdotal response, methylene blue was administered (1.5 mg/kg IV bolus over 1 hour), and ABP again rapidly rose to 135/90, allowing for NE termination 8 hours later. Urine output gradually increased, allowing for the negativization of fluid balance and concurrent recovery of renal function. Haemoglobin levels normalized over a 48-hour period, while albumin remained low (Figure 1). The patient was thereafter discharged home.

3. Discussion

We describe a case of SCLS that responded twice—one time as a rescue for a suspected diagnosis of septic shock, while the

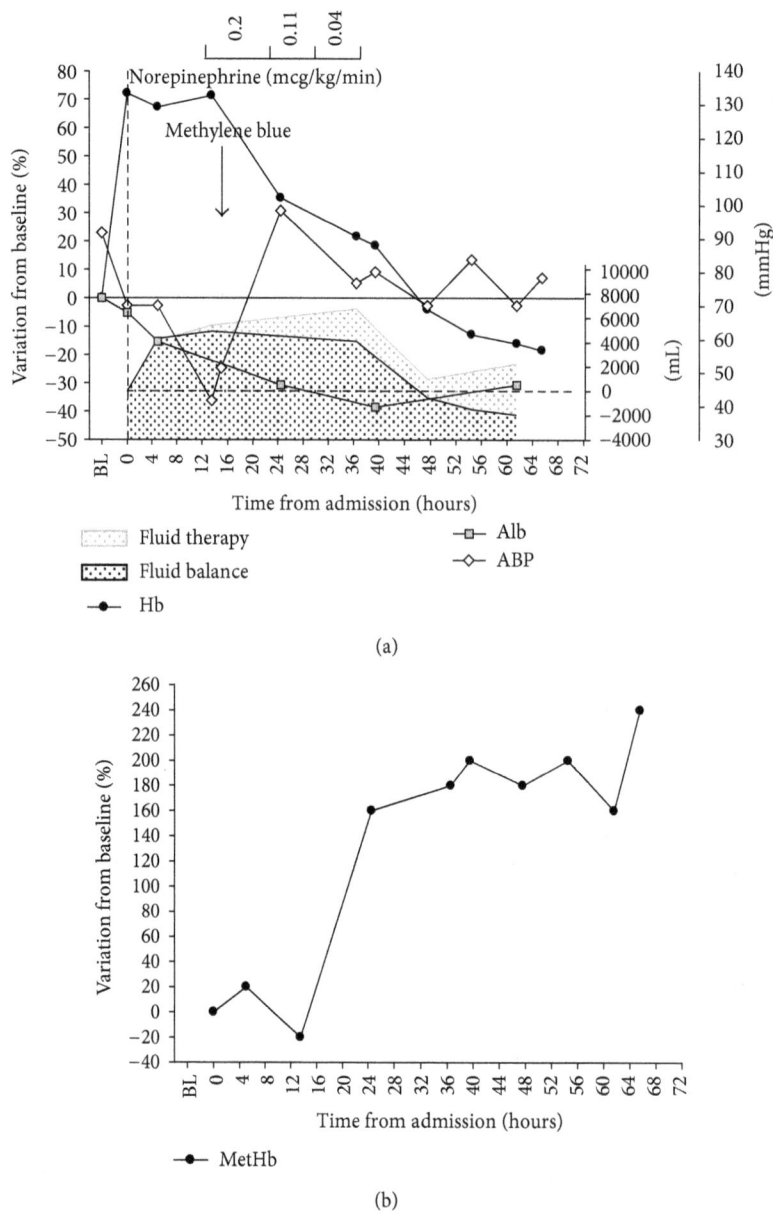

FIGURE 1: (a) Time course of blood pressure, haemoglobin, and albumin levels during the acute episode and effects of therapeutic interventions. (b) Time course of methemoglobin during the acute episode. BL: baseline (3 months before the acute episode), Hb: haemoglobin (% variation form baseline), Alb: albumin (% variation form baseline), ABP: mean arterial blood pressure (absolute value), and MetHb: methaemoglobin (% variation form baseline).

second time intentionally to the administration of methylene blue. In both episodes, the patient had hypotension (with ongoing further reduction during the first 12 hours) and signs of severe haemoconcentration (Hb and Ht about 70% higher than his own baseline normal values) and needed significant amount of NE, despite positive fluid balance of >5 liters in 12 h, in line with the well-known poor response to fluid and vasoactive drugs of SCLS [1]. On the contrary, albumin concentration was not increased, and it further decreased during the first hours, suggesting a shift towards the extracellular space due to increased endothelial permeability. Accordingly, transcapillary escape rate of radio-labeled albumin was found

to be elevated [2] in similar cases. Organ perfusion was inadequate, as highlighted by the reduced urinary output and the increase of plasma lactic acid; however, the absence of a profound metabolic acidosis and the only presence of tachycardia as a sign of SIRS could have raised doubts on the diagnosis of refractory septic shock.

Actual management of the acute shock phase in this condition is based on support of vital functions with IV fluids, including colloids and vasopressors [3]. We avoided albumin administration as extravasation may lead to increased interstitial colloid osmotic pressure, with further reduction of circulating blood volume, and to reduced de novo synthesis

[4]. Infusion of pentastarch or dextrans [5] which could seal the negatively charged endothelial fenestrations [4], were unavailable for clinical use in Italy. Echocardiographic assessment showed signs of both hypovolemia (complete collapse of the inferior vena cava) and loss of systemic vascular resistance (hypotension despite preserved systolic function, as indicated by the normal values of ejection fraction and TAPSE). After about 13 hours of standard treatment, we decided to administer methylene blue and consequently observed the rapid reversal of hypotension, a concomitant gradual reduction of Hb and Ht back to baseline levels, an increase in urine output, a negative fluid balance, and resolution of edema. All these signs are compatible with normalization of endothelial permeability. Albumin levels, however, remained low, likely because the escaped molecules only partially flow back into vessels and are degraded in tissues [6], while the turnover rate for de novo synthesis can take up to 20 days to restore normal values [7]. Meanwhile, during the second episode, we observed a significant increase of methaemoglobin levels.

Despite severe hypotension, the patient was awake and cooperative; moreover, hypoxemia was not present ad admission, and the lung CT scan excluded pulmonary edema. Usually, during SCLS attacks, musculature and connective tissue are the principal target sites of the extravasation of plasma, while the lungs, brain, and kidneys seem to be infrequently involved [8]; as such, we think that the measurement vascular permeability, such as the pulmonary vascular permeability index derived by transpulmonary thermodilution [9], is of limited help in this phase. However, it is quite common that pulmonary edema develops during the recovery phase, as an iatrogenic side effect of the huge amount of intravenous fluid often administered. In this phase, we can speculate that the availability of such an index might potentially be of help for the evaluation of the effects of therapy.

This patient, as the majority of those described in series and case reports, presented a monoclonal gammopathy [10] and elevated VEGF levels [2]; many Clarkson's disease cases predominantly have IgG-κ or IgA-κ monoclonal gammopathy [8]: both multiple myeloma and systemic amyloidosis were excluded via abdominal wall fat pad and bone marrow biopsy. POEMS syndrome (polyneuropathy, organomegaly, endocrinopathy, monoclonal gammopathy, and skin changes), which is almost always associated with IgG-λ or IgA-λ, was excluded by the absence of any sign of polyneuropathy.

The patient was also in long-term treatment with theophylline [11], a drug that increases intracellular cAMP levels. Any possible pathophysiologic interpretation of the response to methylene blue should take these findings into account. In addition to its mitogenic effect, VEGF was shown to increase endothelial permeability, in a process mediated by a NO-dependent increase in cGMP levels [12], the main modulator of increased vascular permeability. Moreover, IL-2 might contribute to the pathogenesis of SCLS [1], based on the fact that IL-2 therapy can develop a leakage syndrome undistinguishable from SCLS [13]. Indeed, increased IL-2 expression was demonstrated on perivascular cells of symptomatic cases of SCLS [14]. Nitric oxide (NO) was suggested

as the mediator of IL-2-induced endothelial permeabilization [15], and inhibition of NO synthesis resulted in reversal of IL-2-induced leakage [16]. Hence, the NO system seems to be a common pathway for both IL-2- and VEGF-mediated endothelial permeabilization. The vascular effects of NO are mainly mediated by the activation of soluble guanylate cyclase (sGC), which leads to the synthesis of cGMP; the latter, in turn, acts on several targets eventually causing smooth muscle relaxation [17] and increased endothelial permeability [18]. cGMP-mediated signalling also contributes to vasopressor hyporesponsiveness [19]. Instead, cAMP (increased by theophylline) counteracts with this pathway, protecting the basal barrier function [18].

The response to methylene blue supports the hypothesis that increased NO levels could be implicated in the pathophysiology of the acute capillary leak phase. Methylene blue (3,7-bis(dimethylamino)-phenothiazin-5-ium chloride) is generally used in the setting of methaemoglobinemia [20] and proved effective in reversing hypotension and restoring the response to vasoactive drugs in many different conditions characterized by increased levels of NO (sepsis, anaphylaxis, severe burns, ischaemia-reperfusion injury and liver failure) [21–25]. Methylene blue opposes NO-induced effects mainly by inhibition of sGC [26–30], ultimately reducing the generation of cGMP. Acute methylene blue administration, unlike drugs that increase intracellular cAMP levels (such as theophylline), aims at decreasing cGMP levels to reduce the severity of supposedly NO-mediated attacks.

Although multiple therapies were administered during the clinical management of the patient, both times we recorded a clear temporal relation between methylene blue administration and reversal of the symptoms, leading us to identify this treatment as the main cause for the change in the clinical course. We did not report direct measures of NO levels in the case we described. Indeed, NO has a very short half-life [31]. However, in septic populations, circulating levels of methaemoglobin proved effective indicators of NO overproduction [32]. Methaemoglobin is generated by the reaction of haemoglobin with NO [33]. In the present case, methaemoglobin levels increased up to 250% their baseline value during the course of the episode. We observed a delay from symptoms appearance and methaemoglobin rise: methaemoglobin generation in the presence of elevated NO may require up to several hours to occur in vitro [34]; under in vivo conditions, this time may even increase, depending on plasma redox state.

At pharmacologic doses methylene blue is a reducing agent via the NADPH-methemoglobin reductase pathway [20]. Methylene blue, when injected intravenously as an antidote, is reduced to leucomethylene blue, which then reduces the heme group from methemoglobin to hemoglobin. However, when given in higher doses, methylene blue may oxidize the ferrous iron of hemoglobin to ferric iron, thus potentially resulting in methemoglobin production. However, the dose we administered in the present case is well within the doses used in the setting of methaemoglobinemia (1-2 mg/kg, repeated up to twice if symptoms of hypoxia fail to subside) [35], thus reducing the possibility that the elevated methaemoglobin levels we recorded were generated by the methylene blue we administered. Elevated levels of methaemoglobin persisted up to the last blood sample taken in the ICU, likely after the effects of methylene blue ended; however, this is not surprising as the elimination half-life of methaemoglobin has been reported to be as high as 15–20 hours [36].

The main limit of the present investigation is its case-report nature. However, the rarity of this condition makes experimental studies difficult to plan, and the incomplete understanding of the underlying mechanisms does not allow for preclinical modeling. Moreover, the hemodynamic response to methylene blue might have simply faced by chance the natural course of the syndrome, which spontaneously reversed. However, the response we observed was similar in two different occasions, and both times it occurred soon after the administration of the drug.

SCLS is a rare yet potentially severe condition, often difficult to recognize and diagnose upon initial presentation. Current therapies are mainly supportive, and the condition is still associated with a 10-year mortality rate of about 30% [1]. We report our experience with a treatment whose safety [37], along with its fluid- and catecholamine-sparing effect deserve consideration and further research.

Abbreviation List

ABP: Arterial blood pressure
cAMP: Cyclic adenosine monophosphate
cGMP: Cyclic guanosine monophosphate
Hb: Hemoglobin
HR: Heart rate
Ht: Hematocrit
NE: Norepinephrine
NO: Nitric oxide
SCLS: Systemic capillary leak syndrome
sGC: Soluble guanilate cyclase
VEGF: Vascular endothelial growth factor.

Authors' Contribution

Michele Umbrello performed the literature search and drafted the first version of the paper, Marco Gardinali and Gaetano Iapichino revised the text for important intellectual content, and Davide Ottolina and Giancarlo Zanforlin collected clinical data and helped to draft the paper.

Funding

This study was carried out by departmental funding only.

References

[1] K. M. Druey and P. R. Greipp, "Narrative review: the systemic capillary leak syndrome," *Annals of Internal Medicine*, vol. 153, no. 2, pp. 90–98, 2010.

[2] W. J. Lesterhuis, A. J. Rennings, W. P. Leenders et al., "Vascular endothelial growth factor in systemic capillary leak syndrome," *The American Journal of Medicine*, vol. 122, no. 6, pp. e5–e7, 2009.

[3] R. P. Dellinger, M. M. Levy, A. Rhodes et al., "Surviving sepsis campaign: international guidelines for management of severe sepsis and septic shock, 2012," *Intensive Care Medicine*, vol. 39, no. 2, pp. 165–228, 2013.

[4] T. E. Woodcock and T. M. Woodcock, "Revised Starling equation and the glycocalyx model of transvascular fluid exchange: an improved paradigm for prescribing intravenous fluid therapy," *British Journal of Anaesthesia*, vol. 108, no. 3, pp. 384–394, 2012.

[5] S. L. Young, Y. K. Sun, W. K. Chin et al., "Two cases of systemic capillary leak syndrome that were treated with pentastarch," *Korean Journal of Internal Medicine*, vol. 22, no. 2, pp. 130–132, 2007.

[6] S. Yedgar, T. E. Carew, R. C. Pittman, W. F. Beltz, and D. Steinberg, "Tissue sites of catabolism of albumin in rabbits," *American Journal of Physiology*, vol. 244, no. 1, pp. E101–E107, 1983.

[7] J. P. Nicholson, M. R. Wolmarans, and G. R. Park, "The role of albumin in critical illness," *British Journal of Anaesthesia*, vol. 85, no. 4, pp. 599–610, 2000.

[8] P. Kapoor, P. T. Greipp, E. W. Schaefer et al., "Idiopathic systemic capillary leak syndrome (Clarkson's disease): the Mayo Clinic experience original article," *Mayo Clinic Proceedings*, vol. 85, no. 10, pp. 905–912, 2010.

[9] X. Monnet, N. Anguel, D. Osman, O. Hamzaoui, C. Richard, and J.-L. Teboul, "Assessing pulmonary permeability by trans-pulmonary thermodilution allows differentiation of hydrostatic pulmonary edema from ALI/ARDS," *Intensive Care Medicine*, vol. 33, no. 3, pp. 448–453, 2007.

[10] W. Zhang, P. W. Ewan, and P. J. Lachmann, "The paraproteins in systemic capillary leak syndrome," *Clinical and Experimental Immunology*, vol. 93, no. 3, pp. 424–429, 1993.

[11] R. M. Droder, R. A. Kyle, and P. R. Greipp, "Control of systemic capillary leak syndrome with aminophylline and terbutaline," *The American Journal of Medicine*, vol. 92, no. 5, pp. 523–526, 1992.

[12] W. G. Mayhan, "VEGF increases permeability of the blood-brain barrier via a nitric oxide synthase/cGMP-dependent pathway," *The American Journal of Physiology*, vol. 276, no. 5, pp. C1148–C1153, 1999.

[13] S. A. Rosenberg, M. T. Lotze, L. M. Muul et al., "Observations on the systemic administration of autologous lymphokine-activated killer cells and recombinant interleukin-2 to patients with metastatic cancer," *The New England Journal of Medicine*, vol. 313, no. 23, pp. 1485–1492, 1985.

[14] M. Cicardi, M. Gardinali, G. Bisiani, A. Rosti, P. Allavena, and A. Agostoni, "The systemic capillary leak syndrome: appearance of interleukin-2-receptor-positive cells during attacks," *Annals of Internal Medicine*, vol. 113, no. 6, pp. 475–477, 1990.

[15] J. B. Hibbs Jr., C. Westenfelder, R. Taintor et al., "Evidence for cytokine-inducible nitric oxide synthesis from L-arginine in patients receiving interleukin-2 therapy," *The Journal of Clinical Investigation*, vol. 89, no. 3, pp. 867–877, 1992.

[16] A. Orucevic and P. K. Lala, "NG-nitro-L-arginine methyl ester, an inhibitor of nitric oxide synthesis, ameliorates interleukin 2-induced capillary leakage and reduces tumour growth in adenocarcinoma-bearing mice," *British Journal of Cancer*, vol. 73, no. 2, pp. 189–196, 1996.

[17] M. Umbrello, A. Dyson, M. Feelisch, and M. Singer, "The key role of nitric oxide in hypoxia: hypoxic vasodilation and energy supply-demand matching," *Antioxidants & Redox Signaling*, vol. 19, no. 14, pp. 1690–1710, 2013.

[18] S. Y. Yuan, "Protein kinase signaling in the modulation of microvascular permeability," *Vascular Pharmacology*, vol. 39, no. 4-5, pp. 213–223, 2002.

[19] J. E. da Silva-Santos, M. R. Terluk, and J. Assreuy, "Differential involvement of guanylate cyclase and potassium channels in nitric oxide-induced hyporesponsiveness to phenylephrine in endotoxemic rats," *Shock*, vol. 17, no. 1, pp. 70–76, 2002.

[20] W. R. Layne and R. P. Smith, "Methylene blue uptake and the reversal of chemically induced methemoglobinemias in human erythrocytes," *Journal of Pharmacology and Experimental Therapeutics*, vol. 165, no. 1, pp. 36–44, 1969.

[21] C. R. G. H. Daemen-Gubbels, P. H. P. Groeneveld, A. B. J. Groeneveld, G. J. Van Kamp, W. Bronsveld, and L. G. Thijs, "Methylene blue increases myocardial function in septic shock," *Critical Care Medicine*, vol. 23, no. 8, pp. 1363–1370, 1995.

[22] J.-C. Preiser, P. Lejeune, A. Roman et al., "Methylene blue administration in septic shock: a clinical trial," *Critical Care Medicine*, vol. 23, no. 2, pp. 259–264, 1995.

[23] A. D. Jaskille, J. C. Jeng, and M. H. Jordan, "Methylene blue in the treatment of vasoplegia following severe burns," *Journal of Burn Care and Research*, vol. 29, no. 2, pp. 408–410, 2008.

[24] H. Koelzow, J. A. Gedney, J. Baumann, N. J. Snook, and M. C. Bellamy, "The effect of methylene blue on the hemodynamic changes during ischemia reperfusion injury in orthotopic liver transplantation," *Anesthesia and Analgesia*, vol. 94, no. 4, pp. 824–829, 2002.

[25] M. Y. Kirov, O. V. Evgenov, N. V. Evgenov et al., "Infusion of methylene blue in human septic shock: a pilot, randomized, controlled study," *Critical Care Medicine*, vol. 29, no. 10, pp. 1860–1867, 2001.

[26] W. Martin, G. M. Villani, D. Jothianandan, and R. F. Furchgott, "Selective blockade of endothelium-dependent and glyceryl trinitrate-induced relaxation by hemoglobin and by methylene blue in the rabbit aorta," *The Journal of Pharmacology and Experimental Therapeutics*, vol. 232, no. 3, pp. 708–716, 1985.

[27] T. M. Griffith, D. H. Edwards, M. J. Lewis, and A. H. Henderson, "Evidence that cyclic guanosine monophosphate (cGMP) mediates endothelium-dependent relaxation," *European Journal of Pharmacology*, vol. 112, no. 2, pp. 195–202, 1985.

[28] L. J. Ignarro, R. G. Harbison, K. S. Wood, and P. J. Kadowitz, "Dissimilarities between methylene blue and cyanide on relaxation and cyclic GMP formation in endothelium-intact intrapulmonary artery caused by nitrogen oxide-containing vasodilators and acetylcholine," *Journal of Pharmacology and Experimental Therapeutics*, vol. 236, no. 1, pp. 30–36, 1986.

[29] C. A. Gruetter, P. J. Kadowitz, and L. J. Ignarro, "Methylene blue inhibits coronary arterial relaxation and guanylate cyclase activation by nitroglycerin, sodium nitrite, and amyl nitrite," *Canadian Journal of Physiology and Pharmacology*, vol. 59, no. 2, pp. 150–156, 1981.

[30] R. J. Gryglewski, A. Zembowicz, D. Salvemini, G. W. Taylor, and J. R. Vane, "Modulation of the pharmacological actions of nitrovasodilators by methylene blue and pyocyanin," *British Journal of Pharmacology*, vol. 106, no. 4, pp. 838–845, 1992.

[31] X. Liu, Q. Yan, K. L. Baskerville, and J. L. Zweier, "Estimation of nitric oxide concentration in blood for different rates of generation: evidence that intravascular nitric oxide levels are too low to exert physiological effects," *The Journal of Biological Chemistry*, vol. 282, no. 12, pp. 8831–8836, 2007.

[32] K. Ohashi, H. Yukioka, M. Hayashi, and A. Asada, "Elevated methemoglobin in patients with sepsis," *Acta Anaesthesiologica Scandinavica*, vol. 42, no. 6, pp. 713–716, 1998.

[33] V. S. Sharma, R. A. Isaacson, M. E. John, M. R. Waterman, and M. Chevion, "Reaction of nitric oxide with heme proteins: studies on metmyoglobin, opossum methemoglobin, and microperoxidase," *Biochemistry*, vol. 22, no. 16, pp. 3897–3902, 1983.

[34] N. Maeda, K. Imaizumi, K. Kon, and T. Shiga, "A kinetic study on functional impairment of nitric oxide-exposed rat erythrocytes," *Environmental Health Perspectives*, vol. 73, pp. 171–177, 1987.

[35] A. Skold, D. L. Cosco, and R. Klein, "Methemoglobinemia: pathogenesis, diagnosis, and management," *Southern Medical Journal*, vol. 104, no. 11, pp. 757–761, 2011.

[36] S. M. Raso, J. B. Fernandez, E. A. Beobide, and A. F. Landaluce, "Methemoglobinemia and CNS toxicity after topical application of EMLA to a 4-year-old girl with molluscum contagiosum," *Pediatric Dermatology*, vol. 23, no. 6, pp. 592–593, 2006.

[37] L. Pasin, M. Umbrello, T. Greco et al., "Methylene blue as a vasopressor: a meta-analysis of randomised trials," *Critical Care and Resuscitation*, vol. 15, no. 1, pp. 42–48, 2013.

12

Clinical and Imaging Resolution of Neonatal Hemochromatosis following Treatment

Ayelet Machtei,[1] Gil Klinger,[1,2] Rivka Shapiro,[2,3] Osnat Konen,[2,4] and Lea Sirota[1,2]

[1] Neonatal Intensive Care Unit, Schneider Children's Medical Center of Israel, 14 Kaplan Street, 49202 Petah Tikva, Israel
[2] The Sackler School of Medicine, Tel Aviv University, Tel Aviv, Israel
[3] Institute of Gastroenterology, Nutrition and Liver Diseases, Schneider Children's Medical Center of Israel, Petah Tikva, Israel
[4] Radiology Department, Schneider Children's Medical Center of Israel, Petah Tikva, Israel

Correspondence should be addressed to Ayelet Machtei; ayelet.malamud@gmail.com

Academic Editor: Ricardo J. Dinis-Oliveira

Neonatal hemochromatosis (NH) is an acute liver disease associated with both hepatic and extrahepatic iron deposition and is a leading cause of neonatal liver transplantation. The concept that NH is an alloimmune disease has led to the emergence of a new treatment approach utilizing exchange transfusion and intravenous immunoglobulin therapy. We present a two-day old neonate with progressive liver dysfunction who was diagnosed with NH. Magnetic resonance imaging confirmed tissue iron overload. Treatment with intravenous immunoglobulins and exchange transfusion led to rapid improvement in liver function. Follow-up physical examination at the age of 8 months showed normal development and near normal liver function. A repeat abdominal magnetic resonance scan at 8 months showed no signs of iron deposition in the liver, pancreas, or adrenal glands. The present report provides further support for the use of exchange transfusion and immunoglobulin therapy in NH and is the first to document resolution of typical iron deposition by magnetic resonance imaging.

1. Introduction

Neonatal hemochromatosis (NH) is a rapidly progressive disease presenting within a few days after birth with fulminant hepatic failure and ensuing multiorgan failure. NH is also known as neonatal iron storage disease or congenital alloimmune hepatitis. For many years the only curative treatment for NH was liver transplantation with survival rates of 50% [1]. Treatment with antioxidants and chelation therapy may improve symptoms but is associated with severe side effects [2]. In recent years the realization that NH is probably an alloimmune disease [3, 4] has led to the emergence of a new treatment approach utilizing exchange transfusion (ET) and intravenous immunoglobulins (IVIG). This has resulted in an improved survival rate and in a dramatic decrease in the need for liver transplantation. The understanding of the pathophysiology of the disease has also led to antenatal treatment with IVIG from 16 weeks' gestation and has been shown to prevent the development of NH in subsequent pregnancies [4]. In the present report we present a full-term newborn with liver dysfunction and multiorgan failure, diagnosed with NH that recovered fully following treatment with IVIG and ET.

2. Case Report

A female neonate was born at 39 weeks of gestation following an uneventful pregnancy. The infant was delivered by vacuum extraction due to a profound deceleration. Apgar scores at birth were 9 and 10 at 1 and 5 minutes, respectively. The infant weighed 2.724 kg (10th percentile) and the initial physical examination was normal. The patient was the first born (and first gestation) to healthy nonconsanguineous Ashkenazi Jews. At the age of two days the mother reported a decreased appetite and subsequently the infant's condition deteriorated rapidly. Physical examination showed pallor, hypothermia (35.9°C), and bradycardia of 70 beats per minute (bpm).

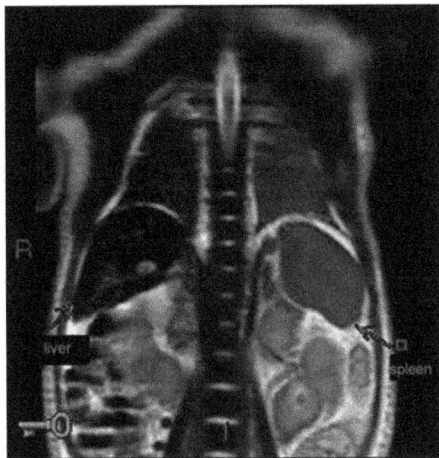

FIGURE 1: Abdominal MRI, coronal view, on day five of life showing low signal intensity of the liver parenchyma with preservation of the signal intensity of splenic parenchyma (T2WI protocol). Calculations of T2* showed rapid decay consistent with iron overload.

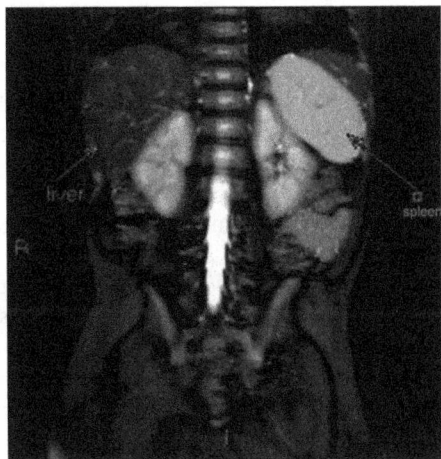

FIGURE 2: Follow-up abdominal MRI, coronal view, at 8 months showing normal intensity of liver parenchyma on T2WI with fat saturation protocol.

The initial laboratory evaluation showed hypoglycemia of 13 mg/dL (normal lower limit of 40 mg/dL). The patient was treated with intravenous boluses of 10% glucose and normal saline and was transferred to the neonatal intensive care unit (NICU). Upon admission to the NICU the infant's vital signs were as follows: temperature of 35.8°C, heart rate of 116 bpm, breath rate of 51 per minute, and blood pressure of 61/33 mm/Hg. Physical examination showed a lethargic infant with glucose level of 19 mg/dL; thus, a second bolus of 10% glucose was administered. During the hypoglycemic episode a critical blood sample was taken (insulin, cortisol, growth hormone, thyroid function, and lactate) and a full sepsis workup (complete blood count, C-reactive protein level, blood culture, and cerebrospinal fluid analysis and culture) was performed. Additional tests drawn included blood chemistry, a coagulation panel, and tests for possible metabolic abnormalities. Treatment with

ampicillin, gentamycin, and acyclovir was initiated. Initial blood tests showed leukocytosis, elevated liver enzymes and creatinine, and evidence of coagulopathy (Table 1). The remaining endocrinological parameters were within normal limits. During the next few days the patient's condition deteriorated. Although she remained normoglycemic, her liver function worsened progressively; coagulation tests showed disseminated intravascular coagulation (DIC) despite treatment with platelets, fresh frozen plasma, and vitamin k. A workup for possible hepatitis causing pathogens turned out negative. The metabolic evaluation was negative (including blood carnitine, acyl carnitine, amino acids, very long chain fatty acids, galactosemia, pyruvate dehydrogenase, E3 deficiency, and congenital disorder of glycosylation). Alpha 1 antitrypsin level was normal, alpha-fetoprotein was high (143,621 ng/mL) compared to normal values [5], iron was 155 μg/dL (normal 40-145), and ferritin was extremely elevated (24,256 ng/mL) compared to standard range (10–291). An abdominal ultrasound showed normal hepatic and bile ducts and a moderate degree of ascites. Because of suspected convulsions the patient underwent a head ultrasound which showed mild cerebral edema and an electroencephalogram that was normal.

Based on the clinical and laboratory findings we suspected NH to be the cause of the infant's condition and performed an abdominal magnetic resonance imaging (MRI) scan and a buccal biopsy. The MRI showed a clear shortening of the T2 signal to 3.5–5.5 ms (normal 25–30 ms) from the liver and pancreas which is characteristic of tissue iron overload (Figure 1). The buccal biopsy was negative for iron staining, as was a repeat biopsy. Treatment was initiated on day 8 with double volume exchange transfusion and IVIG 2 gr/kg as well as with vitamin E 25 IU three times per day. Following treatment, the patient showed rapid clinical and laboratory improvement (Table 1): platelets count (76,000 to 142,000), INR (2.83 to 1.99), ammonia (502 to 149), and creatinine (1.33 to 0.16). The patient was discharged home on day 22 of life.

The infant has continued the follow-up by our Gastroenterology outpatients service. At the age of 8 months the infant was healthy, developing normally, and liver function tests were approaching normal values. A repeat abdominal MRI at the age of 8 months was normal and showed no signs of iron deposition in the liver, pancreas, or adrenal glands as compared to the spleen (Figure 2).

3. Discussion

NH is a rare condition affecting the fetus and newborn that presents during the neonatal period with acute liver failure and ensuing multiorgan failure. Untreated NH is uniformly fatal. No single gene has been recognized as being responsible for the disease [3]. In families with one affected child there is a 70–80% chance of recurrence in subsequent pregnancies [4], a recurrence rate that is not compatible with either an autosomal recessive or dominant inheritance pattern. Mitochondrial inheritance has been suggested but has not been confirmed [1, 2, 6].

TABLE 1: Laboratory values before and after treatment.

	Reference values	Peak value	After treatment
International normalized ratio	0.8–1.20 INR	2.83	1.99
Platelets	150–450 K/micl	76	142
Bilirubin total	0.3–1.2 mg/dL	11	8.4
Bilirubin direct	0.3 mg/dL	3.3	3.8
Aspartate transaminase	25.0–75.0 U/L	727	181
Alanine transaminase	13.0–45.0 U/L	196	114
Albumin	2.8–4.4 g/dL	2.2	2.9
Phosphorus	4.0–6.5 mg/dL	4.3	5.8
C-reactive protein	0.0–0.50 mg/dL	1.552	0.4
Iron	40–145 μg/dL	155	
Ferritin	10.0–291.0 ng/mL	24256	3030
Alpha-fetoprotein	Mean 41,687 ng/mL	143621	94709
Ammonia	0–228 mcg/dL	502	149
Urea	8–26 mg/dL	70	11
Creatinine	0.26–1.01 mg/dL	1.33	0.16

Knisely at al. [7] and Whitington and Malladi [8] suggested that the pattern of recurrence in NH resembles that of gestational alloimmune diseases in which the maternal immune system develops antibodies of the immunoglobulin G class which then cross the placenta and attack the fetal liver (in the current and subsequent pregnancies). In NH this process causes synthetic dysfunction of the different proteins involved in iron homeostasis which results in siderosis.

Patients with NH may present during pregnancy with intrauterine growth retardation, oligohydramnios (or, at times polyhydramnion), and placental edema and are often born prematurely. Within hours or days they develop acute liver failure. Frequently the infants are at first misdiagnosed with overwhelming sepsis. Laboratory abnormalities include hypoglycemia, hypoalbuminemia, and marked coagulopathy. Jaundice with elevated direct and indirect hyperbilirubinemia develops within days. Serum aminotransaminases are disproportionately low for the degree of hepatic injury, while alphafetoprotein levels are very high. Characteristic iron studies show low levels of transferrin that is unusually highly saturated and extremely elevated ferritin levels (150–450 K/micl; [9]). The diagnosis of NH can be difficult to establish because other hepatic disorders may cause liver siderosis or high ferritin levels. The diagnosis is made by exclusion of other causes of neonatal liver failure and by demonstrating extrahepatic siderosis with reticuloendothelial sparing (as seen in hereditary hemochromatosis). Extrahepatic siderosis may be demonstrated by biopsy of the minor salivary glands that are positive in about two thirds of infants with proven NH [9] or by MRI, which demonstrates abnormal iron distribution in about 90% of proven cases. Ferric ions cause shortening of the T1 and, more impressively, of the T2 relaxation times. In NH, tissues that contain iron, such as the liver and pancreas, have a lower intensity signal than that of the normal spleen; although it should be noted that a physiological increase

in iron content of the liver (alone) exists during the third trimester and neonatal period. An MRI can therefore be used for third trimester prenatal diagnosis.

Liver biopsy demonstrates nodular cirrhosis, pronounced fibrosis, and typically significant siderosis. Notably there are no signs of necrosis.

Until recently liver transplantation was considered the only curative treatment for NH with survival rates as high as 50%. Use of an ET for treatment of NH was first reported in 2005 by Rodrigues et al. [1]. In their report of 19 neonates, 17 with NH were treated with ET as a supportive measure. All these treated patients either died or needed subsequent liver transplantation. However, one should note that in this report, ET was given as a last measure to severely compromised patients. Whitington and Hibbard [4] described in 2004 a preventive prenatal treatment for pregnant women whose last pregnancy resulted in an infant or fetus with NH (based on the alloimmune theory). Treatment consisted of IVIG 1 g/kg weekly starting at 18 weeks of gestation (at which point maternal IgG antibodies are actively transported across the placenta). They reported 16 pregnancies that progressed uneventfully and resulted in all infants surviving. High dose immunoglobulin therapy during pregnancy for recurrent NH has since become common practice. In 2009 Rand et al. [10] published the largest series to date of neonates diagnosed with NH and treated by ET at twice the calculated blood volume and/or IVIG 1 g/kg. The ferritin levels were as high as 5509 ng/mL. Twelve subjects (75%) had a good outcome following treatment (poor outcome defined as death or receipt of a liver transplant). Since the initial report, additional reports by Lopriore et al. [11] and Babor et al. [12] have confirmed the effectiveness of ET and IVIG for NH.

The present report includes a newborn diagnosed with NH that presented with untypical severe liver failure. As this infant was the firstborn in her family the patient was only diagnosed after birth, thus adversely affecting the severity of the NH. Our report confirms that even when NH is severe, combined treatment with IVIG and exchange transfusion may achieve complete symptom resolution. The reported infant is the first to demonstrate resolution of iron deposition confirmed by follow-up MRI scan. We add our experience to the accumulating data supporting combined neonatal treatment with IVIG and exchange transfusion.

Abbreviations

NH: Neonatal hemochromatosis
IVIG: Intravenous immunoglobulin
ET: Exchange transfusion
NICU: Neonatal intensive care unit
MRI: Magnetic resonance imaging.

References

[1] F. Rodrigues, M. Kallas, R. Nash et al., "Neonatal hemochromatosis—medical treatment vs. transplantation: the King's experience," *Liver Transplantation*, vol. 11, no. 11, pp. 1417–1424, 2005.

[2] D. M. Flynn, N. Mohan, P. McKiernan et al., "Progress in treatment and outcome for children with neonatal haemochromatosis," *Archives of Disease in Childhood Fetal and Neonatal Edition*, vol. 88, no. 2, pp. F124–F127, 2003.

[3] A. L. Kelly, P. W. Lunt, F. Rodrigues et al., "Classification and genetic features of neonatal haemochromatosis: a study of 27 affected pedigrees and molecular analysis of genes implicated in iron metabolism," *Journal of Medical Genetics*, vol. 38, no. 9, pp. 599–610, 2001.

[4] P. Whitington and J. U. Hibbard, "High-dose immunoglobulin during pregnancy for recurrent neonatal haemochromatosis," *The Lancet*, vol. 364, pp. 1690–1698, 2004.

[5] M. E. Blohm, D. Vesterling-Hörner, G. Calaminus, and U. Göbel, "Alpha 1-fetoprotein (AFP) reference values in infants up to 2 years of age," *Pediatric Hematology and Oncology*, vol. 15, no. 2, pp. 135–142, 1998.

[6] A. Verloes, I. K. Temple, A. Hubert et al., "Recurrence of neonatal haemochromatosis in half sibs born of unaffected mothers," *Journal of Medical Genetics*, vol. 33, no. 6, pp. 444–449, 1996.

[7] A. S. Knisely, G. Mieli-Vergani, and P. Whitington, "Neonatal hemochromatosis," *Gastroenterology Clinics of North America*, vol. 32, no. 3, pp. 877–889, 2003.

[8] P. F. Whitington and P. Malladi, "Neonatal hemochromatosis: is it an alloimmune disease?" *Journal of Pediatric Gastroenterology and Nutrition*, vol. 40, no. 5, pp. 544–549, 2005.

[9] P. Whitington, "Fetal and infantile hemochromatosis," *Hepatology*, vol. 43, no. 4, pp. 654–660, 2006.

[10] E. B. Rand, S. J. Karpen, S. Kelly et al., "Treatment of neonatal hemochromatosis with exchange transfusion and intravenous immunoglobulin," *Journal of Pediatrics*, vol. 155, no. 4, pp. 566–571, 2009.

[11] E. Lopriore, M. L. Mearin, D. Oepkes, R. Devlieger, and P. Whitington, "Neonatal hemochromatosis: management, outcome, and prevention," *Prenatal Diagnosis*, vol. 33, no. 13, pp. 1221–1225, 2013.

[12] F. Babor, B. Hadzik, H. Stannigel, E. Mayatepek, and T. Hoehn, "Successful management of neonatal hemochromatosis by exchange transfusion and immunoglobulin: a case report," *Journal of Perinatology*, vol. 33, no. 1, pp. 83–85, 2013.

13

Disseminated Histoplasmosis and Secondary Hemophagocytic Syndrome in a Non-HIV Patient

Muhammad Kashif,[1] **Hassan Tariq,**[1] **Mohsin Ijaz,**[2] **and Jose Gomez-Marquez**[2]

[1]*Department of Medicine, Bronx Lebanon Hospital Center, 1650 Selwyn Avenue, Suite No. 10 C, Bronx, NY 10457, USA*
[2]*Division of Pulmonary and Critical Care Medicine, Department of Medicine, Bronx Lebanon Hospital Center, 1650 Selwyn Avenue, Suite No. 12 F, Bronx, NY 10457, USA*

Correspondence should be addressed to Muhammad Kashif; mkashif@bronxleb.org

Academic Editor: Mabrouk Bahloul

Histoplasma duboisii, a variant of *Histoplasma capsulatum* that causes "African histoplasmosis," can be resistant to itraconazole, requiring intravenous amphotericin B treatment. Rarely, these patients do not respond to intravenous antifungal therapy, and in such cases, patients may progress to develop secondary hemophagocytic lymphohistiocytosis (HLH). We present a case of a 34-year-old male patient with sickle cell disease who presented with a 5-month history of an enlarging painless axillary mass, persistent low grade fevers, night sweats, weight loss, and anorexia. An excisional biopsy of the right axillary lymph node revealed yeast and granulomas consistent with histoplasma infection. He was started on oral itraconazole. After 4 weeks of therapy, laboratory evaluation revealed worsening anemia, thrombocytopenia, and transaminitis. Due to failure of oral therapy, he was admitted for intravenous amphotericin B treatment. During his hospital course anemia, thrombocytopenia, and transaminitis all worsened. A bone marrow biopsy was done that was consistent with HLH. His clinical status continued to deteriorate, developing multiorgan failure and disseminated intravascular coagulation. He unfortunately had a cardiorespiratory arrest after eight days of admission and passed away.

1. Introduction

Disseminated histoplasmosis (DH) is a chronic granulomatous disease caused by *Histoplasma capsulatum*, usually in immunocompromised patients. It typically responds to treatment with oral antifungal therapy [1, 2]. However, *Histoplasma duboisii, a variant of Histoplasma capsulatum that causes "African histoplasmosis,"* is endemic to tropical and temperate areas of sub-Saharan Western Africa and Madagascar and can be resistant to itraconazole, requiring intravenous amphotericin B treatment [3]. Rarely, these patients do not respond to intravenous antifungal therapy and in such cases, patients may progress to develop secondary hemophagocytic lymphohistiocytosis (HLH) [4, 5]. This diagnosis should be suspected in patients with persistent fever, splenomegaly, cytopenia, hypertriglyceridemia, hypofibrinogenemia, and elevated ferritin level. HLH is associated with a high mortality; hence, early recognition and initiation of treatment is crucial.

2. Case Presentation

A 34-year-old male presented to our outpatient clinic with painless, progressively enlarging right axillary lump that he noticed 5 months prior to presentation. His medical history was significant for sickle cell disease, and his last hospitalization had been 7 years ago for a sickle cell pain crisis. His symptoms included persistent low grade fevers, night sweats, weight loss, and anorexia. He did not have cough, dyspnea, arthritis, chest pain, or abdominal pain. The patient had no sick contacts and no contacts with animals. He had immigrated to United States from Nigeria one year prior to his presentation and had a negative tuberculin skin test. He had never smoked tobacco and had no toxic habits. He had no reported allergies. His medications included folate, iron, and multivitamin supplements.

Physical examination revealed an emaciated man. Vitals showed a fever 100.2 F, pulse rate 88/min, respiratory rate

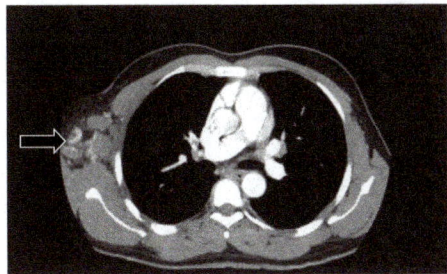

FIGURE 1: Computed tomography showing extensive right axillary lymphadenopathy (arrow).

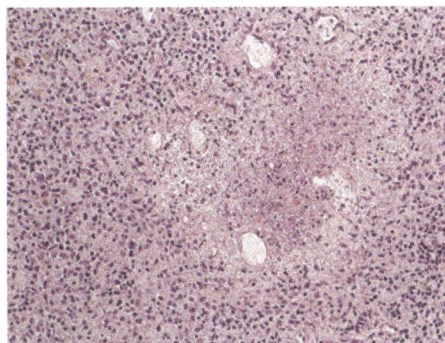

FIGURE 2: Lymph node with necrotizing granuloma comprised of necrotic center surrounded by epithelioid cells and lymphocytes.

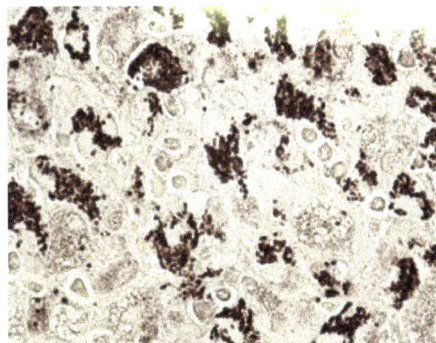

FIGURE 3: Silver stain on lymph node showing large histiocytes containing abundant yeasts (*Histoplasma*).

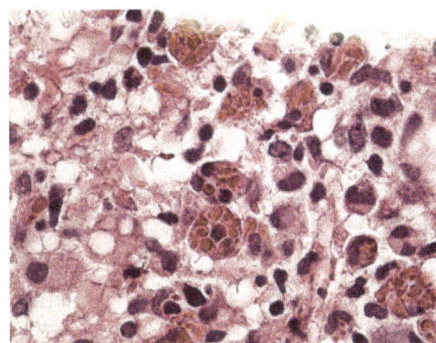

FIGURE 4: Hemophagocytic lymphohistiocytosis: bone marrow showing lymphohistiocytic infiltrate with extensive hemophagocytosis.

18/min, and blood pressure 120/80 mm of hg. He was saturating 95% on ambient air. He had conjunctival pallor and palpable nontender right axillary lymphadenopathy.

Abdominal exam revealed hepatosplenomegaly. There was bilateral air entry on auscultation of lungs with no adventitious sounds. Precordial examination revealed normal heart sounds with no murmur, rub, or gallop.

Computerized tomography (CT) of chest with contrast revealed multiple lung nodules, a large axillary lymph node (Figure 1), and small multiple liver masses. An excisional biopsy of the right axillary lymph node revealed yeast and granulomas consistent with histoplasma infection (Figures 2 and 3). He was started on oral itraconazole. Laboratory evaluation after 4 weeks of treatment revealed worsening anemia, thrombocytopenia, and transaminitis. Due to the failure of oral itraconazole treatment as outpatient, he was admitted for intravenous amphotericin B treatment.

His labs on initial presentation and admission and during hospitalization are summarized in Table 1. Other pertinent laboratory results are shown in Table 2.

The patient was started on liposomal amphotericin B. Hematology was consulted for worsening anemia and thrombocytopenia, and a bone marrow biopsy was performed. His clinical status started to deteriorate on day five of admission, requiring ICU transfer for sepsis with high grade fever, tachycardia, drowsiness, and unilateral alveolar infiltrates on chest radiography. On day six, he developed septic shock and was started on vasopressors. The bone marrow biopsy revealed

a lymphohistiocytic infiltrate with extensive hemophagocytosis consistent with hemophagocytic syndrome (Figure 4). The patient was started on a standard treatment protocol for HLH consisting of dexamethasone and etoposide. Unfortunately, his clinical status continued to worsen, developing multiorgan failure and disseminated intravascular coagulation. He had a cardiopulmonary arrest on day eight and passed away.

3. Discussion

DH is a chronic granulomatous disease caused by the dimorphic fungus *Histoplasma capsulatum* (HC). The fungus is ubiquitous and lives particularly in soil that contains large amounts of bird or bat droppings. It is endemic in the Central and Eastern United States, Central and South America, Africa, Asia, and Australia. It enters the human body through spore inhalation. Immunocompetent patients usually develop a self-limiting disease, manifested by fever, cough, and fatigue [1]. In patients with defective immune systems, the infection can become severe and spread hematogenously to other organs. Disseminated disease manifests as high grade fever, fatigue, weight loss, hepatosplenomegaly, and lymphadenopathy, mimicking the features of tuberculosis [2]. Skin lesions, pancytopenia, and anemia are more common among the immunocompromised. The disease is

TABLE 1: Laboratory values on initial presentation and admission and during hospitalization.

Labs	Initial presentation	On admission Day 1	Days 3-4	Day 8
Hemoglobin (g/dL)	12.3	8.9	6.9	4.9
Hematocrit (%)	38.2	26.6	22	13.7
WBC count (k/uL)	5.6	4.9	7.9	10
Platelet (k/uL)	283	144	92	48
Reticulocyte %		3.7	3.6	
D dimer assay (ng/mL)			4162	26206
Fibrinogen (mg/dL)			254	69
INR	1.2	1.3	2.1	4.9
Activated partial thromboplastin time (seconds)	31	31.3	34	59
LDH	632	777	1466	
Haptoglobin		2	1	
(mL/min)	87	121	87	20
Sodium (mEq/L)	138	136	145	142
Potassium (mEq/L)	4	4.4	4.2	4.4
Chloride (mEq/L)	100	97	112	106
Bicarbonate (mEq/L)	30	29	17	6
Calcium (mg/dL)	10	8.6	8.2	7.7
Phosphorus (mg/dL)		4	4.2	8.5
Glucose (mg/dL)	80	101	110	121
BUN (mg/dL)	14	29	21	36
Creatinine (mg/dL)	0.8	0.9	0.8	3
ALT (unit/L)	70	184	3050	5058
AST (unit/L)	59	214	6171	16637
Alkaline phosphatase (unit/L)	95	139	329	763
Total protein (g/dL)	7.7	5.5	6.4	3.4
Albumin (g/dL)	4.8	3.4		1.8
Total bilirubin (mg/dL)	0.7	1.2	6.3	8.1
Direct bilirubin (mg/dL)	0.3	0.6	5.1	3.1
Lactic acid (mmoles/L)		3	9.6	18
Ammonia (umole/L)			126	
Ferritin (ng/mL)			7493	
Triglycerides (mg/dL)	133	145		135

TABLE 2: Laboratory work-up results.

Test	Result
CD4 + T help cells/UL	496 (53%)
HIV serology	Negative
CMV IgM	Negative
[HTLV-I] and [HTLV-II]	Nonreactive
EBV VCA IgM	<0.91
Serum histoplasma antigen	Negative
Urine histoplasma antigen	Negative
AFB blood culture	Negative
AFB tissue cultures	Negative
Blood cultures and urine cultures	Negative
Blastomyces serology	Negative
Coccidioides serology	Negative
Parvovirus serology	Negative
Echinococcus serology	Negative
Tissue viral culture	Negative
BAL culture	Negative
Hepatitis B surface antigen	Negative
Hepatitis B surface antibody	Positive
Hepatitis C	Negative
Serum Ceruloplasmin (mg/dL)	59
Anti-HEV IgM	Negative
Urine Legionella antigen	Negative
Cryptococcal antigen	Negative
Immunoglobulin G level (mg/dL)	797

Antigen detection appears to be the most sensitive rapid assay, which detects HC in 86–90% of AIDS patients [7]. The sensitivity of the urine histoplasma antigen assay in the immunocompetent patient is not well established, although it is reported to be as high as 80% compared with 82% in the immunosuppressed non-AIDS patient [8]. Polymerase chain reaction assays, blood cultures, and direct microscopic examination of specimens such as bronchial aspirates, bone marrow biopsy, or peripheral blood smear are also utilized [9], with a positive culture being the gold standard for diagnosing DH. In this case the urine and serum histoplasma antigen were negative, requiring histopathology for diagnosis.

Antifungal agents effective for treatment of histoplasmosis include amphotericin B formulations and itraconazole. Amphotericin B formulations are used for patients who have severe pulmonary or disseminated forms of histoplasmosis. Amphotericin B is generally used initially until the patient has shown a favorable response and can take an oral antifungal agent; then itraconazole is given for the remainder of the treatment course. Itraconazole given orally is preferred for patients who have mild-to-moderate histoplasmosis and as a step-down therapy after the initial response to amphotericin B. Depending on the severity of the infection and the immune status, the course of treatment can range from 3 months to 1

milder in the immunocompetent hosts with a higher cure rate [6].

year. Response rate for primary therapy with itraconazole in early studies was 100% for disseminated histoplasmosis [10].

Histoplasma capsulatum var. *duboisii*, which causes African histoplasmosis, is endemic to tropical and temperate areas of sub-Saharan Western Africa and Madagascar and is often resistant to oral therapy with itraconazole [3]. Our patient had migrated from Nigeria, and considering the treatment failure with itraconazole, our suspicion is that he may have had the *duboisii* variant of histoplasmosis. From the onset, treatment with liposomal amphotericin B is recommended in these patients, with favorable clinical outcomes [3].

Hemophagocytic syndrome refers to a wide array of related diseases and can be primary or secondary [11]. Primary HLH syndrome involves a genetic defect caused by mutation of the perforin gene. It includes two categories: familial hemophagocytic lymphohistiocytosis and immune deficiency syndrome, which conversely also includes Chédiak-Higashi syndrome, Griscelli syndrome, X-linked lymphoproliferative syndrome type 1, Wiskott-Aldrich syndrome, severe combined immunodeficiency, and Hermansky-Pudlak syndrome. Secondary HLH is associated with a number of conditions including viral infections (29%), other types of infections (20%), malignancies (27%), rheumatologic disorders (7%), and immune deficiency syndromes (6%) [12]. HLH can occur in all age groups without predilection for race or sex [13].

HLH is believed to be the result of unrestrained macrophage activity. Macrophages serve as antigen presenting cells to lymphocytes for either direct destruction of antigens or antibody development. In the various forms of HLH, macrophages become activated and secrete cytokines. Cytokines, in turn, can cause organ damage when excreted in excessive amounts, resulting in systemic inflammatory response, immune dysregulation, and tissue damage. In addition, chronic antigen stimulation in the setting of viral infections leading to cytotoxic T-cell dysfunction has also been postulated to drive HLH. Natural killer- (NK-) cells function by directly destroying damaged or infected cells, independent of the major histocompatibility complex (MHC). Cytotoxic T-lymphocytes, while being similar to NK-cells, kill autologous cells carrying the foreign antigens associated with MHC Class I. Defects in NK-cell function may vary within the various types of HLH. Genetic forms of HLHs are due to defects in transport, processing, and function of cytotoxic granules in NK-cells and cytotoxic T-lymphocytes [14]. The ineffective antigen removal results in ongoing immune stimulation and inappropriate hemophagocytosis. The diagnosis of HLH requires fulfillment of one or both of the following criteria [11, 15]:

(1) a molecular diagnosis consistent with HLH;

(2) five of these eight findings:

    (i) fever $\geq 38.5^\circ$C,

    (ii) splenomegaly,

    (iii) peripheral blood cytopenia, with at least two of the following: hemoglobin <9 g/dL (for infants <4 weeks, hemoglobin <10 g/dL), platelets <100,000/microL, and absolute neutrophil count <1000/microL;

    (iv) fasting triglycerides >265 mg/dL and/or fibrinogen <150 mg/dL;

    (v) hemophagocytosis in bone marrow, spleen, lymph node, or liver;

    (vi) low or absent NK-cell activity;

    (vii) ferritin >500 ng/mL;

    (viii) elevated soluble CD25 (soluble IL-2 receptor alpha) two standard deviations above age-adjusted laboratory-specific norms.

Serum ferritin level is readily available test; with level above 10,000 μg/L has a sensitivity of 90% and specificity of 96% for the diagnosis of HLH. Flow cytometry can predict the presence of a genetic defect in most cases. When available, comparison of assays measuring IFN-γ, IL-10, and IL-6 may be useful for distinguishing between bacterial sepsis, viral infections, and HLH in febrile patients [16]. Increased levels of serum ferritin, LDH, and liver enzymes are also valuable parameters indicating HLH [11].

There have been 18 reported cases of disseminated histoplasmosis with the hemophagocytic syndrome [4]. Twelve of them occurred in HIV-infected patients and another case involved the development of HLH associated with a vasoocclusive crisis in a patient with hemoglobin Sb+ thalassemia [17]. Infection-associated hemophagocytic syndrome can have a poor outcome. Predictors of a poor outcome include age older than 30 years, the presence of disseminated intravascular coagulation, elevated ferritin level, and anemia with accompanying thrombocytopenia [5].

Management of HLH presents many pitfalls: the condition is rare, it is not considered at onset, recognition can be difficult, and the clinical picture may be misleading [18]. Bone marrow aspiration should be considered early in the evaluation, with patients having pancytopenia, elevated ferritin levels, hypertriglyceridemia, and fever [19]. Early recognition is crucial for reasonable attempt at curative therapy to be made, given that treating an identified infection alone is not enough [15]. Life-threatening hyperinflammation, caused by excessive levels of cytokines, can be treated by corticosteroids which are cytotoxic for lymphocytes and inhibit the expression of cytokines and differentiation of dendritic cells. Most cases of infection-related HLH should be treated aggressively with standard HLH protocols that include dexamethasone, etoposide, and cyclosporine. However, delay in identification and treatment leads to fatal outcomes, as seen in this case. Duration of treatment is 8 weeks in patients with HLH who do not have an identifiable genetic defect [20]. Supportive care with prophylactic antibiotics, blood and platelet transfusions, fluid administration, and electrolyte repletion are all important steps in the treatment of HLH.

4. Conclusions

DH is more common in immunocompromised populations and can be complicated by atypical presentation such as HLH. A travel history to endemic areas is helpful in management.

In the presence of pancytopenia, lymph node and bone marrow biopsies should be utilized early in the course of the evaluation to make the diagnosis of DH and HLH. Treatment involves a combination of antifungal and immunosuppressive therapy. Given the diagnostic difficulties and mortality associated with HLH, there should be a high index of suspicion in cases of disseminated histoplasmosis in sickle cell patients developing pancytopenia and not responding to standard treatment. Patients with infections should be monitored regularly for response since any uncontrolled infection can lead to HLH. A delay in the correct diagnosis of this complication can lead to an adverse outcome.

Abbreviations

ICU: Intensive care unit
CNS: Central nervous system
DH: Disseminated histoplasmosis
HLH: Hemophagocytic lymphohistiocytosis
AIDS: Acquired immunodeficiency syndrome
NK-cells: Natural killer cells.

Authors' Contribution

Muhammad Kashif and Hassan Tariq searched the literature and wrote the paper. Mohsin Ijaz conceived and edited the paper. Jose Gomez-Marquez supervised the patient treatment and critically revised and edited the paper. All authors have made significant contributions to the paper and have reviewed it before submission. All authors have confirmed that the paper is not under consideration for review at any other Journal. All authors have read and approved the final paper.

References

[1] C. A. Kauffman, "Pulmonary histoplasmosis," *Current Infectious Disease Reports*, vol. 3, no. 3, pp. 279–285, 2001.

[2] O. Seriki, W. I. Aderele, A. Johnson, and J. A. Smith, "Disseminated histoplasmosis due to *Histoplasma capsulatum* in two Nigerian children," *Journal of Tropical Medicine and Hygiene*, vol. 78, no. 12, pp. 248–255, 1975.

[3] A. Garcia-Guiñon, J. M. Torres-Rodríguez, D. T. Ndidongarte, F. Cortadellas, and L. Labrín, "Disseminated histoplasmosis by *Histoplasma capsulatum* var. *duboisii* in a paediatric patient from the Chad Republic, Africa," *European Journal of Clinical Microbiology and Infectious Diseases*, vol. 28, no. 6, pp. 697–699, 2009.

[4] P. R. Koduri, V. Chundi, P. DeMarais, B. A. Mizock, A. R. Patel, and R. A. Weinstein, "Reactive hemophagocytic syndrome: a new presentation of disseminated histoplasmosis in patients with AIDS," *Clinical Infectious Diseases*, vol. 21, no. 6, pp. 1463–1465, 1995.

[5] A. Sanchez, A. K. Celaya, and A. Victorio, "Histoplasmosis-associated hemophagocytic syndrome: a case report," *AIDS Reader*, vol. 17, no. 10, pp. 496–499, 2007.

[6] D. Deodhar, F. Frenzen, P. Rupali et al., "Disseminated histoplasmosis: a comparative study of the clinical features and outcome among immunocompromised and immunocompetent patients," *National Medical Journal of India*, vol. 26, no. 4, pp. 214–215, 2013.

[7] C. A. Kauffman, "Diagnosis of histoplasmosis in immunosuppressed patients," *Current Opinion in Infectious Diseases*, vol. 21, no. 4, pp. 421–425, 2008.

[8] L. J. Wheat, T. Garringer, E. Brizendine, and P. Connolly, "Diagnosis of histoplasmosis by antigen detection based upon experience at the histoplasmosis reference laboratory," *Diagnostic Microbiology & Infectious Disease*, vol. 43, no. 1, pp. 29–37, 2002.

[9] C. Andre, J. Badoual, G. Kalifa, and J. Dubousset, "African histoplasmosis. A case," *Archives françaises de Pédiatrie*, vol. 41, no. 6, pp. 429–431, 1984.

[10] L. J. Wheat, A. G. Freifeld, M. B. Kleiman et al., "Clinical practice guidelines for the management of patients with histoplasmosis: 2007 update by the Infectious Diseases Society of America," *Clinical Infectious Diseases*, vol. 45, no. 7, pp. 807–825, 2007.

[11] I. Malinowska, M. Machaczka, K. Popko, A. Siwicka, M. Salamonowicz, and B. Nasiłowska-Adamska, "Hemophagocytic syndrome in children and adults," *Archivum Immunologiae et Therapia Experimentalis*, vol. 62, no. 5, pp. 385–394, 2014.

[12] M. R. George, "Hemophagocytic lymphohistiocytosis: review of etiologies and management," *Journal of Blood Medicine*, vol. 5, pp. 69–86, 2014.

[13] L. Zhang, J. Zhou, and L. Soko, "Hereditary and acquired hemophagocytic lymphohistiocytosis," *Cancer Control*, vol. 21, no. 4, pp. 301–312, 2014.

[14] C. Larroche and L. Mouthon, "Pathogenesis of hemophagocytic syndrome (HPS)," *Autoimmunity Reviews*, vol. 3, no. 2, pp. 69–75, 2004.

[15] Z. Tothova and N. Berliner, "Hemophagocytic syndrome and critical illness: new insights into diagnosis and management," *Journal of Intensive Care Medicine*, 2014.

[16] X.-J. Xu, Y.-M. Tang, H. Song et al., "Diagnostic accuracy of a specific cytokine pattern in hemophagocytic lymphohistiocytosis in children," *Journal of Pediatrics*, vol. 160, no. 6, pp. 984.e1–990.e1, 2012.

[17] E. Kio, A. Onitilo, J. Lazarchick, M. Hanna, C. Brunson, and U. Chaudhary, "Sickle cell crisis associated with hemophagocytic lymphohistiocytosis," *American Journal of Hematology*, vol. 77, no. 3, pp. 229–232, 2004.

[18] S. Rajagopala, U. Dutta, K. S. P. Chandra, P. Bhatia, N. Varma, and R. Kochhar, "Visceral leishmaniasis associated hemophagocytic lymphohistiocytosis—case report and systematic review," *Journal of Infection*, vol. 56, no. 5, pp. 381–388, 2008.

[19] H. M. Madrigal-Jiménez and G. Hernández-Rivera, "Usefulness of bone marrow microscopic examination in HIV-infected patients with pancytopenia," *Gaceta Médica de México*, vol. 142, no. 1, pp. 13–17, 2006.

[20] J.-I. Henter, M. Arico, R. M. Egeler et al., "HLH-94: a treatment protocol for hemophagocytic lymphohistiocytosis. HLH study Group of the Histiocyte Society," *Medical and Pediatric Oncology*, vol. 28, no. 5, pp. 342–347, 1997.

14

Spontaneous Ovarian Hyperstimulation Syndrome in a Triplet Pregnancy

Nisha Rani Agrawal,[1] Garima Gupta,[1] Kusum Verma,[1] and Neeraj Varyani[2]

[1] *Department of Obstetrics and Gynecology, Institute of Medical Sciences, Banaras Hindu University,*
  Uttar Pradesh, Varanasi 221005, India
[2] *Department of General Medicine, Institute of Medical Sciences, Banaras Hindu University,*
  Uttar Pradesh, Varanasi 221005, India

Correspondence should be addressed to Nisha Rani Agrawal, nisharaniagrawal@gmail.com

Academic Editors: C. Diez, M. Doganay, and C. Lazzeri

Ovarian hyperstimulation syndrome (OHSS) is a potentially life-threatening complication, usually iatrogenic after ovulation induction. OHSS is a very rare event in spontaneously conceived pregnancies. Only few cases have been reported in literature to the best of our knowledge. We report a very rare case of spontaneous critical OHSS (according to classification of severity of OHSS as mentioned in Greentop guidelines no. 5, 2006) associated with triplet pregnancy in a 26-year-old woman suffering from severe abdominal pain, distension, and dyspnea. Our case highlights the importance of a strong suspicion for OHSS when a clinical presentation could not be explained by common medical conditions.

1. Introduction

Ovarian hyperstimulation syndrome is a rare and potentially life-threatening complication of ovarian stimulation. OHSS is in almost all cases an iatrogenic complication, the incidence of which is increasing world-wide through an increase in controlled ovarian hyperstimulation cycles.

OHSS has a broad pathophysiologic spectrum ranging from mild illness to severe disease. As many as 33% of in vitro fertilization (IVF) cycles have been reported to be associated with mild forms of OHSS [1]. More severe OHSS has been reported in 3.1–8.0% of IVF cycles [1]. Women without any pharmacological intervention are rarely diagnosed with spontaneous OHSS [2] which needs prompt evaluation and management. Risk factors for OHSS include young age, low body weight, polycystic ovarian syndrome, higher doses of gonadotropins, and previous episodes of hyperstimulation.

Even after an extensive search of literature, we were unable to find the incidence of critical spontaneous OHSS which makes our case even more significant. Symptoms of OHSS do not cease immediately after pregnancy, but may persist or even worsen during days after treatment [3] as in

our case. Misdiagnosis as neoplasm may result in inadvertent interventions. Nevertheless, alternative diagnoses should always be considered, such as complication of an ovarian cyst (torsion, haemorrhage), pelvic infection, intraabdominal haemorrhage, malignancy, ectopic pregnancy, and appendicitis.

Thus knowledge and prompt recognition of ovarian hyperstimulation are essential for its prevention and management.

2. Case Presentation

A 26-year primigravida at 6 weeks of gestation presented with severe abdominal pain, distension, and dyspnea for the past 1 month, which was slow in onset and gradually progressing. The patient conceived spontaneously and denied having ever taken any ovulation inducing agent. Menarche commenced at age of 13 years and subsequently she had oligomenorrhea. She had a history of primary infertility of 8 years for which she was neither investigated nor was on any treatment. There was no history of fever, cough, chest pain, palpitation, jaundice, melena, hematemesis, decreased urine output,

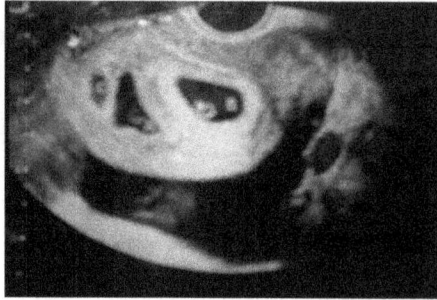

FIGURE 1: Ultra Sonography showing three gestational sacs with gross ascites.

altered bowel habit, antitubercular treatment, joint pain, rashes, photosensitivity, oral ulcers, loss of appetite, vaginal bleeding, treatment for infertility, hyperemesis, headache, visual blurring, weight loss, or tremors. Her past and family history was not significant. On examination she was conscious, oriented, afebrile, pale and ill looking, weight: 78 kg, pulse: 110/min and regular, blood pressure: 126/80 mm Hg, and respiratory rate being 26/min. Icterus, clubbing, cyanosis, and pedal edema were absent. Lymph nodes were not palpable. Thyroid and breast examination were normal. Abdomen was distended with abdominal girth of 97 cm. Tense ascites and fluid thrill were present. There was no organomegaly. Pelvic examination revealed congested cervix. Uterus and ovaries could not be palpated because of tense ascites. Chest examination suggested signs of bilateral pleural effusion.

With this clinical presentation following conditions were considered as provisional diagnosis:

(i) Koch's abdomen,

(ii) Malignancy,

(iii) Collagen vascular disease.

On investigating, patient had anemia (Hb-88 gm/L, Hct-0.27), leucocytosis (14.5×10^9/L) with polymorphs predominance. Her platelet count, chest X-ray, liver, renal, thyroid function tests, EKG, collagen profile, hormonal assays, and coagulation profile were normal. Ascitic tap examination revealed transudative picture. Aspiration cytology was negative for malignant cells and culture was negative for bacteria and fungi. Input output charting was 2.2 L/1.2 L. Abdominal sonography revealed 3 intrauterine gestation sacs of 6wk2d, 6wk3d, and 4wk3d, respectively. Right ovary was enlarged $8.2 \times 7.4 \times 8.3$ cm with multiple large cysts and severe ascites with bilateral pleural effusion was present, suggestive of Ovarian HyperStimulation Syndrome (Figure 1).

A diagnosis of critical OHSS was made. Her management was carefully tailored considering her pregnancy and severity of OHSS. Conservative management was initiated. Body weight, abdominal circumference, input/output, serum electrolytes, ultrasonography, and renal functions were closely monitored on daily basis. Later ultrasound-guided abdominal paracentesis was performed 3 times, in view of respiratory distress and increasing abdominal girth. Medical

termination of pregnancy was done on patient's request at 10 weeks of gestation. Subsequently she developed pyoperitoneum which did not resolve with conservative management. Therefore she underwent exploratory laparotomy for drainage of pyoperitoneum and pus was sent for culture and sensitivity testing. Dense adhesions with septations were present. There was no evidence of uterine or intestinal perforation. Polycystic right ovary of approximately 8 × 6 cm adherent to parietal abdominal wall was present, which reconfirmed our diagnosis of critical OHSS. *E. coli* was grown in pus culture which was sensitive to ceftriaxone. Antibiotics were prescribed accordingly. Following this patient's general condition improved and is in our followup.

3. Discussion

In this case study spontaneous OHSS in association with triplet pregnancy of 6-weeks of gestation was observed which is a very rare occurrence and requires documentation.

In 1996 Olatunbosun et al. [4] first reported case of severe spontaneous OHSS associated with pregnancy and polycystic ovarian disease to result in live births. In this case study patient had polycystic ovaries, thus sharing a common background of excess ovarian follicle growth as in our case study.

The etiology and pathophysiologic characteristics of OHSS are poorly understood. OHSS is a systemic disease resulting from vasoactive products released from hyperstimulated ovaries. It is characterized by increased capillary permeability, leading to leakage of fluid from the vascular compartment, with third space fluid accumulation and intravascular dehydration [5]. Various factors including estrogen, histamine, prostaglandins, aldosterone, renin, and angiotensin II have been implicated in the development of this condition. Recent studies show high renin-like activity and elevated angiotensin II immunoreactivity in both plasma and ascitic fluid (angiotensin II being 6–9 fold higher than plasma) [6]. These findings are in favor of ovarian origin of the elevated renin-like activity and angiotensin II immunoreactivity in ascitic fluid of severe OHSS and suggest a stimulatory role of human chorionic gonadotropin (hCG) on the ovarian renin-angiotensin system during severe OHSS.

One third of the patients developing OHSS after IVF had no previous risk criteria. Exogenous and/or endogenous hCG is suggested as an etiologic factor. Recent studies have revealed the phenomenon of spontaneous OHSS in pregnancy to be caused by a mutation in FSH receptor which tends to recur in subsequent pregnancies [7].

Differential diagnosis includes disorders such as hyperreaction luteinalis, luteomas of pregnancy, and theca lutein cyst.

Management of OHSS is tailored according to its severity. Each case should be classified [8] as in Table 1.

Management guidelines for OHSS as per Green-top Guidelines no. 5 available from http://www.rcog.org.uk/womens-health/clinical-guidance/management-ovarian-hyperstimulation-syndrome-green-top-5 are as follows.

TABLE 1

Grade	Symptoms
Mild OHSS	Abdominal bloating
	Mild abdominal pain
	Ovarian size usually <8 cm
Moderate OHSS	Moderate abdominal pain
	Nausea/vomiting
	Ultrasound evidence of ascites
	Ovarian size usually 8–12 cm
Severe OHSS	Clinical ascites
	Oliguria
	Haemoconcentration >0.45
	Hypoproteinemia
	Ovarian size usually >12 cm
Critical OHSS	Tense ascites
	Haemoconcentration >0.55
	White cell count >25 × 10^9/L
	Oligo/anuria
	Thromboembolism
	Acute respiratory distress syndrome

TABLE 2

Assessment	Measurements
History and Examination	Pain
	Breathlessness
	Hydration
	Weight
	Heart rate, blood pressure
	Cardiovascular
	Abdominal girth, distension, ascites
	Intake and output chart
Investigations	Full blood count
	Haemoglobin, haematocrit, and white cell count
	Urea and electrolytes
	Liver function tests
	Baseline clotting studies
	Pelvic ultrasound (for ascites and ovarian size)
	Chest X-ray or ultrasonography (if respiratory symptoms)
	ECG and echocardiogram (if suspect pericardial effusion)

Hospital admission should be recommended to women with severe OHSS. Women should be kept under review until resolution of the condition. Multidisciplinary assistance should be sought for all women with critical or severe OHSS who have persistent haemoconcentration and dehydration. Features of critical OHSS should prompt consideration of the need for intensive care. Pain relief is best provided with paracetamol and if necessary oral or parenteral opiates. Non-steroidal anti-inflammatory agents are not recommended. Antiemetic drugs used should be those appropriate for the possibility of early pregnancy, such as prochlorperazine, metoclopramide, and cyclizine. Women admitted to hospital with OHSS should be assessed at least daily, with more frequent assessment of those with critical OHSS.

3.1. Inpatient Monitoring of Patients with OHSS as in Table 2. Allowing women to drink according to their thirst represents the most physiological approach to replacing volume. Women with severe OHSS with persistent oliguria and haemoconcentration despite initial colloid volume expansion may need invasive monitoring and should be discussed with an anaesthetist. Diuretics should be avoided as they deplete intravascular volume, although they may have a role with careful haemodynamic monitoring in cases where oliguria persists despite adequate intravascular volume expansion and a normal intra-abdominal pressure. Paracentesis should be considered in women who are distressed due to abdominal distension or in whom oliguria persists despite adequate volume replacement. Paracentesis should be performed under ultrasound guidance to avoid inadvertent puncture of vascular ovaries distended by large luteal cysts. Intravenous colloid replacement should be considered for women who have large volumes of ascitic fluid drained. Pelvic surgery should be restricted to cases with adnexal torsion or coincident problems requiring surgery and only undertaken by an experienced surgeon following careful assessment. Women should be reassured that pregnancy may continue normally despite OHSS, and there is no evidence of an increased risk of congenital abnormalities.

4. Conclusion

Our case highlights the importance of a strong suspicion for OHSS when a clinical presentation could not be explained by common medical conditions. Early identification of OHSS in a patient can improve the quality of life. If left untreated, OHSS can result in serious health complications and even death.

Acknowledgments

This case study was granted approval by Ethical Committee, Institute of Medical Sciences, Banaras Hindu University, Varanasi-221005. The authors N. R. Agrawal, G. Gupta, K. Verma, N. Varyani declare that they have obtained written, informed consent for the publication of the details relating to the patient in this report, all possible steps have been taken to safeguard the identity of the patient, this submission is compliant with the requirements of local research ethics committee, all images, figures and tables are free of copyright, and all authors have approved of the final version before submission.

References

[1] A. Delvinge and S. Rozenberg, "Epidemiology and prevention of ovarian hyperstimulation syndrome (OHSS): a review," *Human Reproduction Update*, vol. 8, no. 6, pp. 559–577, 2002.

[2] A. Ayhan, Z. S. Tuncer, and A. T. Aksu, "Ovarian hyperstimulation syndrome associated with spontaneous pregnancy," *Human Reproduction*, vol. 11, no. 8, pp. 1600–1601, 1996.

[3] M. Ludwig, U. Gembruch, O. Bauer, and K. Diedrich, "Ovarian hyperstimulation syndrome (OHSS) in a spontaneous pregnancy with fetal and placental triploidy: information about the general pathophysiology of OHSS," *Human Reproduction*, vol. 13, no. 8, pp. 2082–2087, 1998.

[4] O. A. Olatunbosun, B. Gilliland, L. A. Brydon et al., "Spontaneous OHSS in four consecutive pregnancy," *Clinical & Experimental Obstetrics & Gynecology*, vol. 23, no. 3, pp. 127–132, 1996.

[5] A. Delbaere, G. Smits, O. Olatunbosun, R. Pierson, G. Vassart, and S. Costagliola, "New insights into the pathophysiology of ovarian hyperstimulation syndrome. What makes the difference between spontaneous and iatrogenic syndrome?" *Human Reproduction*, vol. 19, no. 3, pp. 486–489, 2004.

[6] A. Delbaere, P. J. Bergmann, C. Gervy-Decoster et al., "Increased angiotensin II in ascites during severe ovarian hyperstimulation syndrome: role of early pregnancy and ovarian gonadotropin stimulation," *Fertility and Sterility*, vol. 67, no. 6, pp. 1038–1045, 1997.

[7] U. B. Kaiser, "The pathogenesis of the ovarian hyperstimulation syndrome," *The New England Journal of Medicine*, vol. 349, no. 8, pp. 729–732, 2003.

[8] R. Mathur, I. Evbuomwan, and J. Jenkins, "Prevention and management of ovarian hyperstimulation syndrome," *Current Obstetrics and Gynaecology*, vol. 15, no. 2, pp. 132–138, 2005.

15

Acute Kidney Injury Induced by Systemic Inflammatory Response Syndrome is an Avid and Persistent Sodium-Retaining State

Daniel Vitorio[1] and Alexandre Toledo Maciel[1,2]

[1] *Intensimed Research Group, Adult Intensive Care Unit, Hospital São Camilo, Pompéia, 05024-000 São Paulo, SP, Brazil*
[2] *Intensive Care Unit, Department of Medical Emergencies, Hospital das Clinicas, 05403-001 São Paulo, SP, Brazil*

Correspondence should be addressed to Alexandre Toledo Maciel; alexandre.toledo@imedgroup.com.br

Academic Editor: Nicolas Nin

Acute kidney injury (AKI) is a frequent complication of the systemic inflammatory response syndrome (SIRS), which is triggered by many conditions in the intensive care unit, including different types of circulatory shock. One under-recognized characteristic of the SIRS-induced AKI is its avidity for sodium retention, with progressive decreases in urinary sodium concentration (NaU) and its fractional excretion (FENa). This phenomenon occurs in parallel with increases in serum creatinine, being only transitorily mitigated by diuretic use. In the present case, we report a situation of two consecutive shocks: the first shock is hemorrhagic in origin and then the second shock is a septic one in the same patient. The SIRS and AKI triggered by the first shock were not completely solved when the second shock occurred. This could be viewed as a persistent avid sodium-retaining state, which may be appreciated even during renal replacement therapy (in the absence of complete anuria) and that usually solves only after complete AKI and SIRS resolution. We suggest that decreases in NaU and FENa are major characteristics of SIRS-induced AKI, irrespective of the primary cause, and may serve as additional monitoring tools in its development and resolution.

1. Introduction

Circulatory shock is a pathological condition resulting from the inadequate tissue perfusion and a mismatch between oxygen supply and demand. Systemic inflammatory response syndrome (SIRS) and subsequent multiple organ dysfunction are a frequent end-point of different types of circulatory shock.

Acute kidney injury (AKI) is one of the most frequent organ dysfunctions in the course of SIRS and shock and carries high morbidity/mortality [1]. The pathophysiological mechanisms involved in the genesis of AKI are frequently not related to hypoperfusion and ischemia [2]. Experimental studies have demonstrated that, during endotoxemia, AKI may develop in parallel with increased renal blood flow [3, 4].

We have recently demonstrated that AKI development is associated with decreases in urinary sodium concentration (NaU) [5] and increases in the fractional excretion of potassium (FEK) [6]; both of them are probably related to activa-tion of the sympathetic and renin-angiotensin-aldosterone systems. During AKI recovery, the opposite phenomena seem to occur.

We have also previously reported the NaU profile in the course of AKI secondary to septic shock [7]. In that case, decreases in NaU were a marker of AKI development, increasing only transitorily after loop diuretic administration and remaining in low levels during the entire AKI course (including renal replacement therapy) until almost complete AKI recovery, when it starts to increase again, returning to baseline levels. The aim of the present case report is to describe the behavior of these same urinary parameters in the course of two consecutive shocks: the first shock is hemorrhagic in origin and then the second one is due to sepsis, both triggering an avid sodium retaining state which seems to characterize SIRS-induced AKI independently of its original source.

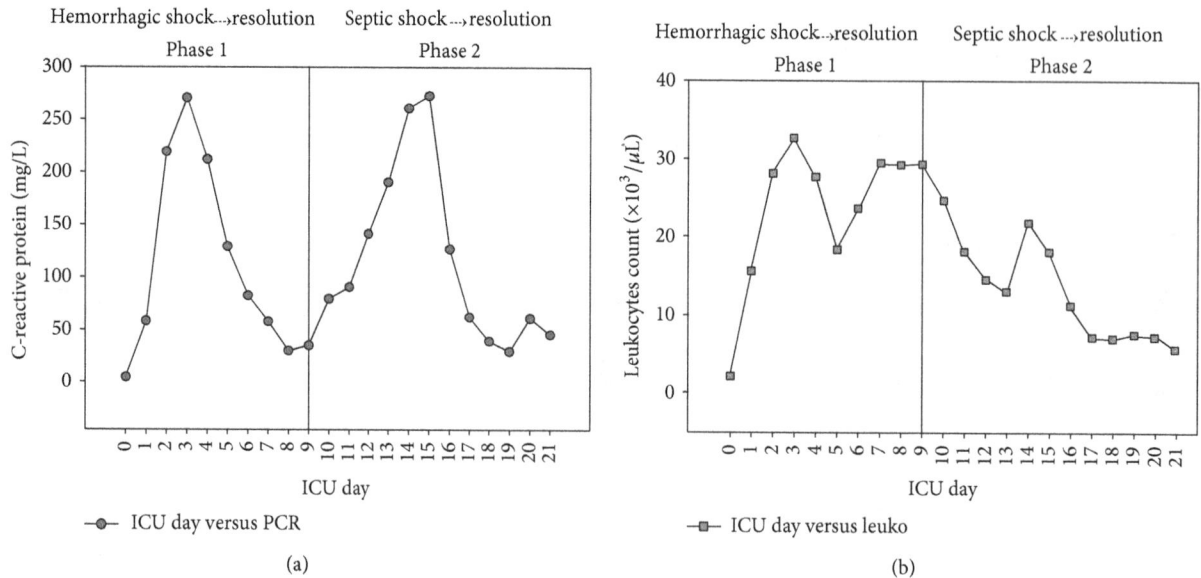

FIGURE 1: Serum C-reactive protein concentration (a) and leukocytes count (b) in the course of hemorrhagic shock development and resolution (phase 1) and subsequent septic shock development and resolution (phase 2). ICU: intensive care unit.

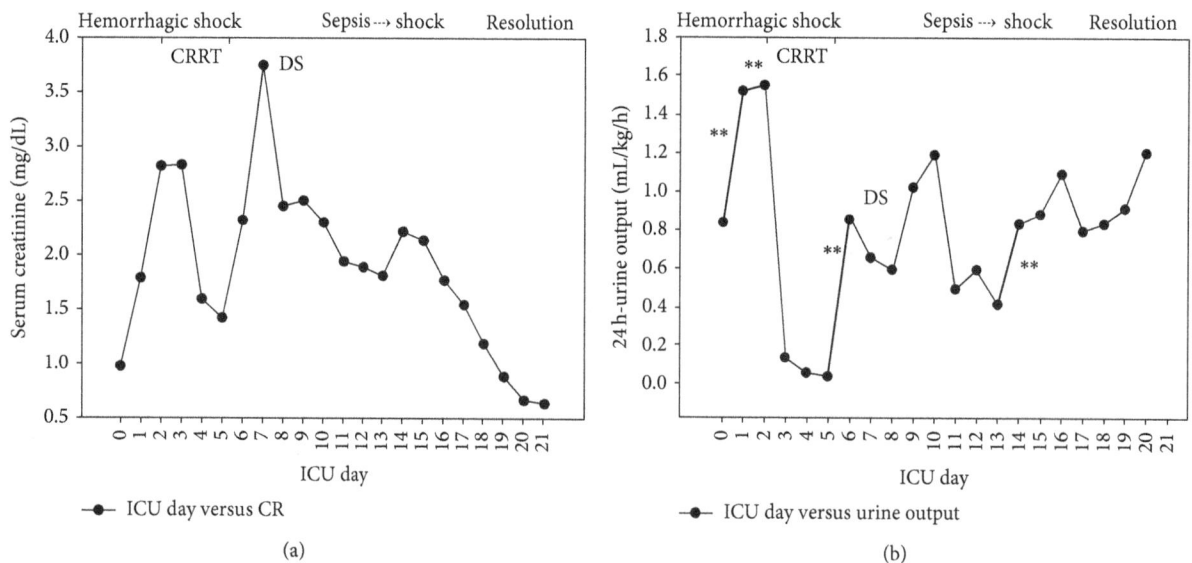

FIGURE 2: Serum creatinine (a) and urine output (b) in the course of hemorrhagic shock and subsequent septic shock. Bold lines with ∗∗ represent the periods in which furosemide was administered. CRRT: continuous renal replacement therapy DS: conventional dialysis. ICU: intensive care unit.

2. Case Presentation

A 63-year-old female patient was admitted to the ICU in the immediate postoperative period (D0) after being submitted to elective percutaneous lithotripsy, nephrostomy, and left double J stent due to a coraliform stone and recurrent previous urinary tract infections. No complications were reported during the surgical procedure. One hour after admission, the patient developed frank hematuria and bleeding through the nephrostomy tube, circulatory shock, and an abrupt fall of the hemoglobin level from 13 to 6 g/dL. After initial resuscitation with fluids, blood, and vasopressors,

she was submitted to embolization of a distal branch of the left renal artery. A subsequent SIRS and multiple-organ dysfunction syndrome developed with abrupt increases in C-reactive protein (CRP—Figure 1(a)), leukopenia followed by leukocytosis (Figure 1(b)), hypothermia (<36°C), metabolic acidosis, hyperlactatemia, need of vasopressors in high doses, mechanical ventilation, and increases in serum creatinine (sCr) (Figure 2(a)).Urine output was maintained with loop diuretic administration (Figure 2(b)). At D2, fever (38.4°C) developed. No infectious agents were retrieved from the cultures at this time. At the end of D2, continuous renal replacement therapy (CRRT) was started due to AKI progression.

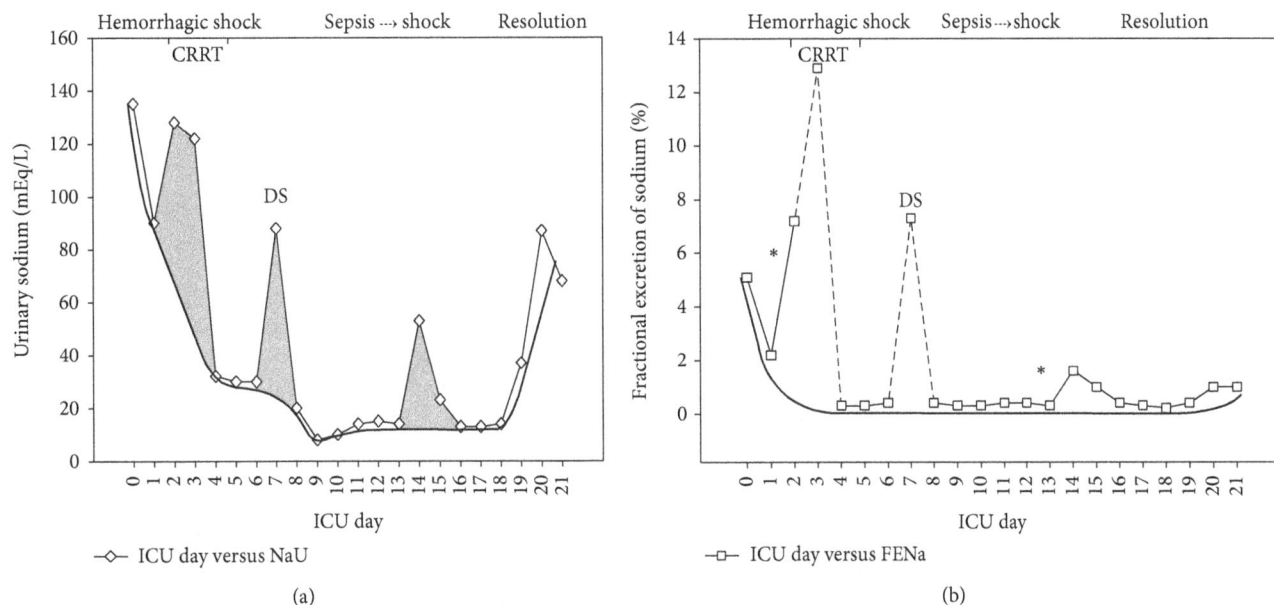

FIGURE 3: Urinary sodium (NaU) (a) and fractional excretion of sodium (FENa) (b) in the course of hemorrhagic shock and subsequent septic shock. Grey areas represent increases in NaU attributable to furosemide administration. The bold lines represent the hypothetical course of NaU and FENa in the absence of diuretic and CRRT interference. The dashed lines represent the period in which FENa is unreliable due to CRRT. ∗ indicates furosemide administration and its influence in FENa. CRRT: continuous renal replacement therapy DS: conventional dialysis. ICU: intensive care unit.

The clinical condition gradually improved with CRRT, and vasopressors were suspended at D5 in parallel with significant decreases in CRP. At D6, furosemide was administered but at D7 a dialysis session was required due to significant increases in serum urea and sCr. From D8 to D13, renal function gradually improved with spontaneous decreases in nitrogenous waste products and better urine output with no more dialysis sessions required—furosemide was administered only at D13 to prevent a positive fluid balance. At D14, new circulatory shock developed with parallel increases in serum CRP (Figure 1(a)) and procalcitonin (PCT) attributable to a urinary tract infection (*Klebsiella pneumoniae* in uroculture). Vasopressors were again required and new deterioration of renal function occurred (Figure 2), but no RRT was required. After 48 hours of antibiotic therapy the shock reverted with norepinephrine withdrawal and progressive decreases in leukocytes count, CRP (Figures 1(a) and 1(b)) and PCT. In parallel, there was renal recovery, with sCr normalization at D21, the day that the patient was discharged from the ICU.

3. Discussion

The above case can be divided in two fundamental parts: the first part (phase 1) that is related to the postoperative hemorrhagic shock and the second part (phase 2) in which the patient has developed a second shock due to a urinary tract infection. In phase 1, AKI developed and rapidly reached an AKIN stage 3 [8] with the need of CRRT. Similar to a previous case report (septic in origin) [7], in the present case, AKI development due to hemorrhagic shock was followed by abrupt decreases in NaU, "artificially" and transitorily

increased with furosemide administration (Figure 3(a)). This initial decrease in NaU could be related to hemorrhagic hypovolemia and renal hypoperfusion (a truly prerenal AKI), but it was rapidly corrected so that we believe that decreases in NaU values in the subsequent days are mainly due to shock-induced SIRS.

Since there was no complete anuria during CRRT, we continued to measure NaU and it remained decreasing daily even after RRT interruption. An increase in NaU may be observed between CRRT and conventional dialysis, but this was attributed again to diuretic use. The lowest NaU values were reached only after RRT was completely removed, suggesting a process that was not directly affected by RRT.

If the increases in NaU due to diuretics were ignored (Figure 3(a)), it may be inferred that AKI development was characterized by progressive decreases in NaU which persisted until late in the course of AKI. However, from a different type of shock, this behavior is very similar to that of our previous case report [7] and emphasizes that low NaU is a common characteristic of SIRS-induced AKI development even in those with persistent AKI and need of CRRT. This argues against the old concept of "persistent" as a synonym for "structural" or "acute tubular necrosis." NaU profile behaved all this period as a progressive "prerenal" AKI and this is probably a reflection of decreases in glomerular filtration rate (GFR) together with an avid capacity of the tubules to retain sodium, which may occur even in the absence of renal hypoperfusion [4].

In the previous case [7], NaU started to recover only when almost normal values of sCr and CRP were reached. In the present case, there was also a peak of CRP and leukocytes around D3 (Figure 1) suggesting an inflammatory

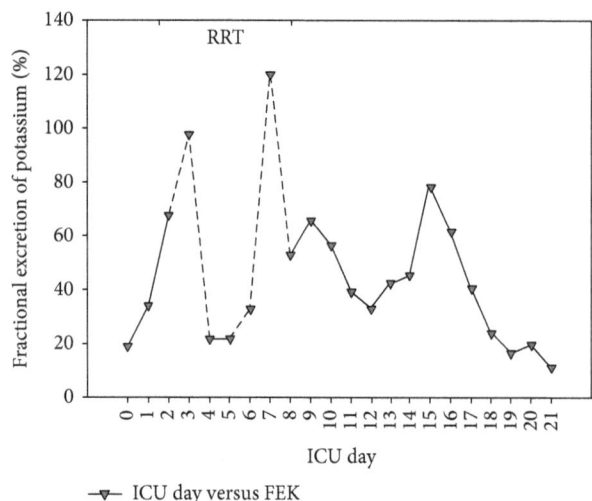

FIGURE 4: Fractional excretion of potassium (FEK) in the course of hemorrhagic shock and subsequent septic shock. Dashed lines represent the period in which FEK is unreliable due to renal replacement therapy (RRT). ICU: intensive care unit.

component triggered by the hemorrhagic shock. CRP was then decreasing, but at D9 a new increase was triggered by sepsis (phase 2). We believe that this phenomenon has prevented AKI recovery to continue so that sCr had a small but new increase at D14 and NaU remained in low levels, "artificially" increasing after furosemide administration (Figure 3(a)) but decreasing again soon after and truly recovering only when the second CRP peak and leukocytosis (the second inflammatory booster) were solved with sepsis treatment. In fact, low NaU levels seem to be tightly related to the presence of SIRS in critically ill patients, infectious [7] or noninfectious [9] in origin. Significant increases in NaU in the last ICU days in the absence of diuretics were probably a combination of increased sodium filtration and decreased tubular sodium reabsorption (SIRS resolution).

The behavior of FENa reaffirms the avid sodium retention that was triggered by shock/SIRS (Figure 3(b)). FENa value decreased abruptly (similar to NaU) and was also only temporarily increased by diuretic use. In addition, FENa interpretation during RRT is unreliable. Again, ignoring the periods of diuretic use and RRT, there was a clear descending curve of FENa with "real" (although discrete) increases only in the late phase of AKI recovery, compatible with less avidity for sodium reabsorption secondary to less activity of sympathetic nervous and renin-angiotensin-aldosterone systems. These two systems seem to have a pivotal role in the AKI genesis [10], interfering in both GFR and electrolyte reabsorption/secretion in the tubules.

Since FENa usually has a low range of variation (except after diuretic), we have proposed the evaluation of FEK [6] in the course of AKI since sodium and potassium usually have opposite behaviors in AKI. Discrete decreases in FENa may be followed by more "visible" increases in FEK. However, similar to FENa, FEK also increases after loop diuretic administration [11]. Hence, interpretation of its value

must be careful. In the present case, FEK value was already increased at ICU admission (around 20%, normal value 10%), suggesting some degree of stress to the kidneys which could be due to the surgical procedure itself (Figure 4). Increases in FEK occurred from D0 to D1 following increases in sCr. This increase was exacerbated by furosemide administration. Fractional excretion values are not real during RRT. Abrupt decreases in FEK in this period were, in our view, only the result of a mathematical coupling with sCr, which decreased abruptly during CRRT. It is noteworthy that the FEK curve was very similar to that of sCr, decreasing and increasing together (Figures 2(a) and 4). This phenomenon did not seem to be merely "mathematical" in the absence of RRT since FENa curve did not follow sCr in the same way. Near-normal values of FEK were only reached at the last ICU days (similar to NaU) and usually after normalization of sCr. We believe, based on this case and our previous studies [5, 6], that both FEK and NaU may begin to change before sCr in AKI development and reach normal values only after complete sCr normalization. Therefore, these parameters have great potential to be valuable tools in AKI monitoring.

4. Conclusion

Circulatory shocks, independently of their origin, trigger similar alterations in the urinary biochemical profile, particularly in NaU, FENa, and FEK. These alterations may precede increases in sCr and remain even after its normalization. Persistent AKI may have a persistent "prerenal" pattern in inflammatory states suggesting that decreases in GFR are followed by preserved global tubular capacity to avidly reabsorb sodium even in advanced stages of AKI. Significant increases in NaU in the absence of diuretics may be a sign not only of AKI resolution but also of SIRS resolution. However, further studies are required to better define the role of these urinary biochemical parameters in the context of SIRS generated by different types of shock.

References

[1] E. A. J. Hoste, J. A. Kellum, N. M. Katz, M. H. Rosner, M. Haase, and C. Ronco, "Epidemiology of acute kidney injury," *Contributions to Nephrology*, vol. 165, pp. 1–8, 2010.

[2] J. Prowle, S. M. Bagshaw, and R. Bellomo, "Renal blood flow, fractional excretion of sodium and acute kidney injury: time for a new paradigm?" *Current Opinion in Critical Care*, vol. 18, no. 6, pp. 585–592, 2012.

[3] C. Langenberg, L. Wan, M. Egi, C. N. May, and R. Bellomo, "Renal blood flow in experimental septic acute renal failure," *Kidney International*, vol. 69, no. 11, pp. 1996–2002, 2006.

[4] C. Langenberg, L. Wan, S. M. Bagshaw, M. Egi, C. N. May, and R. Bellomo, "Urinary biochemistry in experimental septic acute renal failure," *Nephrology Dialysis Transplantation*, vol. 21, no. 12, pp. 3389–3397, 2006.

[5] A. T. Maciel, M. Park, and E. Macedo, "Physicochemical analysis of blood and urine in the course of acute kidney injury in critically ill patients: a prospective, observational study," *BMC Anesthesiology*, vol. 13, article 31, 2013.

[6] A. T. Maciel, M. Park, and E. Macedo, "Fractional excretion of potassium in the course of acute kidney injury in critically ill patients: potential monitoring toll?" *Revista Brasileira de Terapia Intensiva*, vol. 6, no. 2, 2014.

[7] A. Toledo Maciel, D. Vitorio, and L. Delphino Salles, "Urine sodium profile in the course of septic acute kidney injury: insights relevant for kidney function monitoring," *Minerva Anestesiologica*, vol. 80, no. 4, pp. 506–507, 2014.

[8] R. L. Mehta, J. A. Kellum, S. V. Shah et al., "Acute Kidney Injury Network: report of an initiative to improve outcomes in acute kidney injury," *Critical Care (London, England)*, vol. 11, no. 2, article R31, 2007.

[9] A. T. Maciel and D. Vitorio, "Urine biochemistry in the early postoperative period after cardiac surgery: role in acute kidney injury monitoring," *Case Reports in Critical Care*, vol. 2013, Article ID 103450, 4 pages, 2013.

[10] P. Calzavacca, C. N. May, and R. Bellomo, "Glomerular haemodynamics, the renal sympathetic nervous system and sepsis-induced acute kidney injury," *Nephrology, Dialysis, Transplantation*, 2014.

[11] C. G. Musso, J. Reynaldi, M. Vilas, R. de Miguel, N. Imperiali, and L. Algranati, "Fractional excretion of K, Na and Cl following furosemide infusion in healthy, young and very old people," *International Urology and Nephrology*, vol. 42, no. 1, pp. 273–277, 2010.

16

Air Embolism after Endoscopic Retrograde Cholangiopancreatography in a Patient with Budd Chiari Syndrome

Beatriz Wills-Sanin,[1] **Yenny R. Cárdenas,**[2] **Lucas Polanco,**[2]
Oscar Rivero,[2] **Sebastian Suarez,**[2] **and Andrés F. Buitrago**[1]

[1] *Department of Critical Care, University Hospital Fundación Santa Fe de Bogotá, Calle 119 No. 7-75, A.A. 220246, Bogotá, Colombia*
[2] *University Hospital Fundación Santa Fe de Bogotá, Calle 119 No. 7-75, A.A. 220246, Bogotá, Colombia*

Correspondence should be addressed to Andrés F. Buitrago; abuitrag@uniandes.edu.co

Academic Editor: Gerhard Pichler

Endoscopic retrograde cholangiopancreatography is a procedure commonly used for the diagnosis and treatment of various pancreatic and biliary diseases. Air embolism is a rare complication, which may be associated with this procedure. This condition can be manifested as cardiopulmonary instability and/or neurological symptoms. Known risk factors include: sphincterotomy; application of air with high intramural pressure; anatomic abnormalities; and chronic hepatobiliary inflammation. It is important for the health-care staff, including anesthesiologists, interventional gastroenterologists, and critical care specialists, amongst others, to promptly recognize air embolism and to initiate therapy in a timely fashion, thus preventing potentially fatal outcomes. We submit a brief review of the literature and a case report of air embolism which occurred in the immediate postoperative stage of an endoscopic retrograde cholangiopancreatography, performed in a woman with a history of liver transplantation due to Budd Chiari syndrome and biliary stricture.

1. Introduction

Endoscopic retrograde cholangiopancreatography (ERCP) has become a primary tool for the diagnosis and treatment of ductal pancreatic and biliary tree pathology. Due to its complexity and technical demands, the endoscopic technique has a higher rate of complications than other diagnostic procedures [1], some of which include post-ERCP pancreatitis, cholangitis, bleeding or perforation after sphincterotomy. However, endoscopists are familiar with these adverse events, making ERCP a minimally invasive procedure with a good safety profile. Nonetheless, other less common situations—such as air embolism—can result in fatal outcomes. Therefore, it is essential for health professionals to identify risk factors and clinical manifestations of post-ERCP air embolism to improve its management [2].

2. Case Presentation

A 55-year-old female with a history of liver transplant six years ago due to Budd Chiari syndrome is admitted to the emergency room with progressive right-upper-quadrant pain, vomit and diarrhea. Her history included multiple episodes of biliary strictures managed with a self-expanding coated stent implant. At admission, her vital signs were stable, she had adequate oxygen saturation, and she had no fever. Lab reports evidenced elevated alkaline phosphatase and normal bilirubin levels.

To evaluate a probable biliary obstructive syndrome, an abdominal ultrasound and a magnetic resonance cholangiopancreatography were performed (Figure 1), which showed obstruction of the bile duct, secondary expansion, and presence of multiple gallstones. Due to the high risk of

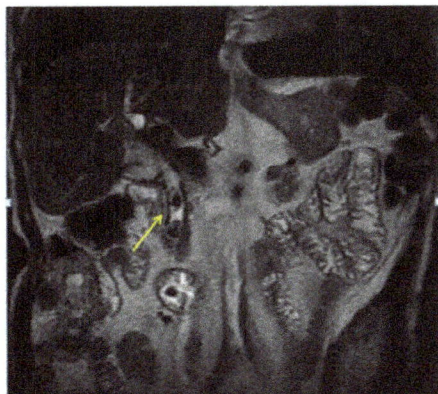

FIGURE 1: *Magnetic resonance* cholangiopancreaticography showing obstructive biliary processes associated with stent dysfunction of the extrahepatic and common bile duct. Intraluminal irregular images (yellow arrow) of low signal intensity on T2-weighted sequences consistent with bile stones are observed; these lead to moderate dilation of the intrahepatic bile duct.

biliary sepsis and probable stent dysfunction, the patient was hospitalized and assessed by interventional gastroenterology, who decided to perform an endoscopic retrograde cholangiography for exchange of biliary stent and stone extraction.

During the procedure, prior papillotomy was identified and biliary stent migration and blockage by small stones were observed. These were removed under guidance with a balloon extractor. Uncoupling between bile duct receptor (8 mm) and donor (20 mm) persisted. Abdominal X-ray confirmed almost complete drainage of contrast media.

In the immediate postoperative period, the patient had hemodynamic collapse with pulseless electrical activity. Life support maneuvers followed and, after 2 minutes, spontaneous circulation was restored. Emergency transthoracic echocardiography revealed IVC collapse, with preserved ejection fraction without signs of cardiac tamponade. A CT angiography was done to rule out massive thromboembolism, which evidenced air embolus in the subsegmental arteries of the apical segment of the right lower lobe (Figures 2 and 3) and gas within the IVC in its hepatic portion (Figure 4).

The patient was admitted to the intensive care unit (ICU) with blood pressure of 76/46 mmHg, mean arterial pressure of 51 mmHg, heart rate of 64 bpm, oxygen saturation of 84%, rhythmic heart sounds, no murmurs, and paleness, requiring high concentrations of vasopressors. Symmetric expansion of chest under controlled assisted ventilation mode was indicated with the following parameters: respiratory frequency 18, 50% FiO_2, PEEP 6, peak pressure 12 cm H_2O, mean pressure 8.4, relationship inspiration: expiration 1 : 2.3, and tidal volume 352 mL. The patient continued receiving medical treatment and, after a favorable clinical outcome, she was discharged of the ICU 48 hours later.

2.1. *Definition and Diagnosis.* Air embolism subsequent to an invasive procedure is a rare adverse event which can lead to serious long-term neurological deficits or cause fatal cardiopulmonary compromise [3].

The symptoms of air embolism associated with ERCP occur or worsen when the patient is repositioned from prone to supine. The diagnosis is confirmed after visualizing air in the vena cava, portal vein, hepatic veins, right atrium, right ventricle, left atrium, left ventricle, or brain using different radiological aids such as transthoracic or transesophageal echocardiography or chest X-ray. However, the diagnosis of an air embolism can be complex, not only because of its rarity and lack of clinical suspicion, but also because the air can be absorbed rapidly from the circulation.

Air embolism may be confused with anesthetic side effects or with an acute ischemic or hemorrhagic event. Clinical manifestations of air embolism can be cardiovascular, including arrhythmia, hypotension, myocardial ischemia, right heart failure, cardiovascular collapse, and/or cardiac arrest. While sudden dyspnea, tachypnea, rales, wheezing, decreased final concentration of expired carbon dioxide, hypoxia, or cyanosis may confirm respiratory compromise. Neurological impairment such as eye deviation, mydriasis, altered state of consciousness during anesthetic recovery, hypertonia, cerebral hypoperfusion, cerebral edema and coma can also be present [4].

2.2. *Pathophysiology.* Air embolism is caused by a direct communication between a source of air and the circulation; it is favored by the pressure gradient that facilitates the passage of air into the circulation. The effect of an air bubble depends on both the flow and the volume of air introduced into the circulation. Venous air embolism occurs when air enters the systemic venous circulation, whereas arterial air embolism can lead to tissue ischemia [5].

Different mechanisms explaining air inlet to the venous system post ERCP have been proposed: (i) intramural dissection by the air blown into the portal vein; (ii) transection of duodenal veins; (iii) fistulas; (iv) portocaval collateral circulation; (v) air directed into the hepatic veins or into the inferior vena cava (IVC); (vi) retrograde flow through the superior vena cava (SVC); (vii) inability of the pulmonary circulation to filter gaseous emboli [6].

Irritation of the bile duct wall also has an important etiologic role in post-ERCP air embolism. Injury may be secondary to endoscopic instrumentation, gallstones, contrast media, stent material, or chronic inflammation. All these factors promote the development of a biliary-venous shunt, serving as a gateway for air.

Other authors have proposed that air embolism may be the result of pressure damage to the biliary tree mucosa caused by the air blown into the cavities. Similarly, preexisting biliovenous shunts can be interrupted by the increased pressure or due to bacteremia. Another mechanism that can explain air embolism after ERCP is the transfer of air through the bile duct wall or sphincter to the adjacent veins. Broken or expanded sutures from a previous surgery could also allow air passage [7].

Rapid entry or large volumes of air entering the systemic venous circulation cause a major strain on the right ventricle. This causes a significant increase in pulmonary arterial pressure, leading to obstruction of right ventricular outflow

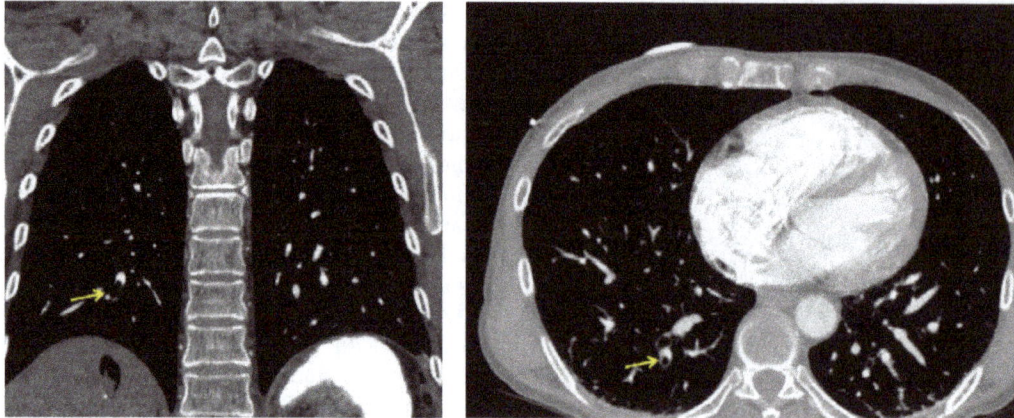

Figure 2: Contrast enhanced coronal and axial chest CT. Subsegmental artery air embolism in apical segment of right lower lobe surrounded by contrast media is observed (yellow arrows).

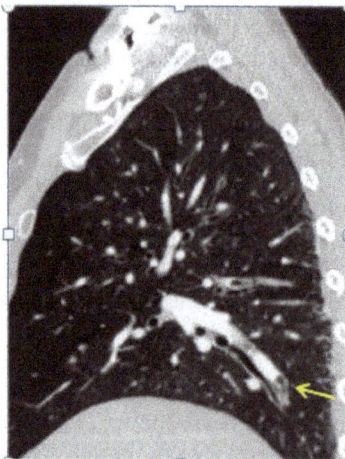

Figure 3: Contrast enhanced sagittal chest CT. Intravascular filling defect with air density bubble in subsegmental artery (yellow arrow) of apical segment of right lower lobe, bronchus is underneath.

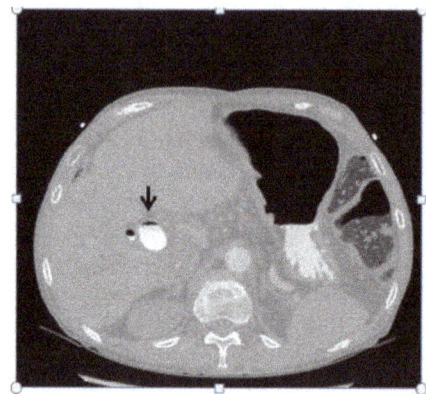

Figure 4: Contrast enhanced axial CT view showing air embolism (black arrow) inside intrahepatic portion of vena cava.

and decreased pulmonary venous return. This results in a decreased left ventricular preload with a consequent decrease in cardiac output, which eventually leads to cardiovascular failure. This was the case of our patient, where collapse of the vena cava led to cardiovascular compromise, which fortunately responded to resuscitation.

Venous air embolism may be limited to the portal venous system, or it may progress into a systemic air embolism via intracardiac or intrapulmonary shunting. It can also be caused by retrograde flow to the cerebral veins through the SVC, or by passage into the left atrium through the pulmonary veins. Since the most common cause of intracardiac shunt is a patent foramen ovale, it is critical to obtain a detailed clinical history in order to anticipate and identify potential complications.

In the case we report herein, several mechanisms may have contributed to the air embolism. First, Budd Chiari and multiple biliary stenosis episodes cause chronic inflammation that may alter gallbladder wall stability and favor the creation of venous dissection and the need of instrumentation

procedures such as sphincterotomy. Other risk factors that may have contributed include a possible gateway through a peripheral or central venous line; prolonged exposure to high pressure blowing air; and mechanical damage during the biliary stent deployment of biliary dilatation [8].

2.3. Risk Factors. Most cases of air embolism related to endoscopy have been associated with ERCP and, of our knowledge, only 27 cases of air embolism after ERCP have been reported. Risk factors included cholangioscopy with air insufflation directed into the bile duct or with high pressure, hepatobiliary surgery, portosystemic shunts, percutaneous biliary drainage, penetrating liver trauma, history of large biliary, metal stent, inflammation of the bile duct or adjacent veins, liver abscesses or tumors, recent liver biopsy, altered papillary anatomy, or surgical blind loop anastomosis (Billroth II or Roux-Y) [9].

2.4. Treatment. To ensure timely management, it is essential to include air embolism in the differential diagnosis of adverse events associated with postoperative ERCP, particularly in patients with known risk factors and acute cardiopulmonary impairment exacerbated in the supine position. If air embolism is suspected, the following steps can have a significant impact on patient outcomes [6].

(1) If possible, immediately stop the procedure.

(2) Administrate high-flow oxygen at 100%, to reduce the air piston size.

(3) Place the patient in lateral decubitus and Trendelenburg position to improve venous return.

(4) Perform an emergency echocardiogram.

(5) If air is detected on the right side of the heart in the echocardiography, insert a central catheter.

(6) Insert a pulmonary artery catheter, if available and if the medical personnel have enough training in its placement and further interpretation.

(7) Decompression with nasogastric suction.

(8) Start hyperbaric oxygen therapy as soon as the patient's condition allows it—subject to availability.

Once the patient is hemodynamically stable, a brain and thoracic CT scan should be considered to confirm the diagnosis.

2.5. Prevention and Prognosis. The use of carbon dioxide (CO_2) in patients without severe lung disease, instead of air insufflation during ERCP, can eliminate the risk of an air embolism, since the CO_2 can be easily absorbed [10]. In the aforementioned case, all endoscopies are done with CO_2.

Ideally, the presence of right-to-left shunt should be ruled out in all patients scheduled for ERCP. However, if patients are subject to this procedure there must be immediate availability and expertise to introduce a pulmonary artery catheter in order to drain air acutely from the right atrium. Another suggestion for high-risk patients is to use a precordial Doppler monitor probe during the procedure to quickly detect the presence of air within the heart or pulmonary circulation.

At present, the development of new noninvasive imaging such as endoscopic ultrasound and magnetic resonance cholangiopancreatography (MRCP) has largely replaced ERCP as a diagnostic tool. This will lessen the adverse effects associated with ERCP, which should be restricted to cases with absolute indications [11]. In the present case, prior MRCP was done which justified an ERCP for biliary stent replacement and gallstone removal.

The clinician should keep in mind that the clinical outcome depends largely on the amount and extent of air migration into the veins and that systemic air embolism is associated with cerebral gas embolism, which can have a fatal prognosis.

3. Conclusion

Although regional or systemic air embolism is a rare complication associated with ERCP, it should be included in the differential diagnosis in patients with cardiac arrest, cardiogenic shock, respiratory failure, or coma. Treatment strategies include administration of 100% oxygen, nasogastric

decompression, placement of the patient in the lateral decubitus and Trendelenburg position, air aspiration via central venous catheter, and hyperbaric oxygen therapy. The outcome in these cases depends on the possibility of establishing an appropriate and early diagnosis in order to start timely measures and reduce mortality.

References

[1] J. Finsterer, C. Stöllberger, and A. Bastovansky, "Cardiac and cerebral air embolism from endoscopic retrograde cholangiopancreatography," *European Journal of Gastroenterology and Hepatology*, vol. 22, no. 10, pp. 1157–1162, 2010.

[2] C.-I. Kwon, S. H. Song, K. B. Hahm, and K. H. Ko, "Unusual complications related to endoscopic retrograde cholangiopancreatography and its endoscopic treatment," *Clinical Endoscopy*, vol. 46, no. 3, pp. 251–259, 2013.

[3] S. Donepudi, D. Chavalitdhamrong, L. Pu et al., "Air embolism complicating gastrointestinal endoscopy: a systematic review," *World Journal of Gastrointestinal Endoscopy*, vol. 5, no. 8, pp. 359–365, 2013.

[4] D. Chavalitdhamrong, S. Donepudi, L. Pu, and P. V. Draganov, "Uncommon and rarely reported adverse events of endoscopic retrograde cholangiopancreatography," *Digestive Endoscopy*, vol. 26, no. 1, pp. 15–22, 2014.

[5] R. A. van Hulst, J. Klein, and B. Lachmann, "Gas embolism: pathophysiology and treatment," *Clinical Physiology and Functional Imaging*, vol. 23, no. 5, pp. 237–246, 2003.

[6] M. A. Mirski, A. V. Lele, L. Fitzsimmons, and T. J. K. Toung, "Diagnosis and treatment of vascular air embolism," *Anesthesiology*, vol. 106, no. 1, pp. 164–177, 2007.

[7] C. G. Lee, H. W. Kang, M. K. Song et al., "A case of hepatic portal venous gas as a complication of endoscopic balloon dilatation," *Journal of Korean Medical Science*, vol. 26, no. 8, pp. 1108–1110, 2011.

[8] C. W. Hammerle, S. Haider, M. Chung et al., "Endoscopic retrograde cholangiopancreatography complications in the era of cholangioscopy: is there an increased risk?" *Digestive and Liver Disease*, vol. 44, no. 9, pp. 754–758, 2012.

[9] J. B. Colton and C. C. Curran, "Quality indicators, including complications, of ERCP in a community setting: a prospective study," *Gastrointestinal Endoscopy*, vol. 70, no. 3, pp. 457–467, 2009.

[10] E. S. Dellon, J. S. Hawk, I. S. Grimm, and N. J. Shaheen, "The use of carbon dioxide for insufflation during GI endoscopy: a systematic review," *Gastrointestinal Endoscopy*, vol. 69, no. 4, pp. 843–849, 2009.

[11] P. B. Cotton, D. A. Garrow, J. Gallagher, and J. Romagnuolo, "Risk factors for complications after ERCP: a multivariate analysis of 11,497 procedures over 12 years," *Gastrointestinal Endoscopy*, vol. 70, no. 1, pp. 80–88, 2009.

17

Acute Respiratory Distress Syndrome in Lemierre's Syndrome

Paul N. Hein,[1] Maida V. Soghikian,[2] and Munveer S. Bhangoo[1]

[1] *Department of Internal Medicine, Scripps Green Hospital, 10666 N Torrey Pines Road (403C), La Jolla, CA 92037, USA*
[2] *Division of Chest and Critical Care Medicine, Scripps Green Hospital, La Jolla, CA 92037, USA*

Correspondence should be addressed to Munveer S. Bhangoo; bhangoo.munveer@scrippshealth.org

Academic Editor: Moritoki Egi

Lemierre's syndrome is an infectious disease defined by the presence of septic thrombophlebitis with associated embolic phenomenon, most commonly to the lungs. Here we present two cases from a single institution of acute respiratory distress syndrome (ARDS) developing as a result of Lemierre's syndrome in previously healthy young adult men. ARDS can occur as a consequence of pulmonary septic emboli and sepsis, both of which are well-described consequences of Lemierre's syndrome. We describe important diagnostic and management considerations in the care of patients with hypoxemic respiratory failure and Lemierre's syndrome. Essential components of management include prompt antibiotic therapy, lung-protective ventilation strategies, and supportive care.

1. Introduction

Lemierre's syndrome is a potentially life-threatening diagnosis characterized by septic thrombophlebitis of the internal jugular vein following an oropharyngeal infection. The most common cause is *Fusobacterium necrophorum*, an anaerobic Gram-negative bacillus species, although other causative organisms have been implicated [1]. Multiorgan system dysfunction occurs as a result of septic emboli. Although relatively uncommon, this condition appears to be rising in prevalence, possibly due to restrictive antibiotic prescribing patterns in primary care settings in patients with upper respiratory infections [2].

This diagnosis should be suspected with the characteristic appearance of multifocal pulmonary infiltrates on chest radiograph. Here we report our experience from a single center of two cases of Lemierre's syndrome between 2010 and 2013. Our patients were previously healthy men who developed ARDS. They required admission to the intensive care unit and respiratory support with mechanical ventilation. These cases highlight the potentially catastrophic consequences of this disease and important management considerations in a critical care setting.

2. Cases

2.1. Case 1. A previously healthy 23-year-old man presented with ten days of sore throat, myalgias, and night sweats. On admission, the patient was febrile and tachycardic. Physical examination revealed posterior oropharyngeal erythema and shotty cervical lymphadenopathy. Chest radiograph revealed multiple patchy diffuse infiltrates (Figure 1(a)). Ultrasound of the neck showed nonocclusive thrombus of the left internal jugular vein extending into the proximal subclavian vein. Given these findings, the diagnosis of Lemierre's Syndrome was suspected. Computed tomography (CT) of the chest confirmed the presence of patchy bilateral cavitary lung nodules and pleural effusions.

Blood cultures later were positive for *Fusobacterium necrophorum* and confirmed the diagnosis. The patient's respiratory status rapidly decompensated five days into the patient's hospital course despite supportive care and prompt initiation of antimicrobial therapy. Repeat chest radiograph demonstrated worsening bilateral pulmonary infiltrates and pleural effusions (Figure 1(b)). Radiographic evidence, PaO_2/FiO_2 ratio of 88 mmHg, and the timeline of decompensation were consistent with diagnosis of severe

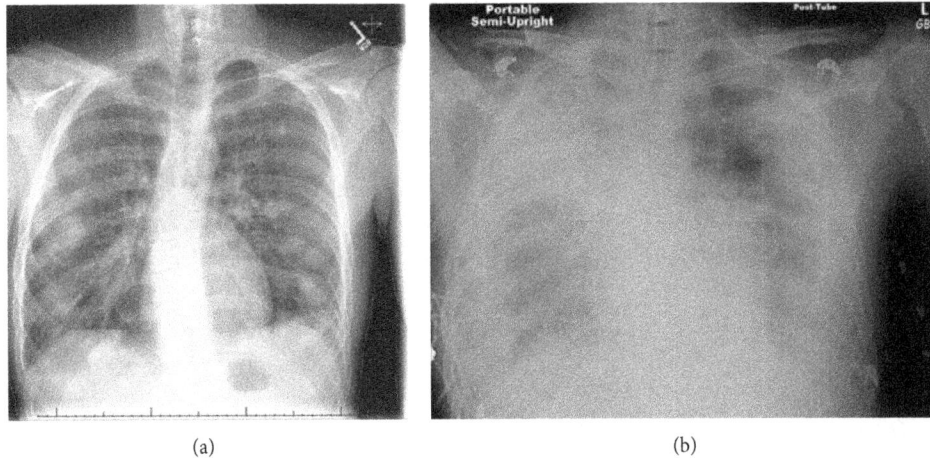

(a)   (b)

FIGURE 1: (a) Case 1 CXR early pulmonary nodules and infiltrates (cavitating on CT). (b) Case 1 CXR developed into dense bilateral infiltrates and ARDS.

ARDS. The patient was intubated and remained on mechanical ventilation for eight days after a seven-day weaning period (Table 1). The highest positive end-expiratory pressure (PEEP) and FiO_2 required to maintain oxygenation were $5\,cmH_2O$ and 40% respectively, and albuterol/ipratropium bromide was given throughout ventilation. In addition, the patient required chest tube drainage of bilateral empyemas. The patient was started on unfractioned heparin to treat the internal jugular vein thrombus. However, he later developed an acute anemia requiring premature discontinuation of anticoagulation.

The patient's hospital course was further complicated by the development of pyomyositis of the right deltoid requiring surgical debridement and drainage. Abdominal imaging revealed a splenic infarct and transthoracic echocardiogram demonstrated a tricuspid valve vegetation consistent with endocarditis. The patient was discharged 23 days after admission and completed four weeks of outpatient treatment with metronidazole and aztreonam.

2.2. Case 2. A 23-year-old man presented to his primary care physician with complaints of four days of fevers, chills, and sore throat. The patient was sent home on azithromycin for suspected bacterial pharyngitis. The patient presented to the emergency room three days later with worsening symptoms. Physical examination revealed fullness and exquisite tenderness to palpation along the left neck as well as tonsillar exudates.

Laboratory evaluation was notable for leukocytosis with bandemia, acute renal failure, and elevated liver enzymes. CT of the chest demonstrated multiple peripheral nodules suspicious for septic emboli and bilateral pleural effusions. CT of the neck demonstrated thrombus and suppurative phlebitis of the left internal jugular vein. The diagnosis of Lemierre's syndrome was confirmed when blood cultures grew out *Fusobacterium necrophorum*. The patient was started on broad-spectrum antibiotic therapy and initiated on unfractioned heparin for treatment of the internal jugular vein thrombus.

The patient developed acute hypoxemic respiratory failure and septic shock requiring vasopressor support three days into his hospitalization. He was emergently intubated on a PEEP of $10\,cmH_2O$ and an FiO_2 of 50% and was given albuterol and ipratropium bromide throughout intubation (Table 1). PaO_2/FiO_2 ratio of $89\,mmHg$, radiographic evidence of bilateral pulmonary infiltrates, and chronological disease progression were consistent with diagnosis of severe ARDS. Repeat CT scan of the chest showed heterogeneous fluid collections of the thorax requiring decortications and chest tube placement. Laboratory evaluation of the pleural fluid was consistent with empyema and hemothorax, at which point anticoagulation therapy was discontinued. The patient required blood product transfusion for acute blood loss anemia. The patient's respiratory status eventually improved and after a weaning period of five days he was extubated fourteen days later.

Twenty-eight days after presentation, the patient was discharged. He completed four weeks of antibiotic therapy of piperacillin/tazobactam and metronidazole. Interestingly, the patient represented to the hospital two years later with streptococcal pharyngitis. Repeat ultrasound of the neck demonstrated stable, chronic DVT in left internal jugular vein. Given that there was no extension of the original thrombus, the patient was discharged home without further anticoagulation.

3. Discussion

We present two cases from a single-center of previously healthy young men with illnesses that progressed rapidly from nonspecific upper respiratory symptoms to severe respiratory failure. In each of these cases, the findings of cavitary lung lesions on radiographic imaging heightened suspicion for embolic phenomena. The presence of internal jugular thrombosis (reported in 59% of cases) further supported the diagnosis of Lemierre's Syndrome. Although no uniform criteria exist for this condition, important components in the diagnosis include (i) a prodromal oropharyngeal illness,

TABLE 1: Summary of relevant case characteristics.

	Case 1	Case 2
Patient characteristics		
Age (years)	23	23
Sex	Male	Male
Duration of stay (hospital/ICU)	23 days/20 days ICU	28 days/23 days ICU
Causative organism	*F. necrophorum*	*F. necrophorum*
Disease characteristics		
Multifocal cavitary pneumonia	Yes	Yes
Mechanical ventilation (duration)	Intubated, 8 days	Intubated, 14 days
Pleural effusions/thoracostomy	Loculated pleural effusion, bilateral thoracostomy	Pleural effusion/hemothorax, bilateral thoracostomy
Renal failure	Yes	Yes
Liver dysfunction	Yes	Yes
Extrapulmonary manifestations	Pyomyositis, splenic infarction, tricuspid valve endocarditis	Peritonsillar abscess
Labs, peak values		
WBC count (k)	20.9	42.4
Hemoglobin/HCT (g/dL)	7.4	6.6
Platelets (trough/peak, k/uL)	60/618	18/1070
INR	2.3	2.9
GFR (mL/min)	28	28
Ventilation		
Max PEEP (cmH$_2$O)	5	10
Max FiO$_2$ (%)	40	50
Patient positioning	Fowler's/Semi-Fowler's	Fowler's/Semi-Fowler's
Inhaled therapies	Albuterol/ipratropium bromide	Albuterol/ipratropium bromide
Weaning time (days)	7	5
Interventions		
Antibiotics	Metronidazole/aztreonam	Metronidazole/Zosyn
Anticoagulation	Heparin (d/c anemia)	Heparin (d/c hemothorax), warfarin on discharge
Blood products	Transfused PRBC's	Transfused PRBC's
Vasopressor	—	Yes
Surgical interventions	Right deltoid abscess drainage/debridement	Unsuccessful peritonsillar abscess drainage

(ii) internal jugular vein thrombophlebitis, (iii) evidence of embolic phenomenon, and (iv) isolation of *Fusobacterium* species [3].

The lungs are the most frequently reported sites of metastasis in Lemierre's syndrome, occurring in 80–90% of patients [3–5]. Multiorgan involvement in this condition is common and occurs as a result of septic emboli. Other reported clinical manifestations include septic arthritis, renal failure, transaminitis, meningitis, abscess formation, and disseminated intravascular coagulation [6].

ARDS is a syndrome defined by hypoxemic respiratory failure associated with noncardiogenic pulmonary edema. The pathogenesis is related to diffuse alveolar damage precipitated by a proinflammatory state [7]. ARDS is most commonly associated with sepsis, most directly due to alveolar inflammation but septic shock-related injury may also be an additional contributory factor in severe cases [8]. The diagnosis requires a PaO$_2$/FiO$_2$ ratio of <300 mmHg with severe disease defined by values below 100 mmHg [9]. Other necessary components include noncardiac pulmonary edema with radiologic evidence of bilateral pulmonary infiltrates.

Based on these criteria, both patients in this series met criteria for severe ARDS. Because patients with Lemierre's syndrome may present to providers with nonspecific, mild respiratory symptoms, the diagnosis may not be considered until an advanced stage of the disease course. Both patients' respiratory status decompensated approximately seven to ten days after the onset of symptoms. This is consistent with one reported case in which ARDS developed eleven days after the onset of symptoms [10]. While ARDS occurring in Lemierre's syndrome has been described in case reports, its incidence in this condition is unknown [10–12]. The potential combination of severe sepsis and pulmonary emboli puts patients with Lemierre's syndrome at high risk of lung injury and hypoxemic respiratory failure. Treatment necessitates a strategy of lung protective ventilation, aggressive antibiotic therapy for treatment of sepsis, and supportive care [13]. While our patients required prolonged courses of mechanical ventilation, their FiO_2 and PEEP requirements to maintain oxygenation were relatively modest. Interestingly, survivors of ARDS associated with Lemierre's syndrome appear to be free of significant long-term pulmonary sequelae, as was the case with our two patients [11].

Prompt initiation of effective antibiotic therapy is likely the most critical component in managing patients with Lemierre's syndrome. Antibiotics should be tailored against *Fusobacterium* species. Metronidazole is an appropriate first-line antibiotic for this condition, although resistant strains are reported [14]. In both cases, delayed recognition of the condition may account for the development of overwhelming sepsis and severe respiratory failure. Ultimately, septic thrombophlebitis in a young person should raise suspicion for Lemierre's syndrome and should warrant an aggressive search for systemic complications including ARDS [15].

4. Conclusion

Lemierre's syndrome is a systemic illness that can progress rapidly from a nonspecific pharyngitis to acute respiratory failure. While direct lung injury from septic emboli is well described, patients also are at risk for developing ARDS. Medical providers in a critical care setting should have a high suspicion for the development of ARDS in a patient with Lemierre's syndrome.

References

[1] J. A. Chirinos, D. M. Lichtstein, J. Garcia, and L. J. Tamariz, "The evolution of Lemierre syndrome: report of 2 cases and review of the literature," *Medicine*, vol. 81, no. 6, pp. 458–465, 2002.

[2] P. D. Karkos, S. Asrani, C. D. Karkos et al., "Lemierre's syndrome: a systematic review," *Laryngoscope*, vol. 119, no. 8, pp. 1552–1559, 2009.

[3] T. Riordan, "Human infection with *Fusobacterium necrophorum* (Necrobacillosis), with a focus on Lemierre's syndrome," *Clinical Microbiology Reviews*, vol. 20, no. 4, pp. 622–659, 2007.

[4] L. H. Hagelskjær, J. Prag, J. Malczynski, and J. H. Kristensen, "Incidence and clinical epidemiology of necrobacillosis, including Lemierre's syndrome, in Denmark 1990–1995," *European Journal of Clinical Microbiology and Infectious Diseases*, vol. 17, no. 8, pp. 561–565, 1998.

[5] S. J. Eykyn, "Necrobacillosis," *Scandinavian Journal of Infectious Diseases. Supplementum*, vol. 62, pp. 41–46, 1989.

[6] T. Riordan and M. Wilson, "Lemierre's syndrome: more than a historical curiosa," *Postgraduate Medical Journal*, vol. 80, no. 944, pp. 328–334, 2004.

[7] J. F. Tomashefski Jr., "Pulmonary pathology of acute respiratory distress syndrome," *Clinics in Chest Medicine*, vol. 21, no. 3, pp. 435–466, 2000.

[8] L. D. Hudson, J. A. Milberg, D. Anardi, and R. J. Maunder, "Clinical risks for development of the acute respiratory distress syndrome," *American Journal of Respiratory and Critical Care Medicine*, vol. 151, no. 2, part 1, pp. 293–301, 1995.

[9] N. D. Ferguson, E. Fan, L. Camporota et al., "The Berlin definition of ARDS: an expanded rationale, justification, and supplementary material," *Intensive Care Medicine*, vol. 38, no. 10, pp. 1573–1582, 2012.

[10] E. F. Cosgrove, S. M. Colodny, and R. R. Pesce, "Adult respiratory distress syndrome as a complication of postanginal sepsis," *Chest*, vol. 103, no. 5, pp. 1628–1629, 1993.

[11] J. M. Cholette, M. Caserta, D. Hardy, and H. V. Connolly, "Outcome of pulmonary function in Lemierre's disease-associated acute respiratory distress syndrome," *Pediatric Pulmonology*, vol. 42, no. 4, pp. 389–392, 2007.

[12] T. Takazono, K. Izumikawa, J. Tsurutani et al., "Lemierre's syndrome followed by acute respiratory distress syndrome successfully rescued by antibiotics and hemoperfusion with polymyxin b-immobilized fiber," *Japanese Journal of Infectious Diseases*, vol. 62, no. 2, pp. 133–136, 2009.

[13] "Ventilation with lower tidal volumes as compared with traditional tidal volumes for acute lung injury and the acute respiratory distress syndrome. The Acute Respiratory Distress Syndrome Network," *The New England Journal of Medicine*, vol. 342, no. 18, pp. 1301–1308, 2000.

[14] I. Brook, "Anaerobic bacteria in upper respiratory tract and head and neck infections: microbiology and treatment," *Anaerobe*, vol. 18, no. 2, pp. 214–220, 2012.

[15] D. Hawes, M. J. Linney, R. Wilkinson, and S. P. Paul, "Lemierre's syndrome: the importance of early detection," *British Journal of Nursing*, vol. 22, no. 18, pp. 1075–1078, 2013.

18

Bronchopleural Fistula Resolution with Endobronchial Valve Placement and Liberation from Mechanical Ventilation in Acute Respiratory Distress Syndrome

Haris Kalatoudis,[1] **Meena Nikhil,**[2] **Fuad Zeid,**[1] **and Yousef Shweihat**[1]

[1]*Pulmonary Department, Byrd Clinical Center, Marshall University School of Medicine, 1249 15th Street, Huntington, WV 25701, USA*
[2]*Internal Medicine Department, Marshall University School of Medicine, 1600 Medical Center Drive, Huntington, WV 25701, USA*

Correspondence should be addressed to Haris Kalatoudis; kalatoudis@marshall.edu

Academic Editor: Kenneth S. Waxman

Patients who have acute respiratory distress syndrome (ARDS) with persistent air leaks have worse outcomes. Endobronchial valves (EBV) are frequently deployed after pulmonary resection in noncritically ill patients to reduce and eliminate bronchopleural fistulas (BPFs) with persistent air leak (PAL). Information regarding EBV placement in mechanically ventilated patients with ARDS and high volume persistent air leaks is rare and limited to case reports. We describe three cases where EBV placement facilitated endotracheal extubation in patients with severe respiratory failure on prolonged mechanical ventilation with BPFs. In each case, EBV placement led to immediate resolution of PAL. We believe endobronchial valve placement is a safe method treating persistent air leak with severe respiratory failure and may reduce days on mechanical ventilation.

1. Introduction

Persistent air leak (PAL) due to alveolopleural or bronchopleural fistulas is associated with an increased length of stay, cost of care, and morbidity [1, 2]. Critically ill patients who develop bronchopleural fistulas (BPF) tend to have prolonged hospital admissions with a poor prognosis [3]. Air leak from BPFs reduces effective minute ventilation and oxygenation [4]. In acute respiratory distress syndrome (ARDS), BPFs can cause incomplete lung expansion, loss of effective tidal volume and positive end expiratory pressure (PEEP), and reduced carbon dioxide elimination [5]. Using endobronchial valves (EBV) should be considered a safe and effective option to treat BPFs [6].

High airway pressure is commonly used in ARDS to ensure continued patency of the fistula; however, this may impair healing and thus closure of the fistula. Endobronchial valves (EBV) are small unidirectional devices that allow air to escape when placed in the segmental or subsegmental airway [7]. This will prevent air from entering the fistula and result in atelectasis and collapse of the fistula. The process

of recovery would lead to fibrosis with resolution of the shunt and eventual extraction of the valve. Consequently, this will increase the effective tidal volume and retained pressure delivered by the mechanical ventilator, hence improving oxygenation and ventilation.

We present three cases that required prolonged mechanical ventilation with persistent bronchopleural fistulas with acute respiratory distress syndrome that were successfully extubated soon after endobronchial valve placement.

We describe three cases where EBV placement facilitated endotracheal extubation in patients with severe respiratory failure on prolonged mechanical ventilation with BPFs.

2. Patient 1

A 32-year-old male presented with worsening dyspnea, fevers, and cough for two weeks. In the ED he developed respiratory failure and was immediately intubated. A chest roentgenogram showed complete left-sided opacification with mediastinal shift to the right. Emergent chest tube diagnosed and relieved a large loculated empyema. It was

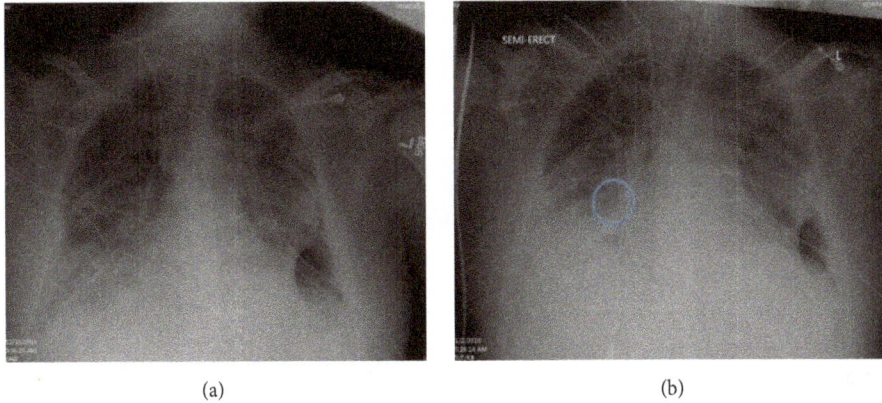

(a)

(b)

FIGURE 1: The left chest roenterogram represent pre-EBV placement. The right chest roenterogram represents post-EBV placement. The circled area depicts the EBV with right middle lobe atelectasis. EBV: endobronchial valve.

further treated with fibrinolytics (tissue plasminogen activator) and dornase alpha since surgery was nonoptional due to multiorgan failure and septic shock. His condition continued to worsen when he developed a right-sided pneumothorax requiring a total of three chest tubes. A large volume air leak persisted despite low tidal volume ventilation with attempts to reduce the peak pressures as well as the plateau pressures. Conservative management failed and he was again deemed not to be a surgical candidate to correct the air leak. On mechanical ventilation day 15, he was evaluated for an endobronchial valve. His respiratory acidosis continued to increase and his PF ratio (PaO2/FiO2) was 150 and decreasing with worsening bilateral infiltrates. Balloon occlusion of the right middle lobe eliminated the air leak. Subsequently, EBV (Spiration Valve Systems, Olympus, USA) implantation completely sealed the BPF. This caused right middle lobe atelectasis (Figure 1). He was liberated successfully from the vent 5 days after the cessation of the leak. He was evaluated 6 weeks later and the EBV was removed without any complications.

3. Patient 2

A 43-year-old female presented with productive cough, hematochezia, fatigue, and weight loss of 15 pounds was found to have a left lower lobe abscess (5 × 2.8 cm) and right middle lobe abscess (4 × 3 cm). She was admitted into the ICU and treated for septic shock due to bilateral pulmonary abscess appropriately. Bilateral spontaneous pneumothorax occurred and she experienced an obstructive cardiac arrest requiring bilateral needle decompression to achieve return of spontaneous circulation. The patient developed bilateral fungal empyema that required chest tube drainage at multiple sites; as a result, a persistent air leak developed on the right side. The patient developed transfusion associated lung injury after she received packed red blood cells. Her lung injury improved but she failed multiple weaning trials that were believed to be secondary to the BPF. Due to multiorgan failure, surgical intervention was deferred to close the BPF. On mechanical ventilation day 11 and following a successful balloon occlusion test, two EBVs (Spiration

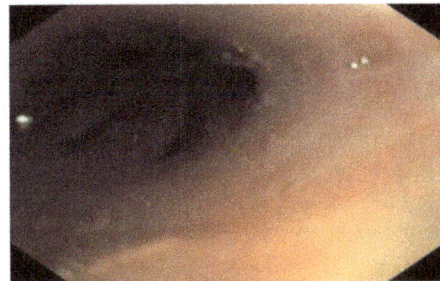

FIGURE 2: One of two endobronchial valves paced within the right middle lobe.

Valve System, Olympus, USA) were placed in the right middle lobe with complete resolution of BPF (Figure 2). The patient was successfully extubated three days later. Patient survived to hospital discharge but was lost to follow-up there after.

4. Patient 3

A 38-year-old female smoker arrived with bilateral infiltrates and severe hypoxic respiratory failure needing mechanical ventilation. An iatrogenic pneumothorax developed that required chest tube placement. She developed an air leak with worsening oxygenation. Bronchoscopy was done with transbronchial biopsies. The biopsy revealed organizing pneumonia. After she was given steroids, the gas exchange improved rapidly; however, she failed weaning trials due to the persistent air leak. On mechanical ventilation day 9, balloon occlusion showed resolution of the leak. Seven EBVs (Spiration Valve System, Olympus, USA) were placed in the right upper and middle lobes. Multiple valves were required in two lobes to occlude all segments to completely abolish the leak. This was most likely due to multiple defects in multiple lobes. She was extubated on day 13. The valves were removed at 4 weeks after the placement without any complications.

She continues to do well after discharge.

5. Discussion

Diagnosis and management of a BPF should occur in a step-wise fashion [8]. Initial treatment with chest tube drainage of pneumothorax with persistent air leak usually continues for a greater period of time when there is underlying pulmonary disease [9]. In the spontaneously breathing patient, surgical intervention can be attempted if the BPF is prolonged. Other options may include Heimlich valve or pleurodesis if the lung remains inflated on chest X-ray [10]. The American College of Chest Physician expert panel recommends that a BPF should be observed for five days prior to intervention, such as EBV placement, in nonsurgical candidates [11]. In patients who require mechanical ventilation, conservative management of BPFs, such as a reduction (or elimination) of PEEP, effective tidal volume, and respiratory rate, help reduce airway pressures in attempts to limit flow through the fistula, thus allowing it to heal. However, in patients who have ARDS, conservative measures are extremely difficult [12]. The main goal is to prevent hypoxia with acceptable ventilation. High frequency ventilation is occasionally applied, but this has limited utility if the lung parenchyma is not normal or BPF is distally located [13]. When conservative measures fail, the next approach is surgical intervention; this leads to closure of 80–95% of BPFs in patients without ARDS [14]. However, most patients who are on mechanical ventilation within the intensive care unit have multiple comorbidities and organ dysfunctions that usually preclude surgical options. The three reported patients were not surgical candidates. Their persistent air leaks affected oxygenation and carbon dioxide elimination and prevented extubation. Patients on mechanical ventilation with severe ARDS and high airway pressures have a very low likelihood of BPF resolution as long as they remain intubated [15]. Closure of the BPFs has helped our patients with mechanical extubation when conservative measures have failed. Although we waited for more than the five recommended days on each patient, an earlier intervention in certain patients with ARDS might be warranted to help shorten the duration of mechanical ventilation. Treating large BPFs early in the course of the disease might alter the outcome in patients with ARDS and reduce hospital length of stay. Preventing loss of PEEP and effective tidal volume can be lung protective by affecting lung recruitment, functional residual capacity, and prevention of atelectasis. This should protect lungs from ventilator-induced lung injury in addition to the benefit of improving oxygenation and carbon dioxide clearance. It should also be noted that our case series indicates safety in implanting the endobronchial valves in patients with ARDS. One other potential benefit is the potential reduction in cost of care. Although a formal financial analysis cannot be performed due to the small number of patients, we believe early intervention can be cost saving too due to reduction in ICU and ventilator days. Larger studies in this group of patients are required to further analyze safety and cost.

6. Conclusion

Data and literature regarding treatment for BPF in patients in the critical care unit with acute respiratory distress syndrome are limited. These cases will add to the literature regarding the application of endobronchial valves for patients with acute respiratory distress syndrome with persistent large volume air leaks who are unable to be weaned off the mechanical ventilator. In our opinion, patients with ARDS and large BPFs should be evaluated early in the course of the disease for intervention to close their fistulas with endobronchial valve placement. This may need to be formally evaluated in a prospective manner.

Authors' Contributions

Yousef Shweihat is the principle investigator. Haris Kalatoudis, Meena Nikhil, and Fuad Zeid are coinvestigators.

References

[1] G. Varela, M. F. Jiménez, N. Novoa, and J. L. Aranda, "Estimating hospital costs attributable to prolonged air leak in pulmonary lobectomy," *European Journal of Cardio-thoracic Surgery*, vol. 27, no. 2, pp. 329–333, 2005.

[2] D. E. Wood, R. J. Cerfolio, X. Gonzalez, and S. C. Springmeyer, "Bronchoscopic management of prolonged air leak," *Clinics in Chest Medicine*, vol. 31, no. 1, pp. 127–133, 2010.

[3] R. R. Kempainen and D. J. Pierson, "Persistent air leaks in patients receiving mechanical ventilation," *Seminars in Respiratory and Critical Care Medicine*, vol. 22, no. 6, pp. 675–684, 2001.

[4] A. K. Mahajan, P. Verhoef, S. B. Patel, G. Carr, and D. K. Hogarth, "Intrabronchial valves a case series describing a minimally invasive approach to bronchopleural fistulas in medical intensive care unit patients," *Journal of Bronchology and Interventional Pulmonology*, vol. 19, no. 2, pp. 137–141, 2012.

[5] D. J. Pierson, "Management of bronchopleural fistula in the adult respiratory distress syndrome," *New Horizons*, vol. 1, no. 4, pp. 512–521, 1993.

[6] A. K. Mahajan, D. C. Doeing, and D. K. Hogarth, "Isolation of persistent air leaks and placement of intrabronchial valves," *Journal of Thoracic and Cardiovascular Surgery*, vol. 145, no. 3, pp. 626–630, 2013.

[7] I. D. Gkegkes, S. Mourtarakos, and I. Gakidis, "Endobronchial valves in treatment of persistent air leaks: a systematic review of clinical evidence," *Medical Science Monitor*, vol. 21, pp. 432–438, 2015.

[8] W. A. Cooper and J. I. Miller Jr., "Management of bronchopleural fistula after lobectomy," *Seminars in Thoracic and Cardiovascular Surgery*, vol. 13, no. 1, pp. 8–12, 2001.

[9] M. Slade, "Management of pneumothorax and prolonged air leak," *Seminars in Respiratory and Critical Care Medicine*, vol. 35, no. 6, pp. 706–714, 2014.

[10] M. Henry, T. Arnold, and J. Harvey, "BTS guidelines for the management of spontaneous pneumothorax," *Thorax*, vol. 58, no. 2, pp. ii39–ii52, 2003.

[11] M. H. Bauman, C. Strange, J. E. Heffner et al., "Management of spontaneous pneumothorax: an American College of Chest

Physicians Delphi Consensus Statement," *Chest*, vol. 119, no. 2, pp. 590–602, 2001.

[12] M. Litmanovitch, G. M. Joynt, P. J. F. Cooper, and P. Kraus, "Persistent bronchopleural fistula in a patient with adult respiratory distress syndrome: treatment with pressure-controlled ventilation," *Chest*, vol. 104, no. 6, pp. 1901–1902, 1993.

[13] M. H. Baumann and S. A. Sahn, "Medical management and therapy of bronchopleural fistulas in the mechanically ventilated patient," *Chest*, vol. 97, no. 3, pp. 721–728, 1990.

[14] S. Sabanathan and J. Richardson, "Management of postpneumonectomy bronchopleural fistulae. A review," *Journal of Cardiovascular Surgery*, vol. 35, no. 5, pp. 449–457, 1994.

[15] M. Lois and M. Noppen, "Bronchopleural fistulas: an overview of the problem with special focus on endoscopic management," *Chest*, vol. 128, no. 6, pp. 3955–3965, 2005.

19

Severe Dextran-Induced Anaphylactic Shock during Induction of Hypertension-Hypervolemia-Hemodilution Therapy following Subarachnoid Hemorrhage

Tohru Shiratori,[1] **Atsushi Sato,**[2] **Masao Fukuzawa,**[3] **Naoko Kondo,**[4] **and Shogo Tanno**[5]

[1]*Division of Intensive Care Unit, Ina Central Hospital, 1313-1 Koshiroukubo, Ina, Nagano 396-8555, Japan*
[2]*Department of Neurosurgery, Ina Central Hospital, 1313-1 Koshiroukubo, Ina, Nagano 396-8555, Japan*
[3]*Department of Dermatology, Ina Central Hospital, 1313-1 Koshiroukubo, Ina, Nagano 396-8555, Japan*
[4]*Department of Anesthesiology, Ina Central Hospital, 1313-1 Koshiroukubo, Ina, Nagano 396-8555, Japan*
[5]*Department of Emergency Medicine, Ina Central Hospital, 1313-1 Koshiroukubo, Ina, Nagano 396-8555, Japan*

Correspondence should be addressed to Tohru Shiratori; ts_62475@inahp.jp

Academic Editor: Chiara Lazzeri

Dextran is a colloid effective for volume expansion; however, a possible side effect of its use is anaphylaxis. Dextran-induced anaphylactoid reaction (DIAR) is a rare but severe complication, with a small dose of dextran solution sufficient to induce anaphylaxis. An 86-year-old female who underwent clipping for a ruptured cerebral aneurysm was admitted to the intensive care unit. Prophylactic hypertension-hypervolemia-hemodilution therapy was induced for cerebral vasospasm following a subarachnoid hemorrhage. The patient went into severe shock after administration of dextran for volume expansion, and dextran administration was immediately discontinued. The volume administered at that time was only 0.8 mL at the most. After fluid resuscitation with a crystalloid solution, circulatory status began to recover. However, cerebral vasospasm occurred and the patient's neurological condition deteriorated. Five weeks after the shock, she was diagnosed with hypersensitivity to dextran by a skin test. When severe hypotension occurs after dextran administration, appropriate treatments for shock should be performed immediately with discontinuation of dextran solution. Although colloid administration is recommended in some guidelines and researches, it is necessary to consider concerning the indication for volume expansion as well as the risk of colloid administration.

1. Introduction

Dextran is a polysaccharide that is frequently used for volume expansion. Possible side effects of dextran infusion include allergic reactions. Anaphylaxis in response to dextran administration has been recognized as rare but life-threatening complication [1, 2]. Symptoms of severe dextran-induced anaphylactic reaction (DIAR) include bronchospasm, severe hypotension, and cardiorespiratory arrest [1, 3, 4].

In a retrospective survey in Sweden for the period from 1970 to 1979, the incidence of fatal DIAR was 0.003% due to dextran 40, which has a molecular weight of 40,000 daltons, and 0.004% due to dextran 70, with a molecular weight of 70,000 daltons [1]. A prospective study for the period of 1981–1986 showed that the incidence of severe DIAR was 0.12% in 5,747 patients undergoing obstetric and gynecologic surgery

and to whom dextran 70 solution was administered [3]. The incidence of DIAR in stroke patients has not been investigated.

Most reactions occur within a few minutes after the beginning of dextran solution infusion [4]. Even a small dose of dextran solution can induce anaphylactic shock [1, 3]. Most people have low titers of dextran-reactive antibody (DRA), and serious DIAR usually occurs in patients with high DRA titers [2]. Appropriate treatment should be initiated rapidly when DIAR is suspected.

2. Case Presentation

An 86-year-old woman was admitted to our hospital because of severe headache and vomiting. She had a history of abdominal total hysterectomy when in her 50s. She had no previous history of allergy to foods or drugs. She had been prescribed benidipine hydrochloride for hypertension, raloxifene hydrochloride for osteoporosis, donepezil hydrochloride for dementia, and sodium ferrous citrate for iron deficiency anemia by her family physician.

On admission, Glasgow Coma Scale was E1V2M4, blood pressure was 224/102 mmHg, and the pulse rate was 69 beats/min. Her pupils were round and equally sized at 3 mm, and her respiratory condition was stable.

Emergent head computed tomography (CT) showed subarachnoid hemorrhage (SAH) with associated large sylvian fissure hematoma extending to the basilar cistern. CT angiography showed rupture of an aneurysm of the middle cerebral artery. She was classified as grade 4 by Hunt and Kosnik's classification and grade 3 by the modified Fisher CT rating scale. Clipping for the ruptured aneurysm was performed on the day of admission to prevent early rebleeding.

On postoperative day 1, she was mechanically ventilated in the intensive care unit using 40% oxygen, and her vital signs were stable. Propofol, ozagrel sodium, and cefazolin sodium were administered intravenously without any problems. Postoperative CT revealed no signs of rebleeding in the immediate vicinity of the ruptured aneurysm. Prophylactic treatment for cerebral vasospasm using hypertension-hypervolemia-hemodilution therapy (triple-H therapy) was induced. The administration of crystalloid solution minimized the development of hypovolemia and reduced the hematocrit level from 37.4% to 28.6%. Colloid solution was additionally administered in order to maintain a central venous pressure greater than 8 mmHg.

The infusion of 10% dextran 40 solution was initiated at a rate of 10 mL/hr. Prior to dextran infusion, blood pressure was 114/64 mmHg, the heart rate was 76 beats/min, and SpO2 was 100%.

Approximately 5 min after initiation of dextran infusion, systolic blood pressure suddenly dropped to 40 mmHg, and the pulse rate increased to 140 beats/min. The patient's face, chest, abdomen, and extremities became flushed and warm. The level of SpO2 remained stable at 100%. Auscultation revealed normal vesicular sound with no rales or crackles. An electrocardiogram showed tachycardia with no change in the ST segment.

Infusion of dextran solution was discontinued immediately. 500 mL sodium acetate solution was administered rapidly and crystalloid administration was continued at a rate of 500 mL/hr. 20 min after the initiation of the shock, systolic blood pressure was restored to 70 mmHg. Continuous infusion of 0.3% dopamine was started peripherally at a rate of 10 mL/hr. Echocardiography revealed normal heart structure compatible with a hyperdynamic state. Peripheral vascular resistance was predicted to be low. Administration of 0.05 mg noradrenaline improved systolic blood pressure, which increased to above 80 mmHg. One g methylprednisolone sodium succinate was also administered. Approximately 40 min after the initiation of the shock, systolic blood pressure rose to above 100 mmHg and the crystalloid administration rate was set at that of 100 mL/hr. While the patient was in shock status, 100% oxygen was administered temporarily. After the recovery from hypotension, the level of

oxygen concentration was gradually decreased to that of 40%. While the patient was in shock, the level of SpO2 was kept at 100%. After these treatments, systolic blood pressure was maintained within the range of 130 mmHg to 160 mmHg with continuous dopamine infusion.

On postoperative day 7, CT revealed cerebral artery spasm and widespread cerebral ischemia in the right cerebral hemisphere with extensive brain swelling. Emergency decompressive hemicraniectomy was performed. Three weeks following hemicraniectomy, cranioplasty was performed and a ventriculoperitoneal shunt was placed. Although the postoperative course was uneventful, the patient's consciousness did not recover.

Five weeks after the shock, we performed a skin test with undiluted 10% dextran solution instead of an examination to detect DRAs.

The patient had been prescribed 3 L oxygen/minute via a face mask for mild congestive heart failure. Before skin test, blood pressure was 102/63 mmHg, the heart rate was 66 beats/min, and SpO2 was 99%. Skin prick test was negative. Approximately 15 min following the skin prick test, intradermal test was conducted with 0.025 mL undiluted 10% dextran solution. Approximately 30 min following the intradermal test, the patient developed a wheezy cough with flares and diffuse wheals on her face and extremities. Blood pressure decreased to 89/58 mmHg, the heart rate increased to 120 beats/min, and SpO2 decreased to 89%. Face mask oxygen was increased to 5 L/minute. Following administration of 200 mL crystalloid solution with 100 mg hydrocortisone and 50 mL of 20% albumin solution, systolic blood pressure recovered to values above 100 mmHg.

The results of the test showed that the patient was hypersensitive to dextran. It was assumed that the patient had suffered a severe anaphylactic reaction to dextran during the induction of the triple-H therapy.

Five months after admission, the patient was discharged to a rehabilitation hospital.

3. Discussion

The initial strategy for treating ruptured aneurysm is to prevent rebleeding. Surgical clipping is the definite treatment for ruptured aneurysms. The second target of treatment is to prevent or control cerebral vasospasm. Cerebral infarction due to cerebral vasospasm after SAH may lead to neurological deterioration [5–8]. Early surgery also permits early treatment for cerebral vasospasm with triple-H therapy when a ruptured aneurysmal sac is separated from the cerebral circulation [5].

Treatment for cerebral vasospasm relies on increasing blood pressure, cardiac output, and blood volume in order to maintain cerebral blood flow through spastic arteries in which the capacity of autoregulation is impaired. While recent researches show less clinical evidence in the triple-H therapy to require normovolemia instead of hypervolemia [5–7], early clinical response to induced hypertension and volume expansion predicts improved outcome in patients with vasospasm after SAH [8]. Triple-H therapy should be induced carefully to reduce the risk of complications.

SAH patients in triple-H therapy require volume expansion with crystalloid or colloid solution. Artificial colloids typically available include dextran and hydroxyethyl starch (HES) that are both widely used drugs for volume expansion [9].

Anaphylactic reaction to dextran is rare, but dextran can induce life-threatening adverse reactions known as DIAR, characterized by bronchospasm, severe hypotension, and cardiovascular collapse [1, 3, 4].

Severe DIAR is an immune complex mediated anaphylactic reaction classified as type III [2]. IgG-DRA is involved in the reaction [4].

DRAs are assumed to be induced by dextran polysaccharides that are derived from dextran contaminants in sugar, dextran in the gastrointestinal tract, dextran in dental plaque, and microbial polysaccharides of pneumococci, *Streptococci*, *Salmonella*, and *Lactobacilli* [1, 2, 10]. The antibody production rate by dextran tends to increase when the molecular weight of dextran is above 90,000 daltons [11]. Although dextran 40 is classified as a small molecule, it can cause a severe anaphylactic reaction [1, 4].

DRA exists at low titers in most people. High DRA titers have been detected in blood samples from patients with severe DIAR. Elevated DRA titers are associated with severe DIAR [1, 2, 9, 12].

Dextran 1, which has a molecular weight of 1,000 daltons, acts as a hapten and inhibits type III allergic reactions due to DRA, which prevents DIAR development. Although the risk of a fatal reaction cannot be completely eliminated by preadministration of dextran 1 in case the patient has a high level of DRA, preadministration of dextran 1 can decrease the incidence of severe DIAR [4, 10, 13–15].

In addition to dextran, HES is also used as a colloid solution for volume expansion. Although there are several case reports on HES-induced anaphylactic reactions [16–19], the incidence of such reactions to HES is extremely low compared with dextran [9, 20, 21]. While DRAs are found in most adults, HES-reactive antibodies are extremely rare [20, 21]. HES is a synthetic polymer derived from amylopectin, a waxy starch of maze. The reason for the low incidence of antibodies to HES is that the structure of HES resembles that of glycogen [20, 21]. Although HES may induce dilution of coagulation factors, HES can be administered instead of dextran in cases where tight hemostasis is completed during operation [22].

Recently, U.S. Food and Drug Administration (FDA) has recommended not to use HES solutions in critically ill adult patients because of the risk of increased mortality and renal injury requiring renal replacement therapy. However, renal injury was not evident in which HES solutions were administered for a short period within seven days according to FDA-analysis in a review of randomized controlled trials [23]. When using HES solutions, the period of HES administration should be limited within seven days and renal function monitoring is necessary.

The development of anaphylactic shock during post-SAH triple-H therapy induction is considered to be ill-timed. According to research reports on animal models [24–29], the direct action of anaphylactic mediators on the cerebral arterial system results in cerebral ischemia and brain injury.

The decrease in cerebral blood flow is greater than what would be expected from the level of severity of arterial hypotension, which is attributed to the rapid and direct action of anaphylactic mediators on cerebral vessels [24, 25]. Even though blood pressure and cardiac output recover following anaphylactic shock, there is a risk of continued cerebral blood flow deterioration [26]. In addition, mast cell activation by anaphylaxis causes a substantial release of vasoactive inflammatory cytokines. Mast cells resident within the cerebral microvasculature act on the basal membrane and damage the blood-brain barrier, resulting in brain edema [24, 27, 28]. When anaphylactic shock occurs in patients suffering from SAH, it is important to take special notice of harmful effects due to anaphylactic shock on cerebral circulation.

The diagnosis of drug allergy is often based on history alone, which is an unreliable indicator of true hypersensitivity [30]. The methods that allow the definitive diagnosis of anaphylaxis include a complete clinical history, clinical manifestations, *in vivo* tests, and some *in vitro* biological tests [31]. Skin tests are the most widely used methods to confirm or exclude sensitization of drugs. Skin tests should be performed 4–6 weeks after the reaction [30, 31].

Although reliable skin test procedures including skin test concentrations for diagnosing drug hypersensitivity are available for some drugs, those for colloids are not presented. Many drugs are undiluted for skin prick test and diluted to 1/10 for intradermal test. Symptoms of skin tests may severely progress in some cases to bronchospasm, hypotension, and anaphylactic shock [30]. Diluted colloid solution should be used for secure intradermal test in critically ill patients who have presented severe anaphylactic symptoms.

When skin tests are not available in cases of poor outcome such as death, *in vitro* biological tests are helpful [32]. Biological tests are also useful for the patients who have the possibility of severe hypersensitivity [31–33].

Consecutive blood measurements of tryptase, which is released from mast cell and has a longer half-life than histamine, are also effective for confirming the occurrence of anaphylaxis [31–33].

Flow cytometry-assisted basophil activation test (BAT) can be utilized in the diagnosis of drug hypersensitivity [31, 34]. However, BAT is an expensive and technically difficult procedure. The recommended time interval between the anaphylactic reaction and BAT test is twelve months [34], which is longer than skin test [31]. Although BAT is the developing diagnostic method for anaphylaxis, it is safe compared with *in vivo* tests. BAT is supposed to be a promising diagnostic method for patients with severe anaphylactic reaction [31, 34].

Initial treatments for anaphylactic shock are extremely important. Guidelines recommend that epinephrine injection, supplemental oxygen, fluid resuscitation, and cardiopulmonary resuscitation should be initiated without delay [33, 35]. Epinephrine is used as a vasoconstrictor in the treatment of anaphylaxis, since prompt epinephrine use prevents the escalation of mediator release in anaphylaxis [35]. Fox et al. observed cerebral blood flow in a patient suffering from anaphylaxis. They reported that the increase of cerebral blood flow following epinephrine administration occurred before complete recovery of arterial blood pressure [36].

Norepinephrine is a vasoconstrictor commonly used to treat hypotension. However, there is a possibility that norepinephrine deteriorates post-SAH cerebral vasospasm in spite of high blood pressure [37]. Although there have been several case reports of DIAR for which epinephrine was not administered [10, 12, 38], epinephrine should have been administered as the first-line vasoactive agent in our case instead of norepinephrine. Supplemental high flow oxygen should be administered while a patient is in shock and 20 mL/kg crystalloid solution should be administered for fluid resuscitation enough to recover from severe hypotension [33, 35]. If hypotension continues, further crystalloid administration may be required [33].

Anaphylaxis must be considered as a possible cause in any case of hypotension [33]. When the patient went into shock, we had little confidence that only a small volume of dextran could cause severe anaphylaxis. However, we suspected anaphylaxis because of the redness of the whole body at onset. If hypotension occurs immediately after initiation of dextran infusion, discontinuation of dextran infusion is critical, since the severity of anaphylaxis increases if dextran infusion is continued as a fluid resuscitation for hypotension. It should be recognized that only a small volume of dextran is sufficient to induce anaphylaxis [1, 10]. Some guidelines and researches recommend the use of colloid solution for fluid resuscitation [35, 39]. Careful consideration is necessary concerning the risk of anaphylaxis due to colloids when administering colloid solutions for volume expansion in critical care patients.

4. Conclusion

In SAH-patients administered colloid solutions for volume expansion, it is important to become aware of and address the complication of colloid solutions, including anaphylaxis. Anaphylactic shock due to colloid used for volume expansion is life-threatening.

In order to recognize the occurrence of DIAR as early as possible, careful observation of the skin and checking of vital signs are necessary when administering dextran solution for the first time. It is critical to discontinue dextran infusion immediately in order to avoid administering the dextran solution as a volume expander after the shock.

When using colloids for post-SAH triple-H therapy, it is also necessary to consider concerning the indication for volume expansion as well as the risk of colloid administration.

Intradermal test should be conducted with diluted concentration in critically ill patients.

When the definitive diagnosis of drug hypersensitivity is required, *in vitro* biological test may be helpful in patients suspected to have severe drug hypersensitivity since allergic symptoms can progress.

References

[1] K. G. Ljungstrom, H. Renck, K. Strandberg, H. Hedin, W. Richter, and E. Widerlöv, "Adverse reactions to dextran in Sweden 1970–1979," *Acta Chirurgica Scandinavica*, vol. 149, no. 3, pp. 253–262, 1983.

[2] H. Hedin and W. Richter, "Pathomechanisms of dextran-induced anaphylactoid/anaphylactic reactions in man," *International Archives of Allergy and Applied Immunology*, vol. 68, no. 2, pp. 122–126, 1982.

[3] J. Paull, "A prospective study of dextran-induced anaphylactoid reactions in 5745 patients," *Anaesthesia and Intensive Care*, vol. 15, no. 2, pp. 163–167, 1987.

[4] C. E. Zinderman, L. Landow, and R. P. Wise, "Anaphylactoid reactions to Dextran 40 and 70: reports to the United States Food and Drug Administration, 1969 to 2004," *Journal of Vascular Surgery*, vol. 43, no. 5, pp. 1004–1009, 2006.

[5] A. Egge, K. Waterloo, H. Sjøholm, T. Solberg, T. Ingebrigtsen, and B. Romner, "Prophylactic hyperdynamic postoperative fluid therapy after aneurysmal subarachnoid hemorrhage: a clinical, prospective, randomized, controlled study," *Neurosurgery*, vol. 49, no. 3, pp. 593–606, 2001.

[6] M. M. Treggiar and Participants in the International Multidisciplinary Consensus Conference on the Critical Care Management of Subarachnoid Hemorrhage, "Hemodynamic management of subarachnoid hemorrhage," *Neurocritical Care*, vol. 15, no. 2, pp. 329–335, 2011.

[7] G. Dabus and R. G. Nogueira, "Current options for the management of aneurysmal subarachnoid hemorrhage-induced cerebral vasospasm: a comprehensive review of the literature," *Interventional Neurology*, vol. 2, no. 1, pp. 30–51, 2013.

[8] J. A. Frontera, A. Fernandez, J. M. Schmidt et al., "Clinical response to hypertensive hypervolemic therapy and outcome after subarachnoid hemorrhage," *Neurosurgery*, vol. 66, no. 1, pp. 35–41, 2010.

[9] D. L. Hepner and M. C. Castells, "Anaphylaxis during the perioperative period," *Anesthesia and Analgesia*, vol. 97, no. 5, pp. 1381–1395, 2003.

[10] R. L. Bernstein, A. D. Rosenberg, E. Y. Pada, and F. F. Jaffe, "A severe reaction to dextran despite hapten inhibition," *Anesthesiology*, vol. 67, no. 4, pp. 567–569, 1987.

[11] E. A. Kabat and A. E. Bezer, "The effect of variation in molecular weight on the antigenicity of dextran in man," *Archives of Biochemistry and Biophysics*, vol. 78, no. 2, pp. 306–318, 1958.

[12] E. M. Berg, S. Fasting, and O. F. M. Sellevold, "Serious complications with dextran-70 despite hapten prophylaxis. Is it best avoided prior to delivery?" *Anaesthesia*, vol. 46, no. 12, pp. 1033–1035, 1991.

[13] K.-G. Ljungström, "Safety of dextran in relation to other colloids—ten years experience with hapten inhibition," *Infusionstherapie und Transfusionsmedizin*, vol. 20, no. 5, pp. 206–210, 1993.

[14] K.-G. Ljungstrom, H. Renck, H. Hedin, W. Richter, and B.-E. Wiholm, "Hapten inhibition and dextran anaphylaxis," *Anaesthesia*, vol. 43, no. 9, pp. 729–732, 1988.

[15] K.-G. Ljungström, "Pretreatment with dextran 1 makes dextran 40 therapy safer," *Journal of Vascular Surgery*, vol. 43, no. 5, pp. 1070–1072, 2006.

[16] D. G. Ebo, A. Schuerwegh, and W. J. Stevens, "Anaphylaxis to starch," *Allergy*, vol. 55, no. 11, pp. 1098–1099, 2000.

[17] M. P. Vercauteren, H. C. Coppejans, and L. Sermeus, "Anaphylactoid reaction to hydroxyethylstarch during cesarean delivery

in a patient with HELLP syndrome," *Anesthesia and Analgesia*, vol. 96, no. 3, pp. 859–861, 2003.

[18] H. J. Kim, S. Y. Kim, M. J. Oh, and J. M. Kim, "Anaphylaxis induced by hydroxyethyl starch during general anesthesia—a case report," *Korean Journal of Anesthesiology*, vol. 63, no. 3, pp. 260–262, 2012.

[19] H. J. Kim, S. Y. Kim, M. J. Oh, and J. M. Kim, "Anaphylaxis induced by hydroxyethyl starch during general anesthesia: a case report," *Korean Journal of Anesthesiology*, vol. 63, no. 3, pp. 260–262, 2012.

[20] H.-J. Dieterich, D. Kraft, C. Sirtl et al., "Hydroxyethyl starch antibodies in humans: incidence and clinical relevance," *Anesthesia and Analgesia*, vol. 86, no. 5, pp. 1123–1126, 1998.

[21] D. Kraft, C. Sirtl, H. Laubenthal et al., "No evidence for the existence of preformed antibodies against hydroxyethyl starch in man," *European Surgical Research*, vol. 24, no. 3, pp. 138–142, 1992.

[22] T. A. Neff, M. Doelberg, C. Jungheinrich, A. Sauerland, D. R. Spahn, and R. Stocker, "Repetitive large-dose infusion of the novel hydroxyethyl starch 130/0.4 in Patients with severe head injury," *Anesthesia and Analgesia*, vol. 96, no. 5, pp. 1453–1459, 2003.

[23] U. S. Food and Drug Administration, *FDA Safety Communication: Boxed Warning on Increased Mortality and Severe Renal Injury, and Additional Warning on Risk of Bleeding, for Use of Hydroxyethyl Starch Solutions in Some Settings*, 2013, http://www.fda.gov/BiologicsBloodVaccines/SafetyAvailability/ucm358271.htm.

[24] G. D. Soufras, G. N. Kounis, and N. G. Kounis, "Brain injury due to anaphylactic shock: broadening manifestations of Kounis syndrome," *International Endodontic Journal*, vol. 47, no. 4, pp. 309–313, 2014.

[25] J. Davidson, F. Zheng, K. Tajima et al., "Anaphylactic shock decreases cerebral blood flow more than what would be expected from severe arterial hypotension," *Shock*, vol. 38, no. 4, pp. 429–435, 2012.

[26] M. A. Kapin and J. L. Ferguson, "Hemodynamic and regional circulatory alterations in dog during anaphylactic challenge," *The American Journal of Physiology*, vol. 249, no. 2, part 2, pp. H430–H437, 1985.

[27] P. J. Lindsberg, D. Strbian, and M.-L. Karjalainen-Lindsberg, "Mast cells as early responders in the regulation of acute blood-brain barrier changes after cerebral ischemia and hemorrhage," *Journal of Cerebral Blood Flow and Metabolism*, vol. 30, no. 4, pp. 689–702, 2010.

[28] Á. Dénes, S. Ferenczi, and K. J. Kovács, "Systemic inflammatory challenges compromise survival after experimental stroke via augmenting brain inflammation, blood-brain barrier damage and brain oedema independently of infarct size," *Journal of Neuroinflammation*, vol. 8, article 164, 13 pages, 2011.

[29] F. Zheng, G. Barthel, O. Collange et al., "Methylene blue and epinephrine: a synergetic association for anaphylactic shock treatment," *Critical Care Medicine*, vol. 41, no. 1, pp. 195–204, 2013.

[30] K. Brockow, L. H. Garvey, W. Aberer et al., "Skin test concentrations for systemically administered drugs—an ENDA/EAACI Drug Allergy Interest Group position paper," *Allergy*, vol. 68, no. 6, pp. 702–712, 2013.

[31] P. Demoly, N. F. Adkinson, K. Brockow et al., "International Consensus on drug allergy," *Allergy*, vol. 69, no. 4, pp. 420–437, 2014.

[32] D. Laroche, P. Gomis, E. Gallimidi, J.-M. Malinovsky, and P. M. Mertes, "Diagnostic value of histamine and tryptase concentrations in severe anaphylaxis with shock or cardiac arrest during anesthesia," *Anesthesiology*, vol. 121, no. 2, pp. 272–279, 2014.

[33] S. J. Kirkbright and S. G. A. Brown, "Anaphylaxis: recognition and management," *Australian Family Physician*, vol. 41, no. 6, pp. 366–370, 2012.

[34] W. J. Song and Y. S. Chang, "Recent applications of basophil activation tests in the diagnosis of drug hypersensitivity," *Asia Pacific Allergy*, vol. 3, no. 4, pp. 266–280, 2013.

[35] F. E. Simons, L. R. Ardusso, M. Bilò et al., "International consensus on (ICON) anaphylaxis," *World Allergy Organization Journal*, vol. 7, no. 1, 2014.

[36] A. J. Fox, I. M. McLaren, and A. R. Naylor, "Cerebral perfusion monitored using transcranial Doppler during acute anaphylaxis," *Anaesthesia*, vol. 54, no. 7, pp. 678–682, 1999.

[37] F. A. Zeiler, J. Silvaggio, A. M. Kaufmann, L. M. Gillman, and M. West, "Norepinephrine as a potential aggravator of symptomatic cerebral vasospasm: two cases and argument for milrinone therapy," *Case Reports in Critical Care*, vol. 2014, Article ID 630970, 5 pages, 2014.

[38] P. Barbier, A.-P. Jonville, E. Autret, and C. Coureau, "Fetal risks with dextrans during delivery," *Drug Safety*, vol. 7, no. 1, pp. 71–73, 1992.

[39] D. O. Cortes, C. Santacruz, K. Donadello, L. Nobile, and F. S. Taccone, "Colloids for fluid resuscitation: what is their role in patients with shock?" *Minerva Anestesiologica*, vol. 80, no. 8, pp. 963–969, 2014.

20

Stenotrophomonas maltophilia Necrotizing Soft Tissue Infection in an Immunocompromised Patient

Oleg Stens,[1] Gabriel Wardi ⓘ,[2,3] Matthew Kinney,[4]
Stephanie Shin,[5] and Demosthenes Papamatheakis ⓘ[3]

[1]*Department of Internal Medicine, Harbor-UCLA Medical Center, Torrance, CA, USA*
[2]*Department of Emergency Medicine, University of California, San Diego, San Diego, CA, USA*
[3]*Division of Pulmonary, Critical Care, and Sleep Medicine, University of California, San Diego, La Jolla, CA, USA*
[4]*Department of Orthopedic Surgery, University of California, San Diego, San Diego, CA, USA*
[5]*Pulmonary and Critical Care Medicine, Sharp Memorial Hospital, San Diego, CA, USA*

Correspondence should be addressed to Gabriel Wardi; gabe.wardi@gmail.com

Academic Editor: Petros Kopterides

Introduction. To report on the first recorded case of necrotizing soft tissue infection (NSTI) in an immunocompromised individual caused by *Stenotrophomonas maltophilia* in the Western Hemisphere and highlight the challenges that medical providers face in promptly diagnosing and treating NSTI in this highly vulnerable patient population. *Case Presentation.* We report a case of NSTI caused by *S. maltophilia* in a neutropenic patient admitted for treatment of acute lymphoblastic leukemia. The patient presented with laboratory and clinical findings atypical for a NSTI that may have confounded its diagnosis and delayed surgical intervention. Despite aggressive medical care and surgical debridement, the patient unfortunately passed away due to overwhelming septic shock. *Conclusions.* Providers should consider atypical organisms as causative in NSTI in immunocompromised patients and recognize that these patients may present without classic clinical and laboratory findings.

1. Background

The term necrotizing soft tissue infection (NSTI) describes an infection caused by bacteria or fungi that spreads rapidly along tissue planes, causing vascular occlusion and necrosis, and carries high mortality even when promptly identified. These infections are rare, with approximately 1000 cases per year reported in the United States, although it is generally felt that the number of cases is underreported and is on the rise [1, 2]. Scoring systems, such as the laboratory risk indicator for necrotizing soft tissue infection (LRINEC), have been developed to help providers differentiate between NSTI and severe cellulitis [3]. However, the interpretation of this score in immunocompromised patients and particularly those with hematologic malignancies is challenging as common laboratory and physical exam findings may be absent. Furthermore, these patients are at high risk for atypical organisms that may require alternative antibiotic regimens in addition to

prompt surgical intervention. To illustrate this, we report a case of an individual with acute lymphoblastic leukemia who developed an NSTI from *Stenotrophomonas maltophilia*, the first case of this being reported in the Western Hemisphere, which illustrates the unique challenges in the identification and management in this patient population.

2. Case Presentation

A 39-year-old otherwise healthy male with newly diagnosed mixed-lineage acute monocytic and B-cell lymphoblastic leukemia was transferred to our institution for initiation of chemotherapy. Prior to transfer, he had received intrathecal methotrexate and oral dexamethasone, as well as vancomycin and cefepime for neutropenic fever and positive blood cultures growing gram-positive cocci. At our institution, the patient was started on GRAALL (Group for Research

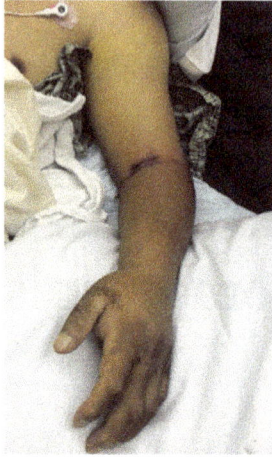

FIGURE 1: Appearance of the patient's arm prior to surgery.

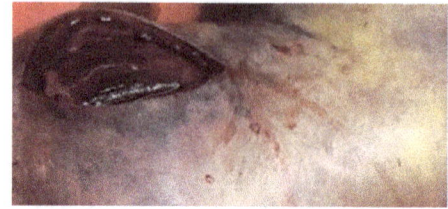

FIGURE 2: Intraoperative photograph showing nonviable tissue from incision made over the biceps muscle.

on Adult Acute Lymphoblastic Leukemia) 2003 chemotherapy. He received cefepime and vancomycin for persistent neutropenic fevers. Eventually, cefepime was switched to meropenem due to development of multifocal pneumonia during his hospital course. Shortly thereafter, liposomal amphotericin was initiated for presumed invasive pulmonary aspergillosis after a bronchoalveolar lavage (BAL) from a diagnostic bronchoscopy revealed a positive galactomannan antigen; however no organisms were seen on gram stain or identified on culture. He was treated with vancomycin for 8 days and meropenem for 17 days, after which he defervesced. Nevertheless, fevers recurred on hospital day 20 and shortly after; blood cultures returned with gram-negative rods at which point vancomycin and cefepime were reinitiated.

Three days later (hospital day 23), the patient reported pain and developed swelling and erythema of his left forearm. On physical examination, the left forearm was swollen, tense, and erythematous, but there were no areas of fluctuance, subcutaneous crepitance, or bullae noted. Duplex ultrasound of the upper extremities showed no evidence of deep vein thrombosis. However, given the acute onset of pain and swelling, orthopedic surgery was consulted for possible necrotizing infection and compartment syndrome. Laboratory testing disclosed a c-reactive protein (CRP) of 12.90 mg/dL, a white blood cell count of less than 0.1×10^9/L, a sodium of 142 mmol/L, a glucose of 110 mg/dL, a hemoglobin of 7.2 g/dL, and a creatinine of 0.96 mg/dL, yielding a LRINEC score of 2 [3]. It was felt, partly due to this low score, that the patient had a severe cellulitis without necrotizing infection or compartment syndrome. Moreover, based on the patient's clinical picture and the available data at the time, invasive testing for compartment syndrome was deemed unnecessary by the orthopedics service. No additional imaging was ordered at this point. Within 10 hours, the swelling and pain had progressed to his entire left upper extremity (Figure 1) and the patient developed hypotension. He was then transferred to the intensive care unit for refractory septic shock and severe metabolic derangement. At this time, laboratory studies were notable for a CRP of 18.80 mg/dL, a white blood cell count of 0.2×10^9/L, a sodium

of 142 mmol/L, a glucose of 116 mg/dL, a hemoglobin of 5.9 g/dL, and a creatinine of 1.06 mg/dL yielding a LRINEC score of 6. The patient continued to clinically decline rapidly despite broadening of his antibiotic regimen (vancomycin, meropenem, gentamicin, and amphotericin B) and was taken to the operating room by the orthopedic surgery service due to concern of a rapidly progressing NSTI.

In the operating room, the entire left upper extremity was prepped, and an initial incision was made over the dorsum of the hand. Exploration of the surrounding tissue revealed necrotic fat, hemorrhagic changes, and gross edema. The expressed fluid was tan but did not have the classic "dishwater" appearance of necrotizing fasciitis, nor was it malodorous. The fascia was thickened and opaque. A counterincision was then made proximally over the biceps muscle in the proximal brachium (Figure 2). This region displayed the same tan drainage with associated fat necrosis, and thrombosed vessels were also appreciated in the subcutaneous tissue. Regions of the thickened, diseased-appearing fascia were excised, revealing that the underlying musculature appeared necrotic, noncontractile, and nonviable.

At this point during the procedure, the anesthesiologist noted that multiple vasopressors were being used to maintain the patient's blood pressure, and there was concern that he was clinically deteriorating. Given the extensive involvement of, essentially, the entire limb and the concern that the bacterial load could not be adequately controlled in this hemodynamically unstable patient, the decision was made to proceed with an emergent glenohumeral amputation. The deltoid muscle remained healthy-appearing and contractile, and thus a lateral-based flap composed of the deltoid and overlying skin and soft tissue was planned. Once the amputation was performed, the wound was copiously irrigated using several liters of normal saline to minimize the remaining bacterial load. Hemostasis was subsequently achieved, a drain was placed, and the flap closure was completed. The patient's hemodynamic status improved during closure, and he was transferred back to the intensive care unit for continued care.

The previously drawn blood culture returned on postoperative day (POD) 0, growing *Stenotrophomonas maltophilia* in both aerobic and anaerobic cultures, at which point trimethoprim-sulfamethoxazole was initiated. Pathology of the surgical specimen confirmed the diagnosis of a NSTI, and multiple tissue cultures grew only *S. maltophilia*. Despite appropriate antibiotic therapy and surgical intervention, the patient remained persistently bacteremic and in refractory shock despite aggressive medical therapy. On POD1, new necrotic skin areas were noted at the surgical site, and cardiothoracic surgery was consulted to evaluate further surgical intervention. The team decided against this, given the patient's very poor prognosis. After discussion with the family, the patient was transitioned to comfort care and passed away shortly thereafter.

3. Discussion

In this article, we present a case of a monomicrobial NSTI caused by *Stenotrophomonas maltophilia* in a neutropenic patient with hematologic malignancy. To our knowledge, this is the first reported case of a NSTI due to *S. maltophilia* in the Western Hemisphere. Sakhnini and colleagues from Israel reported two young women on the same hospital ward dying from fulminant *S. maltophilia* soft tissue infection of the extremities [4]. The key similarities between all three cases include neutropenia (the two women in Israel were neutropenic due to acute myeloid leukemia and aplastic anemia, resp.) and empiric treatment with a carbapenem-class antibiotic prior to the onset of soft tissue infection. We suggest that correctly diagnosing NSTI in immunocompromised patients is particularly challenging, since the causative organisms and the clinical features may differ significantly compared to immunocompetent patients.

NSTIs are classified based on the microbiology of the infection. Type I NSTIs, by far the most common, are polymicrobial, with both aerobic and anaerobic organisms typically present. Type II NSTIs are monomicrobial infections typically associated with gram-positive pathogens like *β*-hemolytic *streptococci* or *S. aureus*. Type III NSTIs are the least common type and are typified by *Clostridium* species, which cause rapidly progressive myonecrosis. Finally some necrotizing infections do not fall within the normal classification system, such as the waterborne agent-related NSTIs (*Aeromonas hydrophila* and *Vibrio vulnificus*) and invasive rhinocerebral fungal infections [5–7]. Prompt diagnosis and surgical intervention are essential to patient survival. Even with early diagnosis, surgical debridement, and aggressive supportive care, mortality remains high, estimated to be over 20% [7]. Unfortunately, there is no single imaging or laboratory study that is both sensitive and specific for NSTIs. The LRINEC score was introduced in 2004 as a method to help providers differentiate between severe cellulitis and NSTIs [3]. Although the original study showed promising positive and negative predictive values for this score [3], follow-up validation studies showed lower sensitivities, challenging the scores ability to distinguish NSTI [8, 9].

In addition to the above, this score may be even more misleading in myelosuppressed patients, since leukocytosis would be absent and anemia could be attributed to impaired erythropoiesis. Furthermore, the characteristic intraoperative finding of a NSTI, "dishwater" discharge, maybe absent in these patients, likely due to profound neutropenia. In our case, the initial LRINEC score of 2 was misleading and provided false reassurance. Moreover, the delay in speciation of the gram-negative rod noted on blood cultures also led to inappropriate antibiotic coverage, despite broad-spectrum antibiotics being provided.

Unfortunately, the diagnosis of NSTIs in immunocompromised populations has been poorly studied. A single-center retrospective study conducted at Brigham & Women's Hospital in Boston found that immunocompromised patients with NSTI were less likely to have significant leukocytosis or purulent drainage at the site of infection, compared to immunocompetent NSTI cases. The immunosuppressed patients NSTI were also more likely to experience delays in diagnosis and initial surgical debridement, which were associated with worse outcomes [10].

S. maltophilia is a waterborne, gram-negative, obligate aerobe bacterium that has been isolated from a variety of sources in the hospital settings. It is an opportunistic healthcare-associated infection closely related to *Pseudomonas* and has high morbidity and mortality in certain patient populations, particularly the immunosuppressed ones. The name *Stenotrophomonas* comes from the Greek language and means "a unit feeding on few substrates" whereas *maltophilia* means "a friend of malt" [11]. *S. maltophilia* has been known to cause a wide range of infections, including pneumonia, bacteremia, endocarditis, and meningitis [12]. Skin and soft tissue infections by *S. maltophilia* including metastatic and primary cellulitis and ecthyma gangrenosum have also been reported, predominantly in patients receiving chemotherapy for hematologic malignancies [13–15]. In our patient, we would favor a primary cellulitis as the source of the infection given that pain and swelling of the left upper extremity preceded clinical deterioration, and there were no other localizing symptoms. Respiratory cultures were negative for the organism. However, we cannot rule out metastatic soft tissue infection from endocarditis as echocardiography was never obtained. Our case report highlights a NSTI due to a microorganism uncommonly associated with such an infection and raises concerns for the breadth of pathogens that can cause such invasive infections on immunosuppressed patients.

Treating infections caused by *S. maltophilia* is challenging because of the organism's inherent resistance to a broad range of antibiotics, including almost all beta-lactams, carbapenems, cephalosporins, and aminoglycosides. Resistance to carbapenems is particularly problematic in the intensive care unit as this class of antibiotic is frequently used when patients fail to respond to other antibiotics that cover gram-negative infections. Trimethoprim-sulfamethoxazole is presently the antibiotic of choice, although ticarcillin-clavulanic acid, minocycline, tigecycline, and certain fluoroquinolones may also be effective [16]. Because of its antibiotic resistance, *S. maltophilia* is not covered by most empiric antibiotic regimens and requires a high level of suspicion to consider this diagnosis and provide proper treatment. More recently, *S. maltophilia* infection has become increasingly common in cancer patients and has been possibly associated with carbapenem antibiotic use, to which it is resistant [17–21].

4. Conclusion

NSTIs in immunocompromised patients present a unique challenge. These patients may not present with the laboratory abnormalities and physical exam findings typically associated with NSTI, leading to a delay in diagnosis and possibly worse outcomes. Moreover, causative organisms may be atypical for NSTI, compared to immunocompetent patients, which may impede appropriate antibiotic therapy. Of these, *S. maltophilia* is becoming increasingly important, based on higher incidence in certain populations. Overreliance on scoring tools such as LRINEC should be avoided, particularly in special patient populations such as the immunocompromised ones and those with hematological malignancies as the patient's underlying disease process may affect results. Potential future research can include targeted prophylactic antibiotic use in certain patient populations that are at higher risk for atypical NSTI. This could include patients with a hematological malignancy or patients who develop new infectious symptoms after receiving carbapenems or other broad-spectrum antibiotics.

Abbreviations

NSTI: Necrotizing soft tissue infection

GRAALL: Group for Research on Adult Acute

                    Lymphoblastic Leukemia

CRP: c-reactive protein

LRINEC: Laboratory risk indicator for necrotizing

                    soft tissue infection

POD: Postoperative day.

Disclosure

This work has not received any funding from any grant or other financial support. It was completed at the University of California, San Diego. It was presented at the American Thoracic Society Annual Meeting in San Francisco 5/2016. This article has not been published or presented or is under consideration at any other journals.

Authors' Contributions

Gabriel Wardi, Matthew Kinney, Stephanie Shin, and Demosthenes Papamatheakis were all involved in the care of the patient and discussion of and creation of the paper. Oleg Stens and Gabriel Wardi drafted the manuscript and all authors contributed substantially to its revision. Oleg Stens and Gabriel Wardi take responsibility for the paper as a whole.

References

[1] S. M. E. Simonsen, E. R. van Orman, B. E. Hatch et al., "Cellulitis incidence in a defined population," *Epidemiology and Infection*, vol. 134, no. 2, pp. 293–299, 2006.

[2] M. A. Malangoni, "Necrotizing soft tissue infections: Are we making any progress?" *Surgical Infections*, vol. 2, no. 2, pp. 145–150, 2001.

[3] C. H. Wong, L. W. Khin, K. S. Heng, K. C. Tan, and C. O. Low, "The LRINEC (Laboratory Risk Indicator for Necrotizing Fasciitis) score: a tool for distinguishing necrotizing fasciitis from other soft tissue infections," *Critical Care Medicine*, vol. 32, no. 7, pp. 1535–1541, 2004.

[4] E. Sakhnini, A. Weissmann, and I. Oren, "Fulminant Stenotrophomonas maltophilia soft tissue infection in immunocompromised patients: An outbreak transmitted via tap water," *The American Journal of the Medical Sciences*, vol. 323, no. 5, pp. 269–272, 2002.

[5] N. Hiransuthikul, W. Tantisiriwat, K. Lertutsahakul, A. Vibhagool, and P. Boonma, "Skin and soft-tissue infections among tsunami survivors in southern Thailand," *Clinical infectious diseases: an official publication of the Infectious Diseases Society of America*, vol. 41, no. 10, pp. e93–e96, 2005.

[6] I. Brook and E. H. Frazier, "Clinical and microbiological features of necrotizing fasciitis," *Journal of Clinical Microbiology*, vol. 33, no. 9, pp. 2382–2387, 1995.

[7] J. S. Ustin and M. A. Malangoni, "Necrotizing soft-tissue infections," *Critical Care Medicine*, vol. 39, no. 9, pp. 2156–2162, 2011.

[8] M. Neeki, F. Dong, C. Au et al., "Evaluating the Laboratory Risk Indicator to Differentiate Cellulitis from Necrotizing Fasciitis in the Emergency Department," *Western Journal of Emergency Medicine*, vol. 18, no. 4, pp. 684–689, 2017.

[9] E. Burner, S. O. Henderson, G. Burke, J. Nakashioya, and J. R. Hoffman, "Inadequate sensitivity of laboratory risk indicator to rule out necrotizing fasciitis in the emergency department," *Western Journal of Emergency Medicine*, vol. 17, no. 3, pp. 333–336, 2016.

[10] E. Z. Keung, X. Liu, A. Nuzhad, C. Adams, S. W. Ashley, and R. Askari, "Immunocompromised status in patients with necrotizing soft-tissue infection," *JAMA Surgery*, vol. 148, no. 5, pp. 419–426, 2013.

[11] M. Denton and K. G. Kerr, "Microbiological and clinical aspects of infection associated with Stenotrophomonas maltophilia," *Clinical Microbiology Reviews*, vol. 11, no. 1, pp. 57–80, 1998.

[12] W.-Y. Teo, M.-Y. Chan, C.-M. Lam, and C.-Y. Chong, "Skin manifestation of Stenotrophomonas maltophilia infection - A case report and review article," *Annals, Academy of Medicine, Singapore*, vol. 35, no. 12, pp. 897–900, 2006.

[13] S. E. Vartivarian, K. A. Papadakis, J. A. Palacios, J. T. Manning Jr., and E. J. Anaissie, "Mocutaneous and soft tissue infections caused by Xanthomonas maltophilia: A new spectrum," *Annals of Internal Medicine*, vol. 121, no. 12, pp. 969–973, 1994.

[14] C. Moser, V. Jønsson, K. Thomsen, J. Albrectsen, M. M. Hansen, and J. Prag, "Subcutaneous lesions and bacteraemia due to Stenotrophomonas maltophilia in three leukaemic patients with neutropenia," *British Journal of Dermatology*, vol. 136, no. 6, pp. 949–952, 1997.

[15] J. I. G. Paez and S. F. Costa, "Risk factors associated with mortality of infections caused by Stenotrophomonas maltophilia: a systematic review," *Journal of Hospital Infection*, vol. 70, no. 2, pp. 101–108, 2008.

[16] A. C. Nicodemo and J. I. G. Paez, "Antimicrobial therapy for Stenotrophomonas maltophilia infections," *European Journal of Clinical Microbiology & Infectious Diseases*, vol. 26, no. 4, pp. 229–237, 2007.

[17] A. Safdar and K. V. Rolston, "Stenotrophomonas maltophilia: Changing spectrum of a serious bacterial pathogen in patients with cancer," *Clinical Infectious Diseases*, vol. 45, no. 12, pp. 1602–1609, 2007.

[18] S. C. Sanyal and E. M. Mokaddas, "The increase in Carbapenem use and emergence of Stenotrophomonas maltophilia as an important nosocomial pathogen," *Journal of Chemotherapy*, vol. 11, no. 1, pp. 28–33, 1999.

[19] S. R. Ansari, H. Hanna, R. Hachem, Y. Jiang, K. Rolston, and I. Raad, "Risk factors for infections with multidrug-resistant Stenotrophomonas maltophilia in patients with cancer," *Cancer*, vol. 109, no. 12, pp. 2615–2622, 2007.

[20] L. S. Elting, N. Khardori, G. P. Bodey, and V. Fainstein, "Nosocomial infection caused by xanthomonas maltophilia: A case–control study of predisposing factors," *Infection Control & Hospital Epidemiology*, vol. 11, no. 3, pp. 134–138, 1990.

[21] G. Aisenberg, K. V. Rolston, B. F. Dickey, D. P. Kontoyiannis, I. I. Raad, and A. Safdar, "Stenotrophomonas maltophilia pneumonia in cancer patients without traditional risk factors for infection, 1997-2004," *European Journal of Clinical Microbiology & Infectious Diseases*, vol. 26, no. 1, pp. 13–20, 2007.

21

Food Protein-Induced Enterocolitis Syndrome Causing Hypovolemic Shock and Methemoglobinemia

Stefan W. Malin ⓘ,[1] **Riad Lutfi,**[2] **Matthew L. Friedman,**[2] **and Alicia M. Teagarden ⓘ**[2]

[1]*Department of Pediatrics, Indiana University School of Medicine, Indianapolis, IN, USA*
[2]*Division of Pediatric Critical Care, Department of Pediatrics, Indiana University School of Medicine, Indianapolis, IN, USA*

Correspondence should be addressed to Stefan W. Malin; malins@iu.edu

Academic Editor: Ricardo Oliveira

A 5-week-old previously healthy male presented with vomiting and diarrhea leading to hypovolemic shock and profound metabolic acidosis. He was subsequently found to have severe methemoglobinemia. The acidosis and shock improved with fluid resuscitation and methemoglobinemia was successfully treated with methylene blue. An extensive workup, including evaluations for infectious and metabolic etiologies, was unremarkable. However, a detailed dietary history revealed a recent change in diet, supporting a diagnosis of food protein-induced enterocolitis syndrome (FPIES). We present this case to highlight the importance of considering FPIES in an infant with vomiting and diarrhea, in the setting of a recent dietary change, leading to profound dehydration, metabolic acidosis, and methemoglobinemia. Diagnosis of FPIES, although difficult to make and one of exclusion, can be potentially life-saving.

1. Introduction

Non-IgE-mediated food allergies can have acute or chronic presentations [1]. Food protein-induced enterocolitis syndrome (FPIES) is a rare, though severe, form of non-IgE-mediated food allergy that can present in infancy with predominant gastrointestinal signs and profound dehydration. Severe methemoglobinemia in the setting of acute intestinal inflammation and increased intestinal nitrites has been described infrequently in FPIES [2]. Methemoglobinemia is a blood disorder in which the ratio of oxidized hemoglobin is altered resulting in a shift in the oxygen hemoglobin dissociation curve. Rapid recognition of FPIES and appropriate therapy is crucial to avoiding recurrent hospitalizations, to unnecessary extensive workup, or in extreme cases, even death.

2. Case Presentation

A five-week-old previously healthy, full-term male initially presented to an emergency department with a two-day history of profound vomiting and diarrhea. He was well appearing and afebrile at the time of presentation; reassurance was given and he was discharged home with close follow-up. At his follow-up appointment, an upper gastrointestinal series (UGI) was obtained that was reassuring. His symptoms persisted, however, so, roughly 24 hours following his UGI, he was taken to another emergency department for worsening gastrointestinal symptoms and lethargy. His initial blood gas showed severe metabolic acidosis with a pH of 6.7, bicarbonate of 3 mmol/L, and base deficit exceeding −30 mmol/L. Intraosseous access was obtained prior to transport to the tertiary care pediatric facility and the child received 20 ml/kg of normal saline during transport.

Upon arrival to the pediatric intensive care unit, the child was lethargic, cyanotic, and mottled with cool extremities. His exam was notable for decreased muscle tone, labored breathing, a soft but distended abdomen, prolonged capillary refill, and a sunken anterior fontanelle. His initial heart rate was 150 beats per minute, blood pressure was 70/30 mmHg, and oxygen saturation was 85% on 2 liters/minute nasal cannula. Intravenous access was obtained and the patient received aggressive isotonic crystalloid resuscitation. He was intubated due to severe acidosis and altered mental status. A broad workup was initiated after stabilization including evaluation for infectious, metabolic, and cardiac causes. His initial labs were also notable for an elevated white blood cell count of 51 k/cumm (normal 6–18), with 38% bands, 5% myelocytes, and 8% metamyelocytes, an ammonia of 211 mCmol/L (normal 11–35), and a lactate of 1.8 mmol/L (normal 0.5–1.6). Stool hemoccult was positive. He was placed on broad-spectrum antibiotics pending blood, urine, cerebrospinal fluid, and stool cultures. An echocardiogram was obtained that demonstrated normal anatomy and function. The child was persistently hypoxemic after intubation despite receiving 100% fraction of inspired oxygen on the ventilator, so an arterial blood gas was obtained and the blood was noted to be dark chocolate colored in appearance (Figure 1). The partial pressure of oxygen was 200 mmHg. Cooximetry was ordered with a serum methemoglobin level, which was greater than 25%, consistent with the diagnosis of methemoglobinemia (>1.5% is considered elevated per laboratory equipment and protocol). After two doses of 1 mg/kg of methylene blue, his serum methemoglobin level decreased to 3.5%. His ammonia level and acidosis corrected with fluid resuscitation. He was extubated roughly 18 hours after presentation.

Multiple subspecialties were consulted to determine the cause of his severe metabolic acidosis and methemoglobinemia, including Metabolism and Gastroenterology. At this point, further history revealed that the infant's formula had been changed multiple times in the days preceding presentation. Malabsorptive causes were considered unlikely due to normal growth prior to presentation and allergic enteritis/proctitis was considered unlikely due to the severity of presentation. Eosinophilic esophagitis was not considered in the differential from gastroenterology because of the diarrhea and severity of the presentation. Infectious enteritis and colitis were initially presumed to be the most likely cause, but a stool culture, ova and parasite exam, rotavirus antigen, and gastrointestinal pathogen PCR test were all negative. The infant was started on hydrolyzed formula (Elecare) and discharged home with follow-up appointments with a pediatric gastroenterologist and an allergist with a presumed diagnosis of FPIES. At the time of his follow-up, roughly 8 weeks after discharge, he was continuing to do well on Elecare and had not had recurrence of his symptoms, and his weight had returned to the 52nd percentile up from the 6th percentile at his initial presentation (Figure 2). His diet has slowly been expanded with the exception of milk; he will have to complete an oral food challenge (OFC) with milk in a controlled office setting prior to its reintroduction.

3. Discussion

Pediatric food allergies are common in the first two years of life and have an estimated prevalence between 3 and 8% [1]. FPIES, a non-IgE-mediated food allergy, had previously been considered a rare disorder, but due to raised awareness, recent studies have estimated its incidence at up to 0.3% of all newborns [1, 3]. Food protein-induced allergic procto-colitis and food protein-induced enteropathy are also non-IgE-mediated food allergies, but they often have subacute

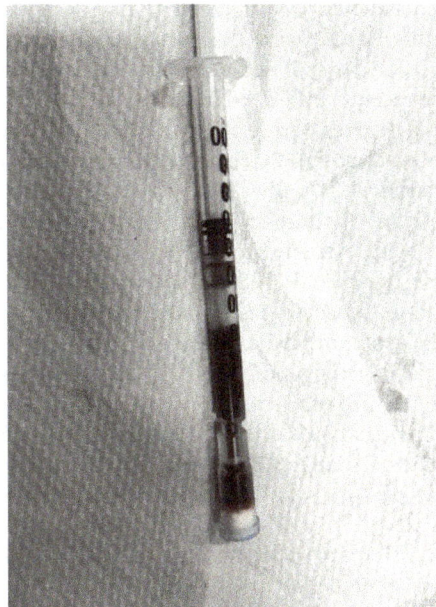

FIGURE 1: This is an arterial blood sample obtained shortly after admission. It was noted to be significantly darker than expected. Cooximetry was obtained and the methemoglobinemia level was reported as greater than 25%.

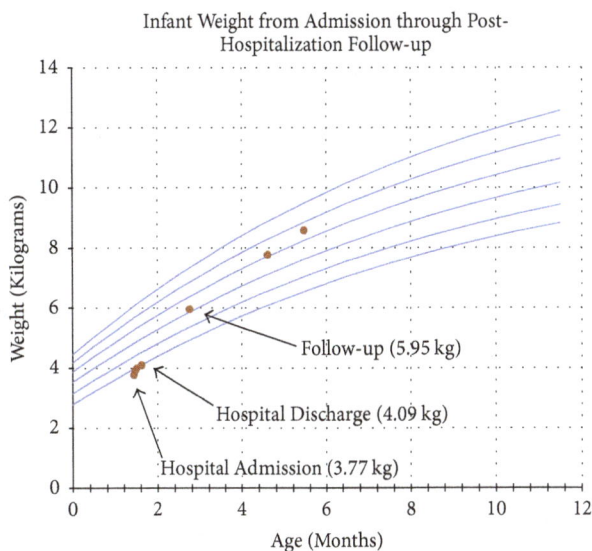

FIGURE 2: This is a copy of the infant's growth chart. The infant was admitted to the PICU and was 3.77 kilograms (kg), which was below his birth weight and at the 6th percentile for age. He was discharged weighing 4.09 kg and at posthospitalization follow-up (6 weeks from discharge) he was 5.95 kg, approximately the 52nd percentile for age.

to chronic presentations ranging from hemoccult-positive stools in healthy infants to chronic diarrhea causing failure to thrive [1]. Differentiation between the various non-IgE-mediated food allergies is made based on clinical history and severity of illness. Occasionally, endoscopies with biopsies are required for diagnosis [1]. FPIES is a severe form of food hypersensitivity reaction that usually presents in infancy and is often difficult to recognize and diagnose [3, 4]. This will hopefully improve, especially considering that the first international evidence-based guidelines for the diagnosis of FPIES were recently published in 2017 [1]. FPIES can present with varying degrees of severity, but at its worst, can present with profuse vomiting, diarrhea, dehydration, and eventual lethargy and shock [4]. At its least severe form, unrecognized FPIES can lead to failure to thrive and potentially multiple admissions with extensive testing and interventions [1, 3]. Increased awareness of FPIES can hopefully lead to improved recognition in subacute cases and need for referral to a tertiary care center in severe cases.

The precise pathogenesis of FPIES has not been clearly defined. T-cells are often considered as a major role player; however, this has come under recent scrutiny [1, 5]. Studies have shown similar CD4 T-cell responses after casein exposure in cow-milk FPIES patients as compared to IgE-mediated allergy to cow's milk and normal subjects [5]. Activation of the innate immune system has recently been identified as a potential role player in FPIES. Monocytes, natural killer cells, neutrophils, and eosinophils, identified by whole blood flow cytometry, were activated in patients with active FPIES exposed to milk proteins [6]. This same pattern was not observed in children who had outgrown their FPIES [6]. Growth of local populations of plasma cells in the intestine has been seen in biopsies following acute FPIES reactions resulting in increased production of IgM and IgA [7]. Only 10–30% of patients will have a positive IgE against the offending food [7]. FPIES often results in a systemic inflammatory response not seen in other non-IgE-mediated food allergies and can present with a profound leukocytosis, margination of leukocytes, and a markedly elevated C-reactive protein [1]. Cytokine profiles in patients with positive OFCs were notable for elevations in IL-2, IL-5, and IL-8, and other cytokines were markedly elevated in patients depending on the severity of their reaction [8]. Despite the fact that the exact etiology is unknown, the end result is severe intestinal inflammation leading to profuse diarrhea and vomiting.

Decreased catalase activity during acute intestinal inflammation leads to increased intestinal nitrites and can cause increased heme molecule oxidation, which leads to methemoglobinemia [3]. Methemoglobin is unable to bind oxygen and shifts the oxygen-dissociation curve to the left [9]. Infants are more at risk for developing methemoglobinemia as fetal hemoglobin is more easily oxidized and their level of cytochrome-b5 reductase does not reach adult values until roughly 4 months of age [9]. In infants with cyanosis and diarrhea, methemoglobinemia should be considered, especially when cyanosis does not improve with supplemental oxygen and arterial blood appears darker than normal [2, 9]. Cooximetry is the most accurate method to reliably measure methemoglobin. Children with severe methemoglobinemia experience marked respiratory distress and altered mental status that would exacerbate with anemia and acidosis leading to further impairment of oxygen delivery and tissue perfusion [9]. Treatment is based on reducing the oxidized iron within the hemoglobin molecule to its ferrous state using 1 mg/kg of intravenous methylene blue [9].

Given that FPIES can present at a very young age, the differential diagnosis for this clinical presentation is varied and includes sepsis, cardiogenic shock, metabolic disorders, and intestinal etiologies. FPIES is a clinical diagnosis, so obtaining a detailed dietary history as part of the evaluation is crucial. Age of presentation, absence of fever, and recurrent episodes of gastrointestinal symptoms are important keys to the diagnosis [1, 10]. Given its variability in presentation, awareness of FPIES and keeping it on the differential is important, even though it is a diagnosis of exclusion.

Treatment of acute FPIES is primarily supportive with fluid resuscitation and close hemodynamic monitoring. Occasionally, vasopressors or inotropes are needed in addition to fluids to treat hypotension. No strong evidence to support the benefit of steroid treatment is available [3]. New, limited evidence has suggested that IV administration of ondansentron (a 5-hydroxytryptamine$_3$ antagonist) as an adjunctive therapy has some benefit in acute presentations [10]. Identifying the causal agent and removing it from the child's diet are crucial and remain the mainstay of treatment. The long-term prognosis for FPIES is good as the majority of children will outgrow their food protein intolerance and catch up with their growth [1, 3]. The age of resolution is variable and depends partly on the offending food substance. For cow milk FPIES, resolution around 1-2 years of age has been reported, although it can take longer than this [10].

In our case report, we discuss the case of an infant presenting with hypovolemic shock, severe metabolic acidosis, and methemoglobinemia due to FPIES. Despite extensive evaluation, no other etiologies were found to explain his symptoms and laboratory findings. Early recognition and aggressive management were key elements for shock reversal. His symptoms and failure to thrive resolved after switching to a hypoallergenic, hydrolyzed formula. FPIES should be suspected in infants who present with diarrhea and methemoglobinemia. As discussed previously, early recognition may prevent excessive diagnostic testing, recurrent hospital admissions, and failure to thrive.

References

[1] P. Biermé, A. Nowak-Wegrzyn, and J.-C. Caubet, "Non-IgE-mediated gastrointestinal food allergies," *Current Opinion in Pediatrics*, vol. 29, no. 6, pp. 697–703, 2017.

[2] K. F. Murray and D. L. Christie, "Dietary protein intolerance in infants with transient methemoglobinemia and diarrhea," *Journal of Pediatrics*, vol. 122, no. 1, pp. 90–92, 1993.

[3] R. W. Coates, K. R. Weaver, R. Lloyd, N. Ceccacci, and M. R. Greenberg, "Food protein-induced enterocolitis syndrome as a cause for Infant hypotension," *Western Journal of Emergency Medicine*, vol. 12, no. 4, pp. 512–514, 2011.

[4] S. K. Mane and S. L. Bahna, "Clinical manifestations of food protein-induced enterocolitis syndrome," *Current Opinion in Allergy and Clinical Immunology*, vol. 14, no. 3, pp. 217–221, 2014.

[5] J. C. Caubet, R. Bencharitiwong, A. Ross, H. A. Sampson, M. C. Berin, and A. Nowak-Węgrzyn, "Humoral and cellular responses to casein in patients with food protein–induced enterocolitis to cow's milk," *The Journal of Allergy and Clinical Immunology*, vol. 139, no. 2, pp. 572–583, 2017.

[6] R. Goswami, A. B. Blazquez, R. Kosoy, A. Rahman, A. Nowak-Węgrzyn, and M. C. Berin, "Systemic innate immune activation in food protein–induced enterocolitis syndrome," *The Journal of Allergy and Clinical Immunology*, vol. 139, no. 6, pp. 1885–1896.e9, 2017.

[7] M. Kimura, Y. Ito, M. Shimomura et al., "Cytokine profile after oral food challenge in infants with food protein-induced enterocolitis syndrome," *Allergology International*, vol. 66, no. 3, pp. 452–457, 2017.

[8] F. R. Greer, M. Shannon, Committee on Nutrition, and Committee on Environmental Health, "Infant methemoglobinemia: the role of dietary nitrate in food and water," *Pediatrics*, vol. 116, no. 3, pp. 784–786, 2005.

[9] K. A. Nelson and M. A. Hosteler, "An infant with methoglobinemia," *Hospital Physician*, vol. 39, no. 2, pp. 31–38, 2003.

[10] S. Mehr, K. Frith, and D. E. Campbell, "Epidemiology of food protein-induced enterocolitis syndrome," *Current Opinion in Allergy and Clinical Immunology*, vol. 14, no. 3, pp. 208–216, 2014.

22

Multiple Transverse Colonic Perforations Associated with Slow-Release Nonsteroidal Anti-Inflammatory Drugs and Corticosteroids

Nobuki Shioya, Shigehiro Shibata, Masahiro Kojika, and Shigeatsu Endo

Department of Critical Care and Emergency, Iwate Prefectural Advanced Critical Care and Emergency Center,
Iwate Medical University, 19-1 Uchimaru, Morioka 020-8505, Japan

Correspondence should be addressed to Nobuki Shioya, fukubuku@xg7.so-net.ne.jp

Academic Editors: A. Banga and M. Doganay

The patient was a 36-year-old woman with sarcoidosis and Sjogren's syndrome, and had been prescribed slow-release diclofenac sodium and prednisolone for the treatment of pain associated with uveitis and erythema nodosum. She was admitted to our emergency center with abdominal pain and distention. A chest X-ray showed free air under the diaphragm on both sides, and an emergency laparotomy was performed for suspected panperitonitis associated with intestinal perforation. Laparotomy revealed several perforations on the antimesenteric aspect of the transverse colon. The resected specimen showed 11 punched-out ulcerations, many of which were up to 10 mm in diameter. The microscopic findings were non-specific, with leukocytic infiltration around the perforations. She showed good postoperative recovery, as evaluated on day 42. The present case highlights the need for exercising caution while prescribing slow-release nonsteroidal anti-inflammatory drugs with corticosteroids to patients with autoimmune diseases, as such treatment may exacerbate intestinal epithelial abnormalities.

1. Introduction

Multiple intestinal perforations, although rare, may be fatal and may be caused by Crohn's disease, Behcet's disease, systemic lupus erythematosus (SLE), medications, infections, and neoplasms. Several autoimmune diseases are associated with changes in the intestinal permeability, and increased colonic permeability induces ulceration and perforation. Sarcoidosis and Crohn's disease share many clinical and immunological features and also have similar pathogenetic mechanisms [1, 2]; Sjogren's syndrome and sarcoidosis also have much in common in terms of the pathophysiology. However, there are no case reports of multiple perforations clearly associated with Sjogren's syndrome and sarcoidosis in the literature. Nonsteroidal anti-inflammatory drugs (NSAIDs) and corticosteroids are commonly prescribed worldwide for a broad spectrum of autoimmune manifestations. NSAIDs are known to damage the surface epithelial cells and increase colonic permeability, and concomitant use of NSAIDs and corticosteroids is known to cause additive damage to the gastrointestinal (GI) tract. Herein, we describe a rare case of multiple localized perforations of the transverse colon associated with coadministration of a slow-release NSAID and low-dose corticosteroid.

2. Case Presentation

A 36-year-old Japanese woman was referred to our critical care and emergency center with mild abdominal distention and epigastric pain of about 10 days duration. She gave a history of having been diagnosed as having bilateral uveitis and erythema nodosum in the lower extremities six months previously. The patient was diagnosed as having Sjogren's syndrome based on a positive Schirmer's test and reduced amount of saliva. During the 2 months prior to hospitalization, the patient suffered from loss of vision, ophthalmoplegia, and painful erythema nodosum nodules in the lower extremities. She had taken prednisolone at the dose of 20 mg/day. The serum albumin and calcium levels were

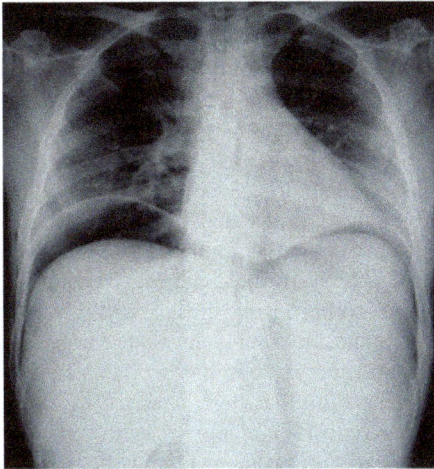

FIGURE 1: Chest radiograph at the initial diagnosis showed bilateral hypodiaphragmatic free air.

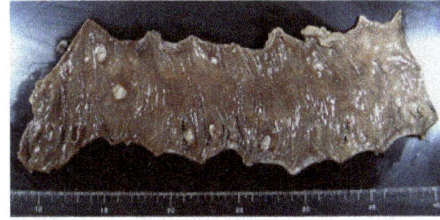

FIGURE 2: Macroscopic findings of resected transverse colonic specimen show multiple perforations. Perforated holes with circular-shape are each from 5 to 10 mm in diameter.

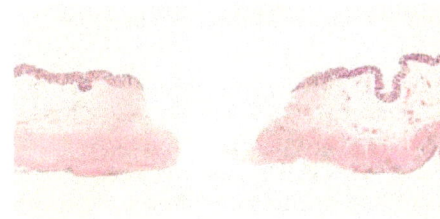

FIGURE 3: Microscopic specimen demonstrates punched-out ulcer. There is active inflammation around the ulcer. (haematoxylin and eosin ×40).

reduced (2.4 mg/dL and 6.7 mg/dL). The serum angiotensin-converting enzyme (ACE) and lysozyme levels were slightly elevated (38.4 IU/l and 23.2 ug/mL, resp.). The tuberculin skin test was the reaction with induration of less than 5 mm in size. Bronchoalveolar lavage contained 61% lymphocytes, with a CD4/CD8 ratio of 4.9, and examination of trans-bronchial lung biopsy (right B8) specimens revealed the presence of noncaseating epithelioid cell granulomas. Microscopic examination of PAS- and acid-fast stained specimens revealed no acid-fast bacilli. Based on these findings, except for the low serum levels of calcium, sarcoidosis had been diagnosed about 4 months previously. She had suffered from pain of progressively increasing severity because of uveitis and erythema nodosum during the 10 days prior to admission. She had been prescribed 75 mg/day of slow-release diclofenac sodium and prednisolone in slowly tapering doses (current dose, 5 mg/day).

At the time of admission to our hospital, her vital signs were as follows: body temperature 36 degrees Celsius, heart rate 81 beats/min, blood pressure 102/45 mm Hg, and respiratory rate 20/min. Physical examination revealed marked abdominal distention, with slight guarding and rebound tenderness. No bowel sounds could be heard on auscultation. She had no history of consumption of contaminated foods or water. There were no clinical features, such as rose spots, tenesmus, mucous/bloody diarrhea, or joint pain. She had sicca syndrome and dry eye, but no oral aphthae or genital ulcers. She had never visited any countries with poor sanitary conditions or tropical areas and had no history of venereal diseases. The pathergy test was negative. The results of blood investigations were as follows: white blood cells 3950/mm³, hemoglobin 10.3 g/dL, and platelet count 73,000/mm³. The serum C-reactive protein level was 3.7 mg/dL. Renal function, hepatobiliary function, serum electrolytes, and the coagulation profile were within normal limits. Radioimmunoassay for hepatitis virus markers in the serum revealed a positive test for hepatitis B surface antigen (HBs Ag) and negative tests for both hepatitis B surface antibody (HBs Ab)

and anti-hepatitis C antibody. Serum tests for rheumatoid factor and HLA-B51 were negative. Both proteinase-3-antineutrophil cytoplasmic antibody (PR3-ANCA) and myeloperoxidase-antineutrophil cytoplasmic antibody (MPO-ANCA) titers were within normal limits (<10 EU). A chest X-ray obtained with the patient upright demonstrated free air under the diaphragm bilaterally (Figure 1). An emergency laparotomy was performed because of suspected panperitonitis caused by intestinal perforation. The abdominal cavity contained approximately 400 mL of fetid fluid. The stomach, duodenum, and small intestine were normal on exploration. There were several perforations on the antimesenteric aspect of the transverse colon. Therefore, a transverse colectomy and loop colostomy were performed. The resected specimen contained a large amount of soft stool and exhibited 11 punched-out ulcerations, many of which measured up to 10 mm in diameter (Figure 2). Microscopic examination revealed nonspecific findings and showed perforation of the intestinal wall with infiltration of the ulcer bed with leukocytes (Figure 3).

Slow-release diclofenac sodium had been discontinued since the time of admission and, subsequently, the corticosteroid was also tapered off and discontinued. On day 14, colonoscopy revealed mild aphthoid ulcers at the anastomotic site, but no evidence of perforation. The patient made good postoperative recovery. Colostomy closure was performed on day 42 without any complications, and the patient was discharged on day 73 of hospitalization.

3. Discussion

Multiple colonic perforations are rare, but life-threatening, and may be caused by inflammatory bowel diseases (Crohn's disease and ulcerative colitis), rheumatological disorders (Behcet's disease, SLE), medications, infectious enterocolitides, such as amebic, typhoidal, and tuberculous colitis, and neoplasms. Our patient did not fulfill the diagnostic criteria for Crohn's disease, Behcet's disease, or SLE. Vasculitis, such as microscopic polyangiitis, was thought to be unlikely because of the normal PR3-ANCA and MPO-ANCA titers and absence of renal function disorder, and in the absence of the histopathological finding of cells infiltrating the walls of small arterioles. Microscopic examination of the resected specimen revealed no pathogens. Infectious enterocolitis was considered to be unlikely because of the absence of rose spots, tenesmus, mucous/bloody diarrhea, and joint pain. Accordingly, mainly the increased topical colonic permeability by the slow-release NSAID was thought to be responsible for the development of the multiple perforations.

NSAIDs exert both local and systemic effects on the GI tract. Local injury to the intestinal mucosa is mainly due to the entry of the NSAIDs, especially slow-release NSAIDs, and their metabolites into the enterohepatic circulation [3]. The NSAID dosing period in our patient was relatively short, and cases of colonic perforation after even short-term diclofenac intake of under one week have been reported [4]. NSAIDs are known to damage the surface epithelial cells and increase the intestinal permeability. NSAIDs can also uncouple mitochondrial oxidative phosphorylation, which impairs the mitochondrial energy production necessary for tight junction complex integrity, leading to increased intestinal inflammation and permeability [5]. Regulation of the intestinal epithelial cell barrier is central to the development of intestinal immunity and inflammation. Tight junctions create a paracellular permeability barrier that is breached when NSAIDs cause GI injury, including increased GI permeability. Intestinal barrier function relies on the tight junctions at the apical contact areas of the intestinal epithelial cells. Tight junctions define cell polarity and regulate the paracellular flow of ions and water, which are crucial functions of acinar cells [6, 7]. In general, the transit time of the drug in the transverse colon is about 4 hours after oral intake. The dissolution rate of slow-release diclofenac sodium is 70% in 8 hours; however, this rate is also influenced by the presence of food [8]. The peak blood concentration of orally ingested slow-release diclofenac sodium is achieved from 6 to 7 hours.

NSAIDs cause numerous side effects, and these drugs together with corticosteroids produce additive damage to the gastrointestinal tract [9–11]. Corticosteroids have powerful immunosuppressive actions, impair the ability to contain a perforation in its early stages, and delay the consecutive healing process [12, 13]. Concomitant use of corticosteroids (odds ratio 4.4–4.7) is one of the risk factors for NSAID-related GI complications [14, 15], which have been recorded to occur 7 times more frequently in patients with perforation than in matched controls [16].

Increased intestinal permeability has also been reported in autoimmune diseases such as IBD, systemic sclerosis, Behçet's syndrome, SLE, ankylosing spondylitis, and juvenile idiopathic arthritis [17–20]. Altered intestinal permeability is a well-described feature of Crohn's disease [1]. Sarcoidosis and Crohn's disease may have shared pathogenetic

mechanisms [2]. There is a report of a case of sarcoidosis with gastrointestinal loss of proteins [21]. Sarcoidosis and Sjogren's syndrome, as autoimmune diseases, often coexist, since both diseases may share the same immunological profile; however, multiple intestinal perforations associated with these autoimmune diseases have not yet been reported. Sarcoidosis is a systemic disease with 90% predilection for the lungs, with gastrointestinal manifestations being rare, although any organ can be involved. The incidence of clinically recognizable gastrointestinal involvement is less than 1.0% [22]. The stomach is the most commonly involved part of the GI tract, and the colon is involved less frequently, and no case of colonic perforation has been reported. Abnormal intestinal permeability has been reported in cases of active pulmonary sarcoidosis [1]. Sjogren's syndrome is a systemic autoimmune exocrinopathy involving the salivary glands, but it can also involve almost every other part of the GI tract. Systemic vasculitic manifestations of Sjogren's syndrome have been reported in approximately 10% of patients [23]. Only one study of multiple colonic ulcers due to vasculitis associated with Sjogren's syndrome has been reported in the Japanese literature [24].

It is considered that slow-release NSAIDs and corticosteroids may cause aggravation of the intestinal epithelial abnormalities in patients with sarcoidosis and Sjogren's syndrome. Close caution must be exercised when both NSAIDs and corticosteroids are prescribed to patients with autoimmune diseases, as these patients are at a higher risk of development of adverse bowel events, such as colonic perforation, than patients without autoimmune diseases.

References

[1] B. Wallaert, J. F. Colombel, A. Adenis et al., "Increased intestinal permeability in active pulmonary sarcoidosis," *American Review of Respiratory Disease*, vol. 145, no. 6, pp. 1440–1445, 1992.

[2] P. A. McCormick, D. P. O'Donoghue, and M. X. FitzGerald, "Crohn's colitis and sarcoidosis," *Postgraduate Medical Journal*, vol. 62, no. 732, pp. 951–953, 1986.

[3] C. Kara, H. Derici, O. Nazll, T. Tansug, and A. D. Bozdag, "Colonic perforation after short-term use of nonsteroidal antiinflammatory drugs: report of two cases," *Techniques in Coloproctology*, vol. 13, no. 1, pp. 75–78, 2009.

[4] L. Schiffmann, S. Kahrau, G. Berger, and H. J. Buhr, "Colon perforation in an adolescent after short-term diclofenac intake," *ANZ Journal of Surgery*, vol. 75, no. 8, pp. 726–727, 2005.

[5] S. Somasundaram, G. Sigthorsson, R. J. Simpson et al., "Uncoupling of intestinal mitochondrial oxidative phosphorylation and inhibition of cyclooxygenase are required for the development of NSAID-enteropathy in the rat," *Alimentary Pharmacology and Therapeutics*, vol. 14, no. 5, pp. 639–650, 2000.

[6] T. Sakaguchi, S. Brand, and H. C. Reinecker, "Mucosal barrier and immune mediators," *Current Opinion in Gastroenterology*, vol. 17, no. 6, pp. 573–577, 2001.

[7] K. R. Groschwitz and S. P. Hogan, "Intestinal barrier function: molecular regulation and disease pathogenesis," *Journal of Allergy and Clinical Immunology*, vol. 124, no. 1, pp. 3–20, 2009.

[8] J. V. Willis, M. J. Kendall, and D. B. Jack, "The influence of food on the absorption of diclofenac after single and multiple oral doses," *European Journal of Clinical Pharmacology*, vol. 19, no. 1, pp. 33–37, 1981.

[9] H. Imaeda, H. Ishii, and M. Goto, "Treatment of peptic ulcer related to rheumatic diseases," *Nippon Rinsho*, vol. 60, no. 8, pp. 1585–1591, 2002.

[10] A. Lanas, "Non-steroidal anti-inflammatory drugs and gastrointestinal bleeding," *Italian Journal of Gastroenterology and Hepatology*, vol. 31, no. 1, pp. S37–S42, 1999.

[11] G. Börsch and G. Schmidt, "What's new in steroid and non-steroid drug effects on gastroduodenal mucosa?" *Pathology Research and Practice*, vol. 180, no. 4, pp. 437–444, 1985.

[12] C. R. Morris, I. M. Harvey, W. S. L. Stebbings, C. T. M. Speakman, H. J. Kennedy, and A. R. Hart, "Epidemiology of perforated colonic diverticular disease," *Postgraduate Medical Journal*, vol. 78, no. 925, pp. 654–659, 2002.

[13] S. Mpofu, C. M. A. Mpofu, D. Hutchinson, A. E. Maier, S. R. Dodd, and R. J. Moots, "Steroids, non-steroidal anti-inflammatory drugs, and sigmoid diverticular abscess perforation in rheumatic conditions," *Annals of the Rheumatic Diseases*, vol. 63, no. 5, pp. 588–590, 2004.

[14] F. L. Lanza, F. K. L. Chan, E. M. M. Quigley et al., "Guidelines for prevention of NSAID-related ulcer complications," *American Journal of Gastroenterology*, vol. 104, no. 3, pp. 728–738, 2009.

[15] J. R. Curtis, F. Xie, L. Chen et al., "The incidence of gastrointestinal perforations among rheumatoid arthritis patients," *Arthritis and Rheumatism*, vol. 63, no. 2, pp. 346–351, 2011.

[16] M. J. S. Langman, L. Morgan, and A. Worrall, "Use of anti-inflammatory drugs by patients admitted with small or large bowel perforations and haemorrhage," *British Medical Journal*, vol. 290, no. 6465, pp. 347–349, 1985.

[17] M. Catanoso, R. Lo Gullo, M. R. Giofré et al., "Gastro-intestinal permeability is increased in patients with limited systemic sclerosis," *Scandinavian Journal of Rheumatology*, vol. 30, no. 2, pp. 77–81, 2001.

[18] I. Fresko, V. Hamuryudan, M. Demir et al., "Intestinal permeability in Behçet's syndrome," *Annals of the Rheumatic Diseases*, vol. 60, no. 1, pp. 65–66, 2001.

[19] P. Picco, M. Gattorno, N. Marchese et al., "Increased gut permeability in juvenile chronic arthritides. A multivariate analysis of the diagnostic parameters," *Clinical and Experimental Rheumatology*, vol. 18, no. 6, pp. 773–778, 2000.

[20] A. Farhadi, A. Banan, J. Fields, and A. Keshavarzian, "Intestinal barrier: an interface between health and disease," *Journal of Gastroenterology and Hepatology*, vol. 18, no. 5, pp. 479–497, 2003.

[21] A. Lindgren, C. P. Engstrom, O. Nilsson, and H. Abrahamsson, "Protein-losing enteropathy in an unusual form of sarcoidosis," *European Journal of Gastroenterology and Hepatology*, vol. 7, no. 10, pp. 1005–1007, 1995.

[22] G. W. Hunninghake, U. Costabel, M. Ando et al., "Statement on sarcoidosis," *American Journal of Respiratory and Critical Care Medicine*, vol. 160, no. 2, pp. 736–755, 1999.

[23] P. Brito-Zerón, M. Ramos-Casals, A. Bove, J. Sentis, and J. Font, "Predicting adverse outcomes in primary Sjögren's syndrome: identification of prognostic factors," *Rheumatology*, vol. 46, no. 8, pp. 1359–1362, 2007.

[24] M. Inoh, M. Tokuda, T. Maruoka et al., "Multiple colonic ulcers in a patient with Sjogren's syndrome," *Ryumachi*, vol. 35, no. 3, pp. 585–588, 1995.

23

Intensive Care in a Patient with Toxic Epidermal Necrolysis

J. Wallenborn[1,2] and M. Fischer[3,4]

[1]Department of Anesthesiology and Intensive Care Medicine, HELIOS Klinikum Aue, Gartenstraße 6, 08280 Aue, Germany
[2]Department of Anesthesiology and Intensive Care Medicine, Universitätsklinikum Carl Gustav Carus,
  Technische Universität Dresden, Fetscherstraße 74, 01307 Dresden, Germany
[3]Department of Dermatology and Venerology, HELIOS Klinikum Aue, Gartenstraße 6, 08280 Aue, Germany
[4]Department of Dermatology and Venerology, Martin-Luther-Universität Halle-Wittenberg, Ernst-Grube-Straße 40,
  06097 Halle, Germany

Correspondence should be addressed to J. Wallenborn; jan.wallenborn@helios-kliniken.de

Academic Editor: Michael J. Cawley

Toxic epidermal necrolysis (TEN) is a serious adverse drug reaction with high lethality, which usually requires intensive-medical care. A 44-year-old man developed generalized exanthema with increasing exfoliation and mucosal involvement after taking allopurinol, ibuprofen, and etoricoxib. The clinical diagnosis of TEN was histologically confirmed. Prednisolone therapy with 3 mg/kg body weight (BW) was not able to prevent further progress to finally 80% of the body surface, and infliximab 5 mg/kg BW was given as a single dose. This prevented further progression of the TEN. Despite marked improvement in skin findings, the ICU stay was prolonged by a complex analgosedation, transient kidney failure, volume management, positioning therapy, and vegetatively impeded weaning. Moreover, there was colonization with multiresistant bacteria (MRSA and VRE). Nonetheless, the patient could be restored to health and was released after four weeks. Infliximab seems to be effective in the treatment of TEN, especially in cases of rapid progression. Moreover, patients with TEN are difficult to handle in intensive-medical care, whereby attention should especially be paid to sufficient pain therapy, and the positioning of the patient is a particular challenge.

1. Introduction

In Europe, between 2.5% and 10.6% of all in-hospital treatment cases are ascribable to adverse drug reactions [1, 2], whereby the skin is affected in only 2–5‰ of the cases. Drug-related exanthemas which require intensive-medical care or which are life-threatening are even less frequent. While nearly all affected patients survive maculopapulous or maculourticarial exanthemas, lethality of up to 10% is reported for hypersensitivity reactions like Drug Rash with Eosinophilia and Systemic Symptoms (DRESS) [3]. Depending on the spread, toxic epidermal necrolysis (TEN) has by far the highest lethality [4]. The intensive-medical care of these patients is very demanding and characterized by various particular features.

2. Case Presentation

Long-term therapy with allopurinol and etoricoxib, with ibuprofen as needed, was initiated due to arthralgia in hyperuricemia in a 44-year-old man, who had been otherwise healthy up to then. Three weeks later, an itchy patch of erythema developed on his back, which spread exanthematically over the entire trunk and extremities during the following 48 hours. Withdrawal of the three cited medications and out-patient administration of prednisolone (1 mg/kg BW/die) could not prevent further progression. On admission to hospital, symmetrically distributed, confluent livid-erythematous exanthema was seen on the trunk and face, with multiple flaccid blisters of amber-colored content. Initially, ca. 50% of the body surface (BOS) was affected. The Nikolski I-Phenomenon was positive. The oral mucosa showed multiple erosions with whitish coating buccal and in the vestibulum oris. The entire prolabium was erosive and covered with scabs. Moreover, there was pronounced conjunctivitis. The SCORTEN [5] on admission was 2 points (Table 1); the risk of mortality was thus 12%. At the time of admission, the CRP was 53.4 mg/l (Norm: <5 mg/l); Leukocytes and procalcitonin were in the normal range. Due to

TABLE 1: Prognosis score for TEN (SCORTEN) [5]. Determination on admission. A point is given for a fulfilled criterion. Rating of mortality: ≤1 points 3%, 2 points 12%, 3 points 35%, 4 points 58%, and ≥5 points 90%.

Parameter SCORTEN	Points
Age ≥ 40	1
Pulse ≥ 120/min	0
Malignoma	0
Affected body surface ≥ 10%	1
Urea > 10 mmol/l	0
Bicarbonate (HCO_3) < 20 mmol/l	0
Glucose > 14 mmol/l	0

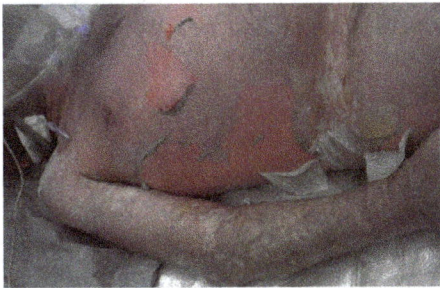

FIGURE 1: Large-area exfoliation in toxic epidermal necrolysis.

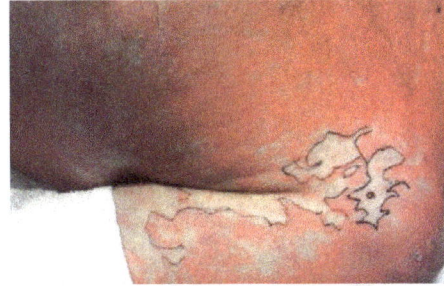

FIGURE 2: Toxic epidermal necrolysis. Cessation of progression after infliximab.

his increasingly worse general condition, the patient was transferred to Intensive Care where initially treatment with prednisolone 3 mg/kg BW was initiated. However, within the following 48 hours, there was additional spread of the exanthema, and finally ca. 80% of the body surface was affected (Figure 1). For this reason, prednisolone was withdrawn and infliximab administered in a single dose of 5 mg/kg BW. This resulted within 6 hours in a complete stop of the exanthema progression (Figure 2). However, during the following days, partial exfoliation was seen within the erythema visible at the start of therapy. Local therapy consisted of application of gels containing polihexanide and bland gauze bandages. Moreover, the patient was bedded on a glass bead bed (Pearls® AFT, Hill-Rom GmbH, Witten, Germany) on Metalline®-Foil. The Air Fluidised Therapy with this special bed supports healing of such pronounced skin lesions by means of micro-climatization, draining of secretions, and marked reduction of shear and friction, as well as pressure on the skin from the covers. Bandages were changed daily by the same team maintaining reverse isolation.

Due to a positive blood culture with proof of *Staphylococcus lugdunensis* and *Staphylococcus epidermidis* with concurrent elevated temperature (39.1°C), systemic antibiotic therapy with tazobactam and clindamycin was started on the 11th day of treatment and continued for 5 days. The PCT remained in the normal range (maximum value: 0.28 µg/l (Norm: <0.5 µg/l)) during the entire hospitalization period. In the regularly performed microbiological skin swabs, methicillin-resistant *Staphylococcus aureus* (MRSA) and vancomycin-resistant Enterococci (VRE) in swabs from the angle of the mouth were found starting on the 15th day of treatment.

Due to severe pain (NAS = 8–10) analgosedation was given during the entire intensive-medical treatment phase, beginning initially with piritramide (Dipidolor®, 5 mg-Boli) and lorazepam (Tavor®, 0.5 mg-Boli). The further course was characterized by prerenal kidney failure and respiratory exhaustion. Maintaining the equilibrium of the fluid house-hold was impeded by the losses via the large skin defects, which were impossible to measure. Efforts were oriented to extensive hemodynamic monitoring (PiCCO advanced) and repetitive albumin measurements. Intubation with controlled respiration in the BiPAP mode was required starting on the 4th day due to involvement of the oral mucosa with increasing difficulty swallowing. The analgosedation was therefore switched to continuous application of sufentanil (Sufenta®: 250 µg/50 ml at 2–8 ml/h) and propofol 2% (Disoprivan®: 1000 mg/50 ml at 4–10 ml/h). After only 48 hours, propofol was replaced by midazolam (Dormicum®: 90 mg/50 ml at 2–8 ml/h) and additional ketamine (Ketanest: 250 mg/50 ml at 4–8 ml/h) to achieve adequate analgesia. Repeated states of restlessness and hypertensive dysregulation up to 210 mmHg both under analgosedation and in the daily withdrawal attempts were terminated with urapidil or ß-blockers and the analgosedation expanded by additional administration of dexmedetomidine (Dexdor®: 1000 µg/50 ml at 1.5–4 ml/h). This unstable state lasted for a total of ten days. Only then could weaning from the respirator be successfully initiated and the analgosedation tapered off. Extubation of the responsive patient under reduced continuing analgosedation was successfully done on the 18th day of treatment. The further course was characterized by intensive physiotherapy to relieve the prominent muscle weakness following long-term sedation and critical-illness polyneuropathy (CIP). Immediately after extubation, the patient could only make weak arm movements; in the course of the first week, the patient could be mobilized to standing and walking.

Under this complex treatment, there was full reepithelization of the skin with postinflammatory hyperpigmentations within four weeks (Figure 3), successful weaning, and mobilization. After reepithelization was complete, neither VRE nor MRSA were found on the skin.

3. Discussion

With a mortality between 39% to 48%, TEN is among the few acute life-threatening skin diseases [4, 6]. Though

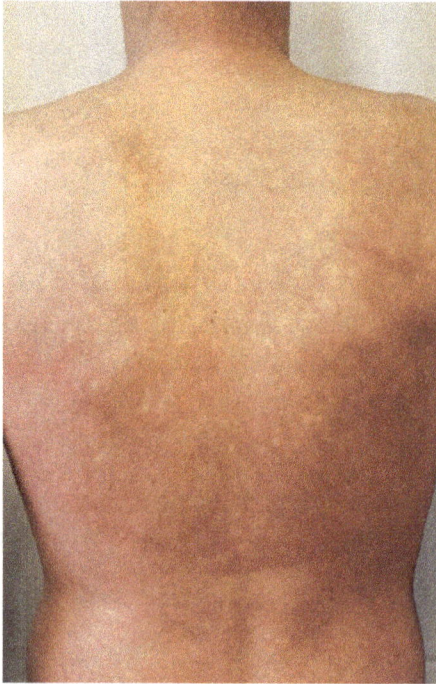

FIGURE 3: Findings on discharge. Complete healing under postinflammatory hyperpigmentations.

many drugs can induce TEN, the most common elicitors are antibiotics, anticonvulsives, nonsteroidal antirheumatics, and allopurinol [4, 6]. The diagnosis is made clinical predominantly. Nonetheless some other dermatoses with epithelial defects (staphylococcal scalded skin syndrome, pemphigus vulgaris, pemphigus foliaceus, acute generalized exanthematic pustulosis, and acute Graft-versus-Host-disease) should be taken into account. Therefore, a histological proof is mandatory.

Various mediators are involved in the apoptotic process of TEN. Granulysin is known to play a major role in inducing necrosis of keratinocytes both in *in vitro* and in a mouse model [6]. Other cytokines, especially tumor necrosis factor-alpha (TNF-α), are also important in the underlying cytotoxicity reaction. For example, TNF-α in high concentrations has been demonstrated in the blister fluid of patients with TEN [7]. Recent studies were also able to show that TNF-α in combination with γ-Interferon effects stimulation of inducible NO-synthase. The resultant NO is cytotoxic for keratinocytes [8]. The good response to the administration of corresponding biologics also illustrates a role of TNF-α in TEN. Since it was first described [9], prompt efficacy of both infliximab and etanercept has been repeatedly described in nearly twenty case reports and smaller case studies [10, 11]. However, no survival advantage for the administration of infliximab in combination with N-acetylcysteine over N-acetylcysteine alone could be demonstrated in a Proof-of-Concept study on ten TEN patients [12]. Here, in addition to the small number of cases, it must also be remembered that the patients in the Proof-of-Concept study were not treated until a relatively late stage of the disease. Medication

administration began on average about seven days after onset of symptoms. At that point, the TNF-α-dependent apoptosis/necrosis has possibly already occurred and can no longer be decisively influenced by the administration of infliximab. This assumption is supported by the clinical experience that although administration of infliximab leads to prompt stopping of further area expansion of TEN, erythematous areas which are already visible may still show exfoliation. Apparently the already-initiated apoptosis cannot be reversed. This points to a particular importance of TNF-α in early and active phases of TEN and thus for early therapy with TNF-α-blockers in TEN.

The stopping of the area expansion observed under infliximab can, independent of overall survival, contribute, in any case, to the reduction of complications and facilitate in-hospital care. The expected cost reductions from new biosimilars to infliximab would also reduce the economic burden of therapy.

The intensive-medical care of TEN patients is particularly complex. Thus, in the present case, the need for analgosedation greatly exceeded the commonly applied substances and dosages [13]. In addition to administration of propofol and sufentanil, the application of ketamine and dexmedetomidine was necessary. This condition still remained during the phase of beginning reepithelization and prolonged the stay in the ICU. The cause of the high need for therapy is unclear, but it does underline the high expense of care for patients with TEN.

Due to the large wound area, there is a high sepsis risk in patients with TEN. The frequency of sepsis is estimated at 20% [14]. Kidney failure is described in 10% of the cases and respiratory failure and pneumonia in 48% of the patients. Interestingly, the bacteria found in the skin swabs of TEN patients with infectious complications have no or only slight predictive value [15], although, as in our case, there is increased skin colonization with multiresistant bacteria [11]. An initial antibiotic prophylaxis therefore does not appear justified. In response to the skin bacteria *Staphylococcus lugdunensis* and *Staphylococcus epidermidis* found in the blood culture, 5-day intravenous antibiotic therapy was administered based on the increased fever and leukocytosis. On the other hand, systemic antibiotic therapy was not given in response to the proven MRSA, but only local antiseptic cleansing and bandages. This makes an intensive-medical difference from burn patients clear. Where damage to deeper skin layers is the starting point for septic complications in burn patients [16], the immunologically caused destruction of the epidermis apparently does not lead to a clinically relevant infection focus for sepsis. This observation has repeatedly elicited discussion of whether treating of patients with large-area exfoliation in normal wards is justified with appropriately intensified care [17]. The answer can only be found as a single-case decision depending on the extent of the wound area. However, the challenges for intensive-medical care outlined here indicate that treatment of TEN patients usually requires intensive therapy (Table 2).

Positioning was in a special bed because of the desired minimal mechanical stress to the skin. This makes positioning on an air cushion with concurrent drainage of secretions

Table 2: Supportive care in TEN.

Local therapy with polihexanide gel and gauze bandages
Reverse isolation
No antibiotic prophylaxis
Sequential microbiological screening, targeted antibiotic therapy for sepsis
Analgosedation
Volume therapy, albumin substitution
In complications: intubation and respiration, renal substitution therapy, sepsis therapy
Positioning therapy
Physiotherapy, ergotherapy, logopedics

and temperature regulation possible. However, the nearly pressure-free positioning leads to the negative effect of loss of depth sensitivity, and, in the case cited, muscular weakness after days of immobilization and onset of CIP were correspondingly pronounced. Intensive physiotherapy supported rapid reconvalescence.

Recent studies [18] pointed out that cyclosporine reduces the mortality of TEN compared with supportive care. Nonetheless TNF-α-blockers like infliximab seem to be effective especially in cases with rapid progression.

References

[1] R. L. Howard, A. J. Avery, S. Slavenburg et al., "Which drugs cause preventable admissions to hospital? A systematic review," *British Journal of Clinical Pharmacology*, vol. 63, no. 2, pp. 136–147, 2007.

[2] J. Sultana, P. Cutroneo, and G. Trifirò, "Clinical and economic burden of adverse drug reactions," *Journal of Pharmacology and Pharmacotherapeutics*, vol. 4, supplement 1, pp. S73–S77, 2013.

[3] P.-D. Ghislain and J.-C. Roujeau, "Treatment of severe drug reactions: Stevens-Johnson syndrome, toxic epidermal necrolysis and hypersensitivity syndrome," *Dermatology Online Journal*, vol. 8, no. 1, article 5, 2002.

[4] M. Mockenhaupt, "Stevens-Johnson syndrome and toxic epidermal necrolysis: Clinical patterns, diagnostic considerations, etiology, and therapeutic management," *Seminars in Cutaneous Medicine and Surgery*, vol. 33, no. 1, pp. 10–16, 2014.

[5] S. Bastuji-Garin, N. Fouchard, M. Bertocchi, J.-C. Roujeau, J. Revuz, and P. Wolkenstein, "Scorten: A severity-of-illness score for toxic epidermal necrolysis," *Journal of Investigative Dermatology*, vol. 115, no. 2, pp. 149–153, 2000.

[6] Y. K. Heng, H. Y. Lee, and J.-C. Roujeau, "Epidermal necrolysis: 60 years of errors and advances," *British Journal of Dermatology*, vol. 173, no. 5, pp. 1250–1254, 2015.

[7] O. Correia, L. Delgado, I. L. Barbosa, F. Campilho, and J. Fleming-Torrinha, "Increased interleukin 10, tumor necrosis factor α, and interleukin 6 levels in blister fluid of toxic epidermal necrolysis," *Journal of the American Academy of Dermatology*, vol. 47, no. 1, pp. 58–62, 2002.

[8] I. Viard-Leveugle, O. Gaide, D. Jankovic et al., "TNF-α and IFN-γ are potential inducers of fas-mediated keratinocyte apoptosis through activation of inducible nitric oxide synthase in toxic epidermal necrolysis," *Journal of Investigative Dermatology*, vol. 133, no. 2, pp. 489–498, 2013.

[9] M. Fischer, E. Fiedler, W. C. Marsch, and J. Wohlrab, "Antitumour necrosis factor-α antibodies (infliximab) in the treatment of a patient with toxic epidermal necrolysis," *British Journal of Dermatology*, vol. 146, no. 4, pp. 707-708, 2002.

[10] A. Paradisi, D. Abeni, F. Bergamo, F. Ricci, D. Didona, and B. Didona, "Etanercept therapy for toxic epidermal necrolysis," *Journal of the American Academy of Dermatology*, vol. 71, no. 2, pp. 278–283, 2014.

[11] L. C. Zárate-Correa, D. C. Carrillo-Gómez, A. F. Ramírez-Escobar, and C. Serrano-Reyes, "Toxic epidermal necrolysis successfully treated with infliximab," *Journal of Investigational Allergology and Clinical Immunology*, vol. 23, pp. 61–63, 2013.

[12] P. Paquet, S. Jennes, A. F. Rousseau, F. Libon, P. Delvenne, and G. E. Piérard, "Effect of N-acetylcysteine combined with infliximab on toxic epidermal necrolysis. A proof-of-concept study," *Burns*, vol. 40, no. 8, pp. 1707–1712, 2014.

[13] http://www.awmf.org/uploads/tx_szleitlinien/001-012l_S3_Analgesie_Sedierung_Delirmanagement_Intensivmedizin_2015-08_01.pdf.

[14] P. D. Mahar, J. Wasiak, B. Hii et al., "A systematic review of the management and outcome of toxic epidermal necrolysis treated in burns centres," *Burns*, vol. 40, no. 7, pp. 1245–1254, 2014.

[15] N. de Prost, S. Ingen-Housz-Oro, T. A. Duong et al., "Bacteremia in Stevens-Johnson syndrome and toxic epidermal necrolysis: epidemiology, risk factors, and predictive value of skin cultures," *Medicine*, vol. 89, no. 1, pp. 28–36, 2010.

[16] L. A. Barajas-Nava, J. López-Alcalde, M. Roqué i Figuls, I. Solà, and X. Bonfill Cosp, "Antibiotic prophylaxis for preventing burn wound infection," *Cochrane Database of Systematic Reviews*, vol. 6, Article ID CD008738, 2013.

[17] I. Hanken, M. Schimmer, and C. A. Sander, "Grundversorgung und medikamentöse Behandlung von Patienten mit toxisch epidermaler Nekrolyse," *Journal der Deutschen Dermatologischen Gesellschaft*, vol. 8, no. 5, pp. 341–347, 2010.

[18] S. Zimmermann, P. Sekula, M. Venhoff et al., "Systemic immunomodulating therapies for Stevens-Johnson syndrome and toxic epidermal necrolysis: a systematic review and meta-analysis," *JAMA Dermatology*, vol. 153, no. 6, pp. 514–522, 2017.

24

Euglycemic Diabetic Ketoacidosis in the ICU

Pablo Lucero ⓘ[1] **and Sebastián Chapela** ⓘ[1,2]

[1]Hospital Británico de Buenos Aires, Intensive Care Services, Argentina
[2]Universidad de Buenos Aires, Facultad de Medicina, Departamento de Bioquimica Humana, Argentina

Correspondence should be addressed to Pablo Lucero; pdlucero@hbritanico.com.ar

Academic Editor: Chiara Lazzeri

Diabetic ketoacidosis (DKA) is an acute complication of diabetes mellitus, both type I and type II, as well as other types with diabetes such gestacional diabetes mellitus. It is characterized by blood glucose levels greater than 250 mg/dL and metabolic acidosis (pH < 7.3 and serum bicarbonate < 15 mEq/dL) with an increased anion gap and the presence of ketone bodies in the blood or urine. Within this pathology, there is a subgroup of pathologies which are characterized by being present with no signs of hyperglycemia, posing a diagnostic challenge due to the absence of the main sign of the pathology and the diversity of their pathophysiology. In this article, we will present 3 clinical cases with 3 different forms of clinical presentation: a case of DKA in pregnancy, a case of DKA associated with the use of sodium-glucose cotransporter 2 (SGLT-2) inhibitors, and a third case related to sepsis, together with a narrative review of the literature on the topic.

1. Introduction

Diabetic ketoacidosis is an acute complication of diabetes. It is diagnosed through laboratory results showing metabolic acidosis with an increased gap and evidence of ketone bodies in the blood or urine. Most of the time, it is present with hyperglycemia. The clinical presentation of this pathology is diverse, going from abdominal pain to sensory deterioration and coma [1].

The pathophysiology of hyperglycemia in diabetic ketoacidosis has 3 cornerstones: an increase in gluconeogenesis, an increase in glycogenolysis and a decrease in peripheral glucose uptake due to a decrease in insulin action in the receptors or a decrease in insulin levels [1]. This prevents glucose from being transported inside the cells and being used as metabolic fuel. On the other hand, there is an increase in lipolysis and fatty acids start being used in the liver, where they are metabolized into ketone bodies, which can be absorbed by most cells [1].

Diabetic ketoacidosis is defined by the presence of blood glucose levels greater than 250 mg/dL, being this the main finding, associated with metabolic acidosis (pH < 7.3 and serum bicarbonate < 15 mEq/dL) with an increased anion gap and the presence of ketone bodies in the blood and/or urine [1]. There are different forms of presentation which differ from the usual presentation described in literature, such as the case of normoglycemic diabetic ketoacidosis. This pathology was first described by Munro in 1973 [2] but, in his work, he studied patients with blood glucose levels under 300mg/dL. Currently, the definition is in line with blood glucose levels under 250mg/dL [1]. 6% of patients show blood glucose levels under 300 mg/dL and around 1% of patients show levels under 180 mg/dL. The most common causes are insulin administration on the way to the hospital and fasting [1]. The diagnosis and treatment of this pathology require a deep pathophysiological knowledge, since it can be triggered by different etiologies. In this review, we will present 3 completely different cases of normoglycemic diabetic ketoacidosis.

2. Clinical Case 1

A 22-year-old woman with a history of diabetes mellitus (diagnosed at 7 years old) is treated with insulin glargine and

TABLE 1: Patients' laboratory results upon admission to the ICU.

	Na+ (mEq/L)	K+ (mEq/L)	Cl (mEq/L)	pH	HCO2 (mEq/L)	BE (mEq/L)	GAP	Δ CL	Ketonemia	Blood Glucose (mg/dL)
CASE 1	137	4.9	102	7.25	10	-14.9	23	-0.75	+	153
CASE 2	142	3.9	108	7.13	2	-23.7	32	1.5	+	165
CASE 3	140	4.8	109	7.28	7.3	-16.8	23	4	+	132

with good adherence to treatment, with hypothyroidism and 2 previous ICU admissions due to diabetic ketoacidosis in which blood glucose levels were greater than 300 mg/dL.

The patient sought consultation due to vomiting and abdominal pain 12 hours after onset. Upon physical examination, the abdomen was distended with diffuse pain and no signs of peritoneal irritation. Laboratory results showed the following values: pH: 7.25; bicarbonate: 10 mEq/dL; BE: -14.9; blood glucose: 153 mg/dL and positive ketonemia. Admission laboratory results are shown in Table 1. Upon diagnosis of normoglycemic diabetic ketoacidosis, in the context of menstrual cycle alterations and with the aim of studying the trigger, beta subunit of human chorionic gonadotropin levels was requested: 98.928 IU/L. A transvaginal ultrasound was performed and showed a gestational sac with an embryo inside. Reanimation was started with parenteral crystalloids administered at 250 mL/h during 24 hrs. It was interspersed isotonic saline solutions and polyelectrolyte solutions. Total income is 7000 ml / 24 hs. Urinary volume is 2750 ml / 24 hs. Positive balance is 4250 ml/24 hs. Continuous insulin infusion was started, as described in literature (receiving a total of 100 IU in 48 hrs). Progress was shown with improvement of the clinical condition and lab monitoring every 8 hours: pH 7.47; bicarbonate of 22 mEq/dL with blood glucose levels in the normal range (< 200 mg/dl). The usual insulin glargine dose was restored and the patient was discharged.

3. Clinical Case 2

A 50-year-old woman, former smoker, with a history of arterial hypertension, dyslipidemia, left side breast cancer which required chemotherapy, radiation therapy and surgery, hypothyroidism, and diabetes mellitus type II, is treated with 10 mg/day of Dapagliflozin, 1000 mg of Metformin every 12 hours, and NPH insulin at 40 and 60 IU. The patient sought consultation due to abdominal pain, diarrhea and fever. Upon admission, the patient was alert, tachypneic, and being with diffuse abdominal pain with no sign of peritoneal irritation. An abdominal ultrasound was requested and showed the gallbladder with multiple gallstones. The complete laboratory results are shown in Table 1. In the context of leukocytosis, acute kidney failure, and severe metabolic acidosis, the patient was admitted to the ICU with a diagnosis of sepsis. Due to the presence of metabolic acidosis with a gap of 32, a ketonemia test was requested. The result was positive and the patient was diagnosed with euglycemic diabetic ketoacidosis.

After starting treatment with a continuous insulin infusion pump and the administration of water, the patient was discharged from the hospital after 5 days.

4. Clinical Case 3

A 74-year-old male patient with a history of arterial hypertension, noninsulin dependent diabetes mellitus medicated with oral hypoglycemic agents, ischemic cardiopathology with stent placement, nonoliguric chronic kidney failure, and cryptogenic liver cirrhosis required a liver transplant and subsequently suffered portal vein thrombosis requiring anticoagulation. The patient sought consultation after 3 days of passing liquid stools, together with emesis. He denied having fever spikes and, on that date, consulted the emergency ward of this institution, to which he was admitted feeling alert, with AT: 130/64, heart rate: 108 beats per minute, and SO2: 97% on room air. Upon physical examination, the patient was alert, tachypneic, and being with dry mucous membranes. Admission laboratory results are shown in Table 1. A ketonemia test was requested and the result was positive. The clinical presentation was interpreted as dehydration secondary to gastrointestinal losses and euglycemic diabetic ketoacidosis. Reanimation was started with crystalloids, a continuous insulin infusion pump, and the administration of intravenous bicarbonate. After 48 hrs, the patient presented DKA resolution criteria.

5. Discussion

Euglycemic diabetic ketoacidosis is a diagnostic challenge for treating physicians, since there is no hyperglycemia. On the other hand, there are many causes of metabolic acidosis in patients in the intensive care unit, although, when analyzing the gap, high gap metabolic acidosis is less frequent than hyperchloremic acidosis [14]. Therefore, knowing this pathology is key when treating patients with diabetes. Moreover, the triggers are varied and, in this study, we presented 3 cases with two different pathophysiological causes.

This pathology is triggered by multiple causes (Table 2). The following pathophysiological mechanisms are common to all causes: a decrease in insulin action or secretion with a decrease in total glucose uptake at a cellular level, an increase in the production of counterregulatory hormones, and a decrease in glucose production by the liver or an increase in the excretion of glucose in the urine [11, 12].

Table 2: Causes of euglycemic diabetic ketoacidosis.

Fasting

Insulin use prior to hospital admission

Pregnancy

Use of SGLT-2

Cocaine abuse

Pancreatitis

Cirrhosis

Use of insulin pump

Sepsis

SGLT-2: type 2 sodium-glucose cotransporter.

The first case deals with a diabetic patient who is pregnant. The reason that normal pregnancy increases blood glucose levels is based on the progressive insulin resistance, which normally occurs. This resistance also explains the worsening of pregestational diabetes during pregnancy. The exogenous insulin loses its effect as the pregnancy progresses. These effects are attributable to the destruction of insulin by the kidney and the action of placental insulinases.

At the beginning of pregnancy, insulin maintains its activity, and its concentration increases due to the hyperplasia of the Beta cells of the pancreatic islets, induced by the high concentrations of placental steroids. As a result of these changes, fasting glycemia decreases. The main effect of insulin in the body is to allow the storage of nutritious substrates to meet energy needs. The provision of food is intermittent while the consumption of energy is constant from where the need for storage arises. The maternal organism stores energies in the form of glucose and fats. In addition, human chorionic gonadotropin causes vomiting, which causes fasting, dehydration, and metabolic acidosis [15].

As pregnancy progresses, the activity of the usual counterregulatory hormones such as human placental lactogen, which is synthesized by the trophoblast and released into the circulation, reduces maternal sensitivity to insulin, increasing postprandial blood glucose levels [10]. Progesterone reduces gastrointestinal motility, increasing glucose uptake [10]. In addition, there is a decrease in insulin sensitivity, particularly in the third trimester, caused by hormonal changes that occur during pregnancy like an increase in estrogen, progestogens, human placental lactogen, and secretion of TNF-α [15]. All these mechanisms induce hyperglycemia in pregnancy. On the other hand, the placenta and the fetus absorb large amounts of glucose, decreasing blood levels when fasting. This leads to an increase in the secretion of maternal fatty acids and their subsequent metabolization in ketone bodies [12].

During late pregnancy, the fetus dramatically increases its glucose-based metabolism and accentuates its anabolic process by growth. On the other hand, the maternal metabolism enters a catabolic process in order to send all the glucose to the fetus through the placenta, using fat as the primary fuel. In the diabetic patient, the decrease in insulin intake profoundly affects the general metabolism, particularly at the level of liver, muscle, and adipose tissue, which are insulin essential action points. The absence of this hormone causes distortion of homeostasis. Plasma levels of glucose, free fatty acids and ketones rise to extreme figures, plasma pH and bicarbonate fall dangerously and there is marked loss of fatty tissue and body mass. If insulin levels are not restored, this case can lead to death.

Finally, the respiratory alkalosis that occurs during pregnancy increases the urinary excretion of bicarbonate, reducing the ability to buffer pH changes caused by the increase in body ketone production [16]. This leads to euglycemic diabetic ketoacidosis in pregnancy.

The incidence rate of diabetic ketoacidosis in all pregnant women with diabetes varies between 0.5 and 3%, being more common in patients with type I diabetes. However, there are more and more cases of patients with type II and gestational diabetes [17, 18]. In a unicentric study in which 223,000 deliveries were analyzed, 14,532 (6.5%) were complicated due to diabetes, just 33 patients presented 40 diabetic ketoacidosis episodes with average blood glucose levels of 380 mg/dL on admission, whereas only 3 cases presented euglycemic diabetic ketoacidosis [18]. The different cases of euglycemic diabetic ketoacidosis in pregnancy, their initial diagnosis, and clinical presentations are analyzed in Table 3. In contrast to most of the cases described in literature, our patient presented with DKA during the first trimester.

The harmful effects of ketoacidosis on the fetus are caused by ketone bodies and glucose passing the placental barrier, dehydration, which leads to decreased placental perfusion and electrolyte imbalance [18]. Fetal acidosis is caused by hyperglycemia, which leads to osmotic diuresis and fetal intravascular volume depletion. Fetal hyperinsulinemia increases oxygen uptake. A decrease in 2,3-DPG increases oxygen affinity for hemoglobin, reducing the amount of oxygen available to the fetus and generating hypoxia [17]. The electrolyte disturbance can not only generate maternal arrhythmias with a subsequent decrease in placental perfusion, but also generate fetal arrhythmias and risk of cardiorespiratory arrest [18]. Although there are no studies that show the long-term consequences for the fetuses born alive, neurodevelopmental alterations were observed. In contrast to other pregnancy complications, a hasty delivery with DKA would be harmful to the fetus. Therefore, it is recommended to stabilize the mother first [19]. Some studies state that fetal mortality in patients with DKA can reach 9% [15] and perinatal mortality is between 9 and 35% [17]. However, there are also authors who argue that ketoacidosis is not associated with a higher mortality rate during the first trimester, nor with a higher rate of malformations [20].

The mainstay of treatment does not differ from the treatment for hyperglycemic ketoacidosis, that is, hydration and insulin. The difference is that, in order to maintain blood glucose levels, the amount of glucose administered must be higher and, in the case of pregnant patients, care should be taken to maintain blood glucose levels suitable for fetal welfare. There is evidence in literature showing that a value of 250 mg/dL (Baha M. 2014) or values between 100 and 150 mg/dL would accomplish this [20].

The second case is associated with the use of sodium-glucose cotransporter 2 (SGLT-2) inhibitors. The incidence

TABLE 3: Cases of euglycemic DKA in pregnancy reported in literature.

Author and Year	Age of the Patient	Gestational Week	Obstetric History	History of Diabetes	Blood Glucose upon Admission	pH upon Admission	Triggering Factor
Darhambulla, 2012 [3]	30 years old	33	Pregnancy: 2 Borns: ?	Recently diagnosed gestational diabetes	95 mg/dL	7.17	Urinary tract infection
Cardonell, 2016 [4]	33 years old	35	Pregnancy: 3 Borns: 2	Diabetes type II	134 mg/dL	7.02	Unknown. During delivery
Chico, 2008 [5]	29 years old	24	Pregnancy: 2 Borns: 1	Diabetes type I	93 mg/dL	7.22	Unknown. During delivery
Franke, 2001 [6]	23 years old	32	Unknown	Recently diagnosed gestational diabetes	127 mg/dL	7.2	Influenza A infection
Kamalakannan, 2003 [7]	28 years old	36	Pregnancy: 5 Borns:?	Diabetes type I	234 mg/dL	7.1	Vomiting and poor treatment adherence
Karpate, 2013 [8]	25 years old	37	Pregnancy: 1 Borns: 0	None	102 mg/dL	N/A	Fasting
Napoli, 2011 [9]	26 years old	34	Pregnancy: 3 Borns: 2	Diabetes type I	211 mg/dL	7.25	Altered food intake
Oliver, 2007 [10]	29 years old	28	N/A	Diabetes type I	205 mg/dL	7.15	Bronchial pneumonia
Rivas, 2016 [11, 12]	39 years old	32	Pregnancy: 2 Borns: 1	None	225 mg/dL	7.15	Emesis
Tarif, 2007 [13]	37 years old	35	Pregnancy: 5 Borns: 4	Gestational diabetes	78 mg/dL	7.32	Emesis and diarrhea

rate of diabetic ketoacidosis in patients treated with SGLT-2 inhibitors varies between 0.16 and 0.76 cases per 1000 patients per year [21, 22]. In a review of literature, 46 cases of diabetic ketoacidosis associated with the use of SGLT-2 were found and, in 70% of the cases, the ketoacidosis was euglycemic [23]. The main mechanism of action is the inhibition of glucose uptake in proximal tubules, increasing glycosuria [24]. In addition, SGLT-2 inhibitors significantly increase plasma glucagon levels through a decrease in paracrine inhibition of insulin and possibly due to the inhibition of glucose transport into pancreatic α cells by SGLT-2 [22]. At the same time, they decrease 3-hydroxybutyrate and acetoacetate elimination at the kidney level [24–28]. Moreover, when blood glucose levels decrease, patients that are being treated with insulin decrease its administration. Therefore, counterregulatory hormone effects predominate, resulting in a lower inhibition of lipolysis and lipogenesis and, thereby, triggering euglycemic ketoacidosis [29–31]. Case reports include the 3 drugs of the gliflozin class: Dapagliflozin [24, 25, 29–35], Canagliflozin [26–28, 31–33, 36, 37], and Empagliflozin [38–40].

The last case deals with a patient with diabetic ketoacidosis associated with dehydration. During fasting, when hepatic glycogen is consumed, there is no source of glucose release into the bloodstream; however, lipolysis and the generation of ketone bodies are increased [41]. Dehydration is also a factor that contributes to the development of euglycemia [42].

Luethi et al. [43] analyzed blood glucose levels, arterial blood gases, and ketonemia and ketonuria in 60 critically ill patients. 63% of the patients developed some degree of ketosis (β-hydroxybutyric levels greater than 0.6 mmol/L). In 12% of the patients, it was severe (greater than 3 mmol/L), and 33 % developed ketonuria (which was only severe in 2% of the patients). The prevalence of ketosis was the same in those who presented glucose peaks greater than 180 mg/dL and those who did not [1]. It is interesting to observe that, in this study [44], only 2 patients out of the 60 developed ketoacidosis based on the criteria set forth by the Joint British Diabetes Society [45] and none of them did, based on the ADA's criteria [11].

Finally, another possible cause of euglycemic ketoacidosis is the administration of insulin before being admitted to the hospital [42]. Other causes are pancreatic lesions developed during pancreatitis due to alcohol consumption, associated with the fasting required by this condition, which would explain the development of euglycemic ketoacidosis [42]. Furthermore, cocaine abuse causes an increase in the secretion of cortisol and noradrenaline by the adrenal gland, in addition to the anorexigenic effects of this drug, which lead to fasting [46].

6. Conclusion

Euglycemic diabetic ketoacidosis is a diagnostic challenge, not only due to the absence of its most important sign, which is hyperglycemia, but also due to its varied triggers. Knowing the different contexts in which it can occur will allow us to suspect euglycemic diabetic ketoacidosis and begin rapid and adequate treatment of the precipitating cause, as well as aggressive hydration, glucose homeostasis through insulin administration, and the adjustment of electrolyte imbalances. A delay results in serious complications both in the fetus (in the case of gestational diabetes) and in the patient, increasing in-hospital morbidity and mortality.

References

[1] A. E. Kitabchi, G. E. Umpierrez, J. M. Miles, and J. N. Fisher, "Hyperglycemic crises in adult patients with diabetes," *Diabetes Care*, vol. 32, no. 7, pp. 1335–1343, 2009.

[2] J. F. Munro, I. W. Campbell, A. C. McCuish, and L. J. Duncan, "Euglycaemic diabetic ketoacidosis," *British Medical Journal*, vol. 2, no. 5866, pp. 578–580, 1973.

[3] B. Franke, D. Carr, and M. H. Hatem, "A case of euglycaemic diabetic ketoacidosis in pregnancy," *Diabetic Medicine*, vol. 18, no. 10, pp. 858-859, 2001.

[4] D. Kamalakannan, V. Baskar, D. M. Barton, and T. A. M. Abdu, "Diabetic ketoacidosis in pregnancy," *Postgraduate Medical Journal*, vol. 79, no. 934, pp. 454–457, 2003.

[5] S. J. Karpate, H. Morsi, M. Shehmar, J. Dale, and C. Patel, "Euglycemic ketoacidosis in pregnancy and its management: case report and review of literature," *European Journal of Obstetrics & Gynecology and Reproductive Biology*, vol. 171, no. 2, pp. 386-387, 2013.

[6] A. Napoli, M. Framarino, A. Colatrella et al., "Eating disorders and diabetic ketoacidosis in a pregnant woman with type 1 diabetes: A case report," *Eating and Weight Disorders*, vol. 16, no. 2, pp. e146–e149, 2011.

[7] R. Oliver, P. Jagadeesan, R. J. Howard, and K. Nikookam, "Euglycaemic diabetic ketoacidosis in pregnancy: An unusual presentation," *Journal of Obstetrics & Gynaecology*, vol. 27, no. 3, p. 308, 2007.

[8] M. Rivas M, P. Belmar Z, P. Durruty A, L. Sanhueza M, and G. López S, "Cetoacidosis diabética normoglicémica en el embarazo: Caso clínico," *Revista Médica de Chile*, vol. 144, no. 10, pp. 1360-1364, 2016.

[9] N. Tarif and W. Al Badr, "Euglycemic diabetic ketoacidosis in pregnancy," *Saudi Journal of Kidney Disease and Transplantation*, vol. 18, no. 4, pp. 590–593, 2007.

[10] B. M. Sibai and O. A. Viteri, "Diabetic ketoacidosis in pregnancy," *Obstetrics & Gynecology*, vol. 123, no. 1, pp. 167–178, 2014.

[11] A. A. Abdin, M. Hamza, M. S. Khan, and A. Ahmed, "ase Report Euglycemic Diabetic Ketoacidosis in a Patient with Cocaine Intoxication," *Case Reports Crit Care*, vol. 2016, 2016.

[12] F. Le Neveu, B. Hywel, and J. N. Harvey, "Euglycaemic ketoacidosis in patients with and without diabetes," *Practical Diabetes*, vol. 30, no. 4, pp. 167–171, 2013.

[13] V. N. Baş, S. Uytun, and Y. A. Torun, "Diabetic euglycemic ketoacidosis in newly diagnosed type 1 diabetes mellitus during Ramadan fasting," *Journal of Pediatric Endocrinology and Metabolism*, vol. 28, no. 3-4, pp. 333–335, 2015.

[14] P. M. Gauthier and H. M. Szerlip, "Metabolic acidosis in the intensive care unit," *Critical Care Clinics*, vol. 18, no. 2, pp. 289–308, 2002.

[15] M. G. Dalfrà, S. Burlina, G. Sartore, and A. Lapolla, "Ketoacidosis in diabetic pregnancy," *The Journal of Maternal-Fetal and Neonatal Medicine*, vol. 29, no. 17, pp. 2889–2895, 2016.

[16] S. N. Bryant, C. L. Herrera, D. B. Nelson, and F. G. Cunningham, "Diabetic ketoacidosis complicating pregnancy," *Journal of Neonatal-Perinatal Medicine*, vol. 10, no. 1, pp. 17–23, 2017.

[17] M. d. Veciana, "Diabetes ketoacidosis in pregnancy," *Seminars in Perinatology*, vol. 37, no. 4, pp. 267–273, 2013.

[18] J. A. Parker and D. L. Conway, "Diabetic Ketoacidosis in Pregnancy," *Obstetrics and Gynecology Clinics of North America*, vol. 34, no. 3, pp. 533–543, 2007.

[19] M. A. Carroll and E. R. Yeomans, "Diabetic ketoacidosis in pregnancy," *Critical Care Medicine*, vol. 33, no. 10, pp. S347–S353, 2005.

[20] R. M. Goldenberg, L. D. Berard, A. Y. Cheng et al., "SGLT2 Inhibitor–associated Diabetic Ketoacidosis: Clinical Review and Recommendations for Prevention and Diagnosis," *Clinical Therapeutics*, vol. 38, no. 12, pp. 2654–2664.e1, 2016.

[21] H. Qiu, A. Novikov, and V. Vallon, "Ketosis and diabetic ketoacidosis in response to SGLT2 inhibitors: Basic mechanisms and therapeutic perspectives," *Diabetes/Metabolism Research and Reviews*, vol. 33, no. 5, p. e2886, 2017.

[22] J. A. Levine, S. L. Karam, and G. Aleppo, "SGLT2-I in the Hospital Setting: Diabetic Ketoacidosis and Other Benefits and Concerns," *Current Diabetes Reports*, vol. 17, no. 7, 2017.

[23] J. Rosenstock and E. Ferrannini, "Euglycemic diabetic ketoacidosis: a predictable, detectable, and preventable safety concern with SGLT2 inhibitors," *Diabetes Care*, vol. 38, no. 9, pp. 1638–1642, 2015.

[24] J. Adachi, Y. Inaba, and C. Maki, "Euglycemic diabetic ketoacidosis with persistent diuresis treated with canagliflozin," *Internal Medicine*, vol. 56, no. 2, pp. 187–190, 2017.

[25] D. A. Kelmenson, K. Burr, Y. Azhar, P. Reynolds, C. A. Baker, and N. Rasouli, "Euglycemic Diabetic Ketoacidosis With Prolonged Glucosuria Associated With the Sodium-Glucose Cotransporter-2 Canagliflozin," *Journal of Investigative Medicine High Impact Case Reports*, vol. 5, no. 2, p. 232470961771273, 2017.

[26] M. Jazi and G. Porfiris, "Euglycemic diabetic ketoacidosis in type 2 diabetes treated with a sodium-glucose cotransporter-2 inhibitor," *Canadian Family Physician*, vol. 62, no. 9, pp. 722–e517, 2016.

[27] S. Maraka, A. E. Kearns, N. E. N. Kittah, and D. T. O'Keeffe, "Recurrent euglycemic diabetic ketoacidosis after discontinuation of sodium-glucose cotransporter 2 inhibitor," *Diabetes Research and Clinical Practice*, vol. 118, pp. 77-78, 2016.

[28] S. Ullah, N. Khan, H. Zeb, and H. Tahir, "Metabolic ketoacidosis with normal blood glucose: A rare complication of sodium–glucose cotransporter 2 inhibitors," *SAGE Open Medical Case Reports*, vol. 4, p. 2050313X1667525, 2016.

[29] H. Storgaard, J. I. Bagger, F. K. Knop, T. Vilsbøll, and J. Rungby, "Diabetic Ketoacidosis in a Patient with Type 2 Diabetes After Initiation of Sodium-Glucose Cotransporter 2 Inhibitor Treatment," *Basic & Clinical Pharmacology & Toxicology*, vol. 118, no. 2, pp. 168–170, 2016.

[30] S. Pujara and A. Ioachimescu, "Prolonged Ketosis in a Patient With Euglycemic Diabetic Ketoacidosis Secondary to Dapagliflozin," *Journal of Investigative Medicine High Impact Case Reports*, vol. 5, no. 2, p. 232470961771004, 2017.

[31] F. Brown and T. McColl, "Euglycemic Diabetic Ketoacidosis Secondary to Dapagliflozin Use: A Case Report," *The Journal of Emergency Medicine*, vol. 54, no. 1, pp. 109–111, 2018.

[32] M. Ahmed, M. J. McKenna, and R. K. Crowley, "Diabetic keto-acidosis in patients with type 2 diabetes recently commenced on sglt-2 inhibitors: An ongoing concerN," *Endocrine practice : official journal of the American College of Endocrinology and the American Association of Clinical Endocrinologists*, vol. 23, no. 4, pp. 506–508, 2017.

[33] S. Dizon, E. J. Keely, J. Malcolm, and A. Arnaout, "Insights Into the Recognition and Management of SGLT2-Inhibitor-Associated Ketoacidosis: It's Not Just Euglycemic Diabetic Ketoacidosis," *Canadian Journal of Diabetes*, vol. 41, no. 5, pp. 499–503, 2017.

[34] M. Kim, "Euglycemic diabetic ketoacidosis with SGLT2 inhibitors in lean type 2 diabetes," *Integrative Obesity and Diabetes*, vol. 2, no. 4, 2016.

[35] A. L. Peters, E. O. Buschur, J. B. Buse, P. Cohan, J. C. Diner, and I. B. Hirsch, "Euglycemic diabetic ketoacidosis: a potential complication of treatment with sodium-glucose cotransporter 2 inhibition," *Diabetes Care*, vol. 38, no. 9, pp. 1687–1693, 2015.

[36] J. S. Kum-Nji, A. R. Gosmanov, H. Steinberg, and S. Dagogo-Jack, "Hyperglycemic, high anion-gap metabolic acidosis in patients receiving SGLT-2 inhibitors for diabetes management," *Journal of Diabetes and its Complications*, vol. 31, no. 3, pp. 611–614, 2017.

[37] Alehegn Gelaye, Abdallah Haidar, Christina Kassab, Syed Kazmi, and Prabhat Sinha, "Severe Ketoacidosis Associated with Canagliflozin (Invokana): A Safety Concern," *Case Reports in Critical Care*, vol. 2016, Article ID 1656182, 3 pages, 2016.

[38] N. Candelario and J. Wykretowicz, "The DKA that wasn't: A case of euglycemic diabetic ketoacidosis due to empagliflozin," *Oxford Medical Case Reports*, vol. 2016, no. 7, pp. 144–146, 2016.

[39] P. D. Farjo, K. M. Kidd, and J. L. Reece, "A case of euglycemic diabetic ketoacidosis following long-term empagliflozin therapy," *Diabetes Care*, vol. 39, no. 10, pp. e165–e166, 2016.

[40] W. Ogawa and K. Sakaguchi, "Euglycemic diabetic ketoacidosis induced by SGLT2 inhibitors: Possible mechanism and contributing factors," *Journal of Diabetes Investigation*, vol. 7, no. 2, pp. 135–138, 2016.

[41] J. Prater and J. Chaiban, "Euglycemic diabetic ketoacidosis with acute pancreatitis in a patient not known to have diabetes," *Endocrine Practice*, vol. 1, no. 2, pp. e88–e91, 2015.

[42] N. Luethi, L. Cioccari, M. Crisman, R. Bellomo, G. M. Eastwood, and J. Mårtensson, "Prevalence of ketosis, ketonuria, and ketoacidosis during liberal glycemic control in critically ill patients with diabetes: an observational study," *Critical Care*, vol. 20, no. 1, 2016.

[43] M. W. Savage, K. K. Dhatariya, A. Kilvert et al., "Joint British Diabetes Societies guideline for the management of diabetic ketoacidosis," *Diabetic Medicine*, vol. 28, no. 5, pp. 508–515, 2011.

[44] S. Darbhamulla, N. Shah, and P. Bosio, "Euglycaemic ketoacidosis in a patient with gestational diabetes," *European Journal of Obstetrics & Gynecology and Reproductive Biology*, vol. 163, no. 1, pp. 118–119, 2012.

[45] B. L. Cardonell, B. A. Marks, and M. H. Entrup, "Normoglycemic Diabetic Ketoacidosis in a Pregnant Patient with Type II Diabetes Mellitus Presenting for Emergent Cesarean Delivery," *A & A case reports*, vol. 6, no. 8, pp. 228–229, 2016.

[46] M. Chico, S. N. Levine, and D. F. Lewis, "Normoglycemic diabetic ketoacidosis in pregnancy," *Journal of Perinatology*, vol. 28, no. 4, pp. 310–312, 2008.

25

Fatal Cerebral Air Embolism: A Case Series

Rashmi Mishra,[1] Pavithra Reddy,[2] and Misbahuddin Khaja[1]

[1]Division of Pulmonary and Critical Care Medicine, Bronx Lebanon Hospital Center Affiliated to Icahn School of
  Medicine at Mount Sinai, 1650 Grand Concourse, Bronx, NY 10457, USA
[2]Department of Medicine, Bronx Lebanon Hospital Center Affiliated to Icahn School of Medicine at Mount Sinai,
  1650 Grand Concourse, Bronx, NY 10457, USA

Correspondence should be addressed to Rashmi Mishra; rashmi_mishra1987@yahoo.com

Academic Editor: Kenneth S. Waxman

Cerebral air embolism (CAE) is an infrequently reported complication of routine medical procedures. We present two cases of CAE. The first patient was a 55-year-old male presenting with vomiting and loss of consciousness one day after his hemodialysis session. Physical exam was significant for hypotension and hypoxia with no focal neurologic deficits. Computed tomography (CT) scan of head showed gas in cerebral venous circulation. The patient did not undergo any procedures prior to presentation, and his last hemodialysis session was uneventful. Retrograde rise of venous air to the cerebral circulation was the likely mechanism for venous CAE. The second patient was a 46-year-old female presenting with fever, shortness of breath, and hematemesis. She was febrile, tachypneic, and tachycardic and required intubation and mechanical ventilation. An orogastric tube inserted drained 2500 mL of bright red blood. Flexible laryngoscopy and esophagogastroduodenoscopy were performed. She also underwent central venous catheter placement. CT scan of head performed the next day due to absent brain stem reflexes revealed intravascular air within cerebral arteries. A transthoracic echocardiogram with bubble study ruled out patent foramen ovale. The patient had a paradoxical CAE in the absence of a patent foramen ovale.

1. Introduction

The introduction of air into cerebral arterial or venous circulation called cerebral air embolism (CAE) can lead to severe neurologic deficits and possible death. It may be iatrogenic secondary to central venous catheter (CVC) placement or removal, endoscopy, hysteroscopy, laparoscopy, and defibrillator placement [1–4]. Cases of CAE have been reported after hemodialysis despite the safeguards associated with modern hemodialysis machines [5]. We report two cases of CAE. The first was a case of CAE one day after an uneventful hemodialysis session, and the second was a case of CAE occurring after the patient underwent esophagogastroduodenoscopy (EGD), laryngoscopy, and CVC placement.

2. Case Presentation

Case 1. The patient was a 55-year-old male who presented to the hospital with multiple episodes of vomiting, loss of consciousness, and repeated falls over the last day. He denied any chest pain, palpitations, or injury to his head. His medical history was significant for hypertension, diabetes mellitus, and end-stage renal disease. He received hemodialysis through his left forearm arteriovenous fistula one day prior to presentation. On presentation, the patient was hypotensive, with blood pressure of 90/50 mm Hg, was hypoxic, with an oxygen saturation of 88% of room air, had a heart rate of 79 beats per minute, and was afebrile. On physical exam, he was alert and oriented, with negative respiratory and cardiovascular exams. Neurological exam did not show any focal neurologic deficits. Laboratory data were significant for thrombocytopenia with a platelet count of $122 \times 10^3/\mu L$ and a hemoglobin level of 17.3 g/dL. He underwent a CT scan of his head, which showed foci of gas in the cavernous sinus, anterior sagittal sinus, left side of the face, and left temporalis muscle (Figure 1). He had not undergone any other procedures before presentation, and, by

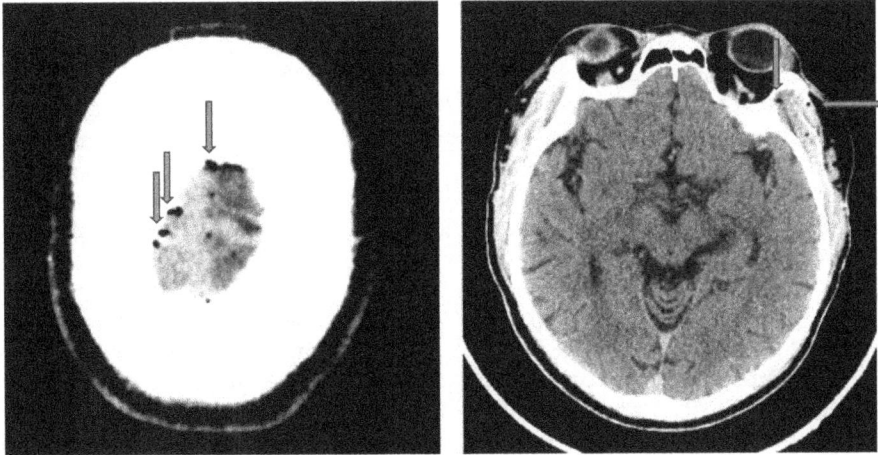

FIGURE 1: Case 1 CT scan of head: axial cuts showing foci of gas in cerebral vein and left temporal muscle (blue arrows).

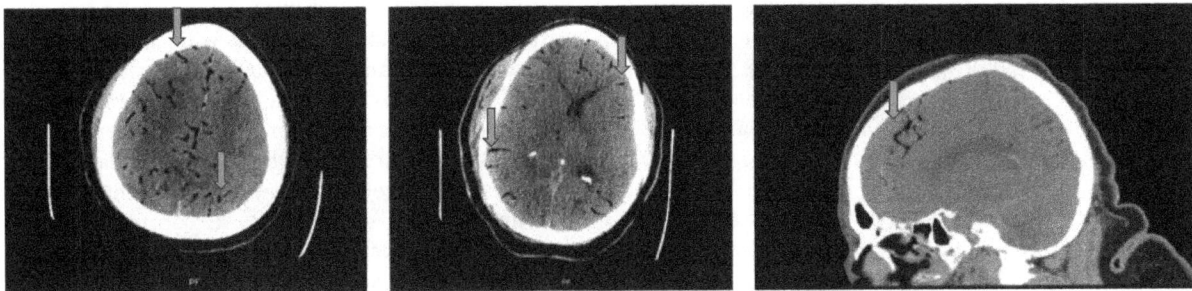

FIGURE 2: Case 2 CT scan of head: axial and sagittal cuts showing foci of gas in bilateral cerebral arteries (blue arrows).

history, his hemodialysis had been uneventful. The patient's condition deteriorated rapidly; he became comatose and had a cardiac arrest. He was successfully resuscitated within five minutes. After resuscitation, the patient developed shock requiring vasopressor support. He was started on intravenous piperacillin-tazobactam and vancomycin for possible sepsis. In the presence of high pulmonary pressures and without any evidence of paradoxical air embolism, a bubble study to look for a patent foramen ovale was not performed. Adequate oxygenation was maintained throughout his hospital stay. He was not a candidate for transfer to another center for possible hyperbaric oxygen therapy due to his tenuous hemodynamic status. The patient's further course was complicated by hematemesis due to a Mallory-Weiss tear diagnosed by endoscopy. Sepsis work-up was negative. As his prognosis was poor, he was transferred to hospice care where he expired.

Case 2. The patient was a 46-year-old female who presented to the emergency room with a one-day history of fever, shortness of breath, hematemesis, and abdominal pain. Her past medical history included hypertension, chronic systolic congestive heart failure, atrial fibrillation with implantable cardioverter-defibrillator (ICD) placement and accessory pathway ablation two weeks prior to presentation, and coronary artery disease. Vital signs included fever, with a temperature of 39.3°C, tachypnea, and tachycardia. Worsening tachypnea and tachycardia necessitated endotracheal

intubation for acute respiratory failure. An orogastric tube was placed and drained 2500 mL of bright red blood. Flexible laryngoscopy and EGD did not reveal an upper airway or upper gastrointestinal (GI) source of bleeding. The patient eventually required placement of a CVC for administration of fluids, blood products, and vasopressors. She was admitted to the medical intensive care unit with a working diagnosis of hemorrhagic shock secondary to an upper GI bleed and sepsis secondary to healthcare-associated pneumonia. She was started on esomeprazole and octreotide drips and empiric antibiotics. On the second day after admission, neurologic examination without sedation revealed absent brain stem reflexes. CT scan of the head performed revealed extensive intravascular air within numerous cerebral arteries bilaterally, diffuse cerebral edema, and tonsillar herniation (Figure 2). A transthoracic echocardiogram with bubble study ruled out a patent foramen ovale. Bedside apnea testing confirmed brain death. Autopsy revealed severe dilated cardiomyopathy with no obvious cause of CAE.

3. Discussion

Cerebral air embolism can be a potentially lethal complication. It can occur iatrogenically, secondary to CVC placement or removal, endoscopy, hysteroscopy, laparoscopy, or defibrillator placement, among other reported causes [1–4]. It has been reported in relation to hemodialysis by Hysell [5].

In the past, CAE with a demonstrable air column in the hemodialysis circuit has been reported [6]. Use of a hemodialysis catheter outside of hemodialysis and declotting of hemodialysis access have also been reported as causes of CAE [7, 8]. With the advent of modern hemodialysis, there are safety measures in hemodialysis machines to protect against CAE, but it may still occur. Microbubbles have been noted in hemodialysis circuits. They may originate in arterial luer lock connector at negative pressure or from remnant bubbles due to insufficient priming, but in some cases, the source remains unknown. These may not be picked up as air by the dialysis circuit. Blood flow rate and negative arterial pressure correlate with the microbubble rate as per a recent observational study [9]. The microbubbles get lodged in the capillaries and cause tissue ischemia, inflammatory response, and complement activation. Furthermore, obstruction of microcirculation and tissue damage occur due to platelet aggregation and clot formation [10].

Iatrogenic CAE related to CVC has been widely reported. In a systematic review of iatrogenic CAE related to CVC, the most common locations for emboli, in decreasing order of frequency, are in the subarachnoid space, cerebral parenchyma, and venous sinus. The most common neurologic symptoms reported were focal neurologic deficits, coma, seizures, encephalopathy, and headache. The time to symptom onset has been reported to be very acute, with the median time to onset reported by the review being one minute [11]. Iatrogenic CAE has been reported with CVC placement, manipulation, and removal [12–15]. The risk of air embolism is higher in conditions with decreased central venous pressure like hypovolemia, deep inspiration, or patient in upright position [15].

CAE secondary to endoscopy and other GI procedures, such as endoscopic retrograde cholangiopancreatography, have also been previously reported. It is thought that air insufflation required for EGD creates pressure gradient favoring passage of air into the vasculature [16, 17].

The mechanism for entrance of air into the cerebral venous circulation is thought to be through retrograde rise. Air, once it enters the venous circulation, can rise in an upright patient to the cerebral venous circulation at a speed greater than the venous blood flow due to its low specific gravity [18]. The rise of air depends further on factors like bubble size, central vein diameter, and cardiac output [19]. Loss of consciousness, seizures, and possible death can occur as a result of the CAE [20]. Retrograde cerebral venous air embolism to the sagittal sinus and cortical veins has been reported in association with CVC disconnection and the use of a CVC in a mobile patient [12, 13]. If the patient is recumbent, air can enter the heart and pass into the ventricle and lungs, causing dyspnea, cough, chest tightness, and arrhythmias [20].

Arterial CAE, on the other hand, may occur if air passes from the venous into the arterial circulation. This may occur due to the presence of a right-to-left shunt, such as a patent foramen ovale. In the absence of an obvious right-to-left shunt, pulmonary arteriovenous malformations may cause paradoxical CAE. Inability of the pulmonary vasculature to filter out emboli due to the presence of a large volume venous embolism or the use of anesthetic agents may also cause paradoxical CAE [4, 14]. Animal studies show that lung, which can act as a physiologic filter, can become overwhelmed above 0.3 mL/kg/min, but exact filtering capacity of human lung is unknown [21]. Pathologic dilation of pulmonary vessels or pulmonary AV malformations may occur in chronic liver disease or in patients with hereditary hemorrhagic telangiectasia [22]. Our patient with arterial CAE did not have history suggestive of either. Intrapulmonary arteriovenous malformations closed at rest, but which can open during exercise or other hyperdynamic conditions, are present in more than 90% of humans. These intrapulmonary anastomoses can be affected by oxygen tension and by body positioning. Once these pathways open, these pathways can be closed by $FiO_2 = 1.0$ during submaximal-through-maximal exercise in most healthy humans [23].

The treatment of venous CAE consists of volume resuscitation to increase venous pressure in order to prevent continued entry of air into the venous circulation. Adequate oxygenation should be attained, with an increase in the fraction of inspired oxygen (FiO2) of inspired gas. Increasing the FiO2 also helps to decrease the size of the air embolus by increasing the gradient for nitrogen. Hyperbaric oxygen therapy is not the first line of therapy for venous CAE. If there is evidence of neurologic deficits, it may be considered [4].

The treatment of arterial CAE consists of supportive treatment. Endotracheal intubation, ventilation, and administration of oxygen to maintain and improve oxygenation and decrease the size of gas bubbles are recommended. Suppression of seizures with benzodiazepines or barbiturates should be performed. Hyperbaric oxygen therapy helps by raising ambient pressure around the gas bubble and increasing the gradient for nitrogen out of the bubble and for oxygen into the bubble. Hemoconcentration may occur with gas embolism, which can cause increased viscosity and compromise microcirculation. Normovolemia should be attained with infusion of colloids. Use of anticoagulation and corticosteroids is not recommended [4].

Our first patient presented the next day after undergoing hemodialysis with symptoms of syncope, recurrent falls, and vomiting. Initially, he was alert and able to provide history. In the venous CAE case reported by Brouns et al., the patient also had syncope one day prior to the development of coma [12]. Other cases have also reported delayed symptoms after retrograde venous CAE [24]. The arterial needle, prepump arterial tubing segment, and inadvertently opened end of a CVC are common sites of air entry [20]. In our patient, the mechanism of air entry into the venous circulation is unclear. Microbubbles during hemodialysis may be a possible explanation. Once air entered the venous circulation, retrograde cerebral venous air embolism seems to be the mechanism of the CAE.

Our second patient underwent multiple procedures including laryngoscopy, endoscopy, and placement of a CVC, any of which could have caused the CAE. Due to the absence of a patent foramen ovale, the mechanism for the paradoxical CAE was likely the inability of the pulmonary circulation to filter out the air embolus from the venous circulation.

4. Conclusion

Sudden cardiac and cerebral dysfunction in mechanically ventilated patients with risk factors should suggest CAE, especially in the setting of invasive endoscopic procedures and/or CVC placement, which are common in any intensive care unit. Also, CAE is uncommon in the era of modern hemodialysis, but this may still occur, as is evident from the first case. The first case is also interesting in that the patient showed delayed symptoms after his hemodialysis session. CAE should be considered in the differential diagnosis of hemodialysis patients presenting with neurologic symptoms at any time. These cases bring to light the need for awareness among physicians regarding the possibility of this complication following routine medical procedures.

Abbreviations

CAE: Cerebral air embolism
CVC: Central venous catheter
EGD: Esophagogastroduodenoscopy
CT: Computed tomography.

Competing Interests

None of the authors has a financial relationship with a commercial entity that has an interest in the subject of the manuscript.

References

[1] F. A. Groenman, L. W. Peters, B. M. P. Rademaker, and E. A. Bakkum, "Embolism of air and gas in hysteroscopic procedures: pathophysiology and implication for daily practice," *Journal of Minimally Invasive Gynecology*, vol. 15, no. 2, pp. 241–247, 2008.

[2] J. L. M. C. Azevedo, O. C. Azevedo, S. A. Miyahira et al., "Injuries caused by Veress needle insertion for creation of pneumoperitoneum: a systematic literature review," *Surgical Endoscopy*, vol. 23, no. 7, pp. 1428–1432, 2009.

[3] M. G. Bongiorni, A. De Cori, E. Soldati et al., "Iatrogenic risk of permanent pacemaker and defibrillator implantation," *Giornale Italiano di Cardiologia*, vol. 10, pp. 395–406, 2009.

[4] C. M. Muth and E. S. Shank, "Gas embolism," *The New England Journal of Medicine*, vol. 342, no. 7, pp. 476–482, 2000.

[5] M. K. Hysell, "Cerebral air embolism after hemodialysis," *Journal of Emergency Medicine*, vol. 49, no. 1, pp. e27–e28, 2015.

[6] M. K. Ward, M. Shadforth, A. V. L. Hill et al., "Air embolism during haemodialysis," *The British Medical Journal*, vol. 3, no. 5766, pp. 74–78, 1971.

[7] A. S. L. Yu and E. Levy, "Paradoxical cerebral air embolism from a hemodialysis catheter," *American Journal of Kidney Diseases*, vol. 29, no. 3, pp. 453–455, 1997.

[8] J. P. Santos, Z. Hamadeh, and N. Ansari, "Cerebrovascular accident secondary to paradoxical embolism following arteriovenous graft thrombectomy," *Case Reports in Nephrology*, vol. 2012, Article ID 183730, 3 pages, 2012.

[9] S. Wagner, C. Rode, R. Wojke, and B. Canaud, "Observation of microbubbles during standard dialysis treatments," *Clinical Kidney Journal*, vol. 8, no. 4, pp. 400–404, 2015.

[10] M. Barak and Y. Katz, "Microbubbles: pathophysiology and clinical implications," *Chest*, vol. 128, no. 4, pp. 2918–2932, 2005.

[11] J. Pinho, J. M. Amorim, J. M. Araújo et al., "Cerebral gas embolism associated with central venous catheter: systematic review," *Journal of the Neurological Sciences*, vol. 362, pp. 160–164, 2016.

[12] R. Brouns, D. D. Surgeloose, I. Neetens, and P. P. De Deyn, "Fatal venous cerebral air embolism secondary to a disconnected central venous catheter," *Cerebrovascular Diseases*, vol. 21, no. 3, pp. 212–214, 2006.

[13] F. Ploner, L. Saltuari, M. J. Marosi, R. Dolif, and A. Salsa, "Cerebral air emboli with use of central venous catheter in mobile patient," *The Lancet*, vol. 338, no. 8778, p. 1331, 1991.

[14] H. Eum da, S. H. Lee, H. W. Kim et al., "Cerebral air embolism following the removal of a central venous catheter in the absence of intracardiac right-to-left shunting: a case report," *Medicine*, vol. 94, no. 13, article e630, 2015.

[15] W. H. Boer and R. J. Hene, "Lethal air embolism following removal of a double lumen jugular vein catheter," *Nephrology Dialysis Transplantation*, vol. 14, no. 8, pp. 1850–1852, 1999.

[16] S. Park, J. Y. Ahn, Y. E. Ahn et al., "Two cases of cerebral air embolism that occurred during esophageal ballooning and endoscopic retrograde cholangiopancreatography," *Clinical Endoscopy*, vol. 49, no. 2, pp. 191–196, 2016.

[17] A. V. Pandurangadu, J. A. P. Paul, M. Barawi, and C. B. Irvin, "A case report of cerebral air embolism after esophagogastroduodenoscopy: diagnosis and management in the emergency department," *Journal of Emergency Medicine*, vol. 43, no. 6, pp. 976–979, 2012.

[18] C. J. Schlimp, T. Loimer, M. Rieger, M. B. Schmidts, and W. Lederer, "Pathophysiological mechanism and immediate treatment of retrograde cerebral venous air embolism," *Intensive Care Medicine*, vol. 32, no. 6, p. 945, 2006.

[19] C. J. Schlimp, T. Loimer, M. Rieger, W. Lederer, and M. B. Schmidts, "The potential of venous air embolism ascending retrograde to the brain," *Journal of Forensic Sciences*, vol. 50, no. 4, pp. 906–909, 2005.

[20] H. Bregman, J. T. Daugirdas, and T. S. Ing, "Complications during hemodialysis," in *Handbook of Dialysis*, J. T. Daugirdas and T. S. Ing, Eds., pp. 148–168, Little, Brown, New York, NY, USA, 1994.

[21] B. D. Butler and B. A. Hills, "Transpulmonary passage of venous air emboli," *Journal of Applied Physiology*, vol. 59, no. 2, pp. 543–547, 1985.

[22] W. E. Hopkins, A. D. Waggoner, and B. Barzilai, "Frequency and significance of intrapulmonary right-to-left shunting in end-stage hepatic disease," *The American Journal of Cardiology*, vol. 70, no. 4, pp. 516–519, 1992.

[23] A. T. Lovering, J. E. Elliott, K. M. Beasley, and S. S. Laurie, "Pulmonary pathways and mechanisms regulating transpulmonary shunting into the general circulation: an update," *Injury*, vol. 41, no. 2, pp. S16–S23, 2010.

[24] M. Yesilaras, O. D. Atilla, E. Aksay, and T. Y. Kilic, "Retrograde cerebral air embolism," *The American Journal of Emergency Medicine*, vol. 32, no. 12, pp. 1562.e1–1562.e2, 2014.

26

A 32-Year-Old Female with AIDS, *Pneumocystis jiroveci* Pneumonia, and Methemoglobinemia

Guillermo J. Giangreco,[1] **Dean Campbell,**[2] **and Mark J. Cowan**[2]

[1] *Baltimore-Washington Medical Center, Glen Burnie, MD 21061, USA*

[2] *University of Maryland School of Medicine, Baltimore, MD 21201, USA*

Correspondence should be addressed to Mark J. Cowan; mark.cowan@verizon.net

Academic Editors: C. Diez, M. Egi, and C. Mammina

We report a case of methemoglobinemia with significant hemoglobin desaturation in a young female with AIDS who was being treated for *Pneumocystis jiroveci* pneumonia. A review of the etiology, pathophysiology, and treatment of methemoglobinemia is presented.

1. Background

Methemoglobinemia is the presence of a significant amount of oxidized iron (Fe^{3+}, met-Hgb) within hemoglobin (Hgb) in the blood, rendering it unable to bind oxygen. It is caused by a number of medications and toxins and can quickly degrade oxygen transport sufficiently enough to cause or aggravate severe tissue hypoxemia. Its hallmark features are hemoglobin desaturation out of proportion to blood partial pressure of oxygen and "chocolate brown" blood. Definitive diagnosis can be made quickly and easily with co-oximetry, but must be suspected, as co-oximetry is not routinely performed in patients. It is important to recognize, as correction of the pathologic hemoglobin redox state with methylene blue is simple, rapid, effective, and lifesaving. We present a case of methemoglobinemia secondary to primaquine, which was successfully treated with methylene blue and discontinuation of the drug.

2. Case Presentation

A 32-year-old female with a history of intravenous drug abuse and AIDS (last CD_4 count = 26/mm^3) was admitted to a local hospital for cough, fever, and respiratory distress. Initial blood cultures grew gram-positive cocci in clusters, and endocarditis was suspected. Vancomycin was started, but a transthoracic echocardiogram was nondiagnostic, and the patient was transferred to our institution for further evaluation.

The patient was unmarried and had been HIV positive for three years. She had no history of opportunistic infections and had been in good health for the past year taking no medications. She smoked one pack of cigarettes/day, used heroin intravenously 3–5 times/week, and denied alcohol use. She reported an intolerance to sulfa drugs.

On arrival, we found a slender female in moderate to severe respiratory distress. Temperature was 99.2°F, respiratory rate of 35/min, blood pressure 110/62 mmHg, and heart rate 140/minute. Oxygen saturation measured by pulse oximetry was 88% on a 100% nonrebreather mask. She could speak only in short sentences. Cardiac examination revealed tachycardia without murmur. Lung examination revealed coarse crackles throughout. Abdomen was benign and the extremities were without cyanosis or edema. Skin showed evidence of chronic intravenous needlesticks without cellulitis. The remainder of the physical examination was unremarkable.

Arterial blood gases obtained on presentation showed a pH of 7.51, pCO_2 of 33 mmHg, and a pO_2 of 59 mmHg with a saturation of 89% on room air. White blood cell count was 4,300 cells/μL, hemoglobin was 10.4 g/dL, and the hematocrit was 35%. Electrolytes were within normal limits; serum LDH

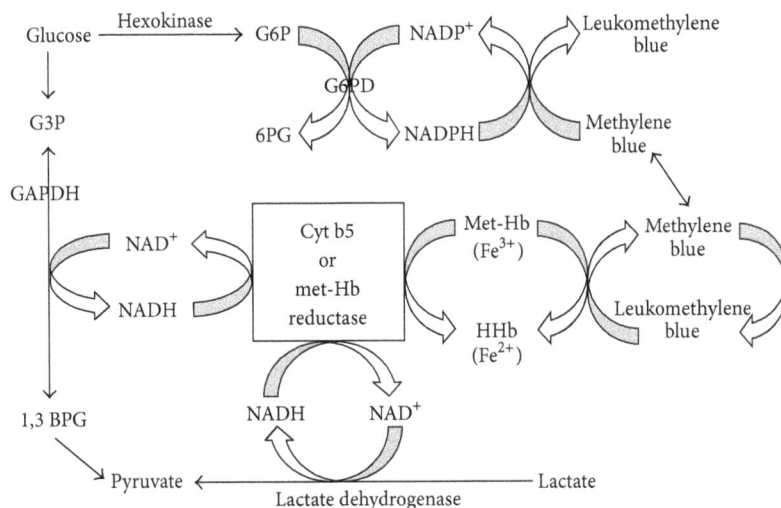

FIGURE 1: Biochemical pathways of hemoglobin reduction. NAD Nicotine adenine dinucleotide, GAPDH: glyceraldehyde-3-phosphate dehydrogenase, G3P: glyceraldehyde-3-phosphate, 1,3 BPG: 1,3 bisphosphoglycerate, cyt: cytochrome, and metHB: methemoglobin. Adapted from [6].

was 654 IU/L. Chest X-ray showed diffuse bilateral airspace disease with an upper lobe predominance. G6PD level was normal.

She was started on empiric gatifloxacin, primaquin, clindamycin, and prednisone for community-acquired pneumonia, with coverage for *Pneumocystis jiroveci*. The patient respiratory status worsened despite noninvasive ventilation, and she required intubation and mechanical ventilation on hospital day 5. A diagnostic bronchoscopy with bronchoalveolar lavage was performed, demonstrating *Pneumocystis jiroveci* cysts. Gatifloxacin was discontinued, and the patient experienced improvement of her hypoxemia over the next day (FIO_2 of 60% and PEEP of +8). On day 7, she developed moderate digital and perioral cyanosis and an increasing lactic acid level (7.3 mmol/L). ABG showed pH 7.42, pCO_2 33, with a saturation of only 86% despite a pO_2 of 165. Co-oximetry revealed a carboxyhemoglobin level of 1.6% and a methemoglobin level of 20.1%. She received methylene blue 100 mg IV and was switched from primaquin to intravenous pentamidine. Methemoglobin did not recur. She ultimately died from complications of multiorgan system failure (MOSF) on hospital day 12.

3. Discussion

Met-Hgb is Fe^{3+} in the heme moiety of Hgb. Normally, met-Hgb is produced at low levels by oxidative stress in the blood at a rate of 3% per day [1]. Fe^{+3} is rapidly and efficiently reduced to normal (Fe^{+2}) via the cytochrome b5 reductase pathway (see Figure 1 for the heme redox cycle), normally keeping met-Hgb levels <1% [2]. Backup reduction is provided by nicotinamide adenine dinucleotide phosphate (NADPH)-met-Hgb reductase, which in turn requires the glucose-6-phosphatase (G6P)/glutathione reductase system to maintain NADPH levels. This pathway typically accounts

for only 5% of met-Hgb reduction, as it is primarily used in reducing oxidant xenobiotics rather than met-Hgb [3]. Met-Hgb will not normally increase to clinically significant levels unless production is increased (acquired disease), or reduction is decreased (hereditary disease) [4, 5].

The inherited types of methemoglobinemia are associated with enzymatic deficiencies in pathways that reduce met-Hgb to Hgb, or with an abnormal Hgb (M type) that resists reduction. Due to the chronic nature of the inherited type, compensatory mechanisms such as increased red blood cell mass and cardiac output have time to develop, and thus patients are characteristically cyanotic but asymptomatic [1, 5]. Table 1 lists the causes of inherited met-Hgb.

Acquired met-Hgb results from exposure to drugs, pollutants, and toxins, which are also listed in Table 1. The common causative agents in hospitalized patients include local anesthetics, sulfa antibiotics, dapsone, primaquin, nitrates, and metoclopramide. These generally induce methemoglobinemia by increasing the oxidation rate of Hgb by 100-fold or greater, overwhelming the blood's reductase systems and driving NADPH to very low levels [1, 3, 5]. Dapsone is an antimicrobial and anti-inflammatory agent that has also been shown to cause methemoglobinemia. Met-Hgb levels as high as 55% have been reported in patients after dapsone overdose [15, 16]. Primaquin is more likely to cause met-Hgb when the daily dose exceeds 60 mg [17].

Mild cyanosis is characteristic of methemoglobinemia. Only about 1.5 g/dL (10–15%) of met-Hgb is needed to produce detectable cyanosis, and up to 70% met-Hgb can be relatively well tolerated if the amount of Hgb is adequate, and there has been enough time to develop compensatory mechanisms. Met-Hgb levels of 25–50% can cause headache, confusion, and chest pain [18]. More problematic is acquired met-Hgb in a critically ill patient. Cyanosis can easily be missed or overlooked in ICU patients for a variety of reasons: poor illumination of the room, dark skin, and incorrect

TABLE 1: Causes of methemoglobinemia.

Congenital
Abnormal hemoglobin
    Hemoglobin M_{Boston}
    Hemoglobin $M_{Hyde\ Park}$
    Hemoglobin M_{Iwate}
    Hemoglobin $M_{Milwaukee}$
    Hemoglobin $M_{Ratnagiri}$
    Hemoglobin M_s
    Hemoglobin $M_{Saskatoon}$
Enzyme deficiency
    Cytochrome b5/NADH reductase deficiencies (Types I–IV)
    G6PD deficiency
    NADPH-flavin reductase deficiency
Acquired
Anti-infectives
    Chloroquine
    Dapsone
    Nitrofurans
    Primaquine
    Rifampin
    Sulfanilamide (topical)
    Sulfonamides
    Sulfoxone
Chemicals
    Acetanilide
    Alloxan
    Aniline derivatives
    Aromatic amines
    Arsine
    Bivalent copper
    Chlorates
    Chromates
    Dimethyl sulfoxide
    Dimethyltoluidine
    Ferricyanide
    Hydroxylamine
    Naphthalene
    Phenacetin
    Toluidine
    Phenols
Drugs
    Acetaminophen (metabolites)
    Clofazimine
    Flutamide
    Methylene blue (high dose)
    Isosulfan blue
    Metoclopramide
    Nitric oxide
    Nitrous oxide
    Paraquat
    Phenazopyridine
    Phenytoin

TABLE 1: Continued.

    Rasburicase
    Resorcinol
    Sodium valproate
    Sulfasalazine
Environmental/occupational
    Automobile exhaust fumes
    Inks
    Nitrites
    Paints
    Propellants
    Room deodorizer
    Varnishes
Foods
    Menthol
    Fava beans
    Vegetables (spinach, beets, and carrots)
    Well water
Local anesthetics
    Benzocaine
    Bupivacaine
    Lidocaine
    Prilocaine
    Tetracaine (lozenges)
Nitrates
    Alkyl nitrate
    Amyl nitrate
    Bismuth subnitrate
    Butyl nitrate
    Dinitrophenol
    Isobutyl nitrate
    Nitrobenzene
    Nitroglycerin
    Nitrophenol
    Nitroprusside
    Silver nitrate
    Trinitrotoluene

Adapted from [7–14].

attribution of the cyanosis to another cause [19]. In addition to decreasing the amount of normal Hgb available to deliver oxygen to the tissues, the presence of met-Hbg increases the O_2-Hgb affinity within the affected multimer, left shifting the Hgb dissociation curve. This further decreases oxygen delivery by decreasing oxygen offloading in peripheral tissues [19, 20]. Many critically ill patients are already either hypoxemic or have insufficient oxygen delivery and are frequently exposed to drugs capable of inducing met-Hgb. An otherwise well tolerated level of met-Hgb can manifest symptoms and signs which reflect body-wide inadequate oxygen delivery including myocardial ischemia/infarction, hemodynamic instability, lactic acidosis, ischemic bowel, and stroke. We suspect that drug-acquired met is underappreciated in the ICU setting and may contribute to adverse clinical outcomes.

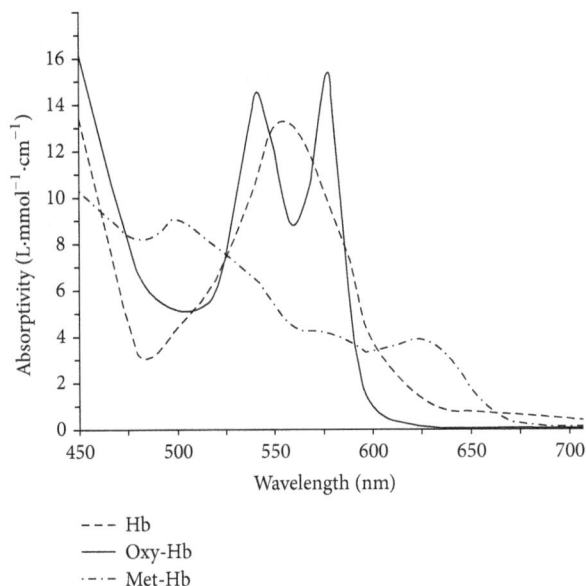

FIGURE 2: Absorbance as a function of wavelength for oxyhemoglobin, reduced hemoglobin, and methemoglobin. Transmission pulse oximetry utilizes absorbance at two wavelengths (here red 660 nm and infrared 910 nm) to determine the oxygen saturation of an arterial pulsation of blood into the skin. Adapted from [25].

Pulse oximetry, especially in combination with arterial blood gas analysis, is useful in the diagnosis of methemoglobinemia. The absorption spectrum of met-Hgb overlaps with that of oxyhemoglobin at 660 and 910 nm, the wavelengths used in most pulse oximeters (Figure 2), and so direct measurement of met-Hgb with pulse oximetry is impossible [21]. However, there are features that should raise the concern for the presence of met-Hgb. In the presence of met-Hgb, the measured O_2 saturation will be decreased from that predicted by the PaO_2 and a normal oxygen-Hgb dissociation curve. A rule of thumb is that the saturation, as measured by pulse-oximetry, will drop by one half of the met-Hgb concentration between 3 and 20%. Thus, a patient with 98% saturated arterial hemoglobin who develops a met-Hgb level of 10% can be expected to have pulse oximetry of 93% [22]. With higher levels of met-Hgb (>30%), the pulse oximetry tends to plateau around 85%, irrespective of true oxygen content or met-Hgb levels, and the arterial blood is characteristically chocolate brown in color [22, 23]. Definitive measurement of met-Hgb requires co-oximetry, a test which is not performed routinely in most ICUs, and must be ordered specifically. Co-oximetry uses multiple wavelengths of light to correctly distinguish met-Hgb from oxyhemoglobin, deoxyhemoglobin, and carboxyhemoglobin [22, 24].

Initial treatment consists of discontinuation of the offending drug. Methylene blue, a dye that acts to transport an electron from NADPH to hemoglobin, may be administered at a rate of 1-2 mg/kg for 5 minutes to hasten met-Hgb reduction, although in theory other antioxidants such as vitamin C (risk of renal stones and hyperoxaluria), tocopherol, or N-acetyl cysteine may also be beneficial, and have been utilized in

occupational and congenital diseases [18, 19]. Of note, due to a severe hemolytic reaction, methylene blue therapy is contraindicated in G6PD deficient patients. Methylene blue is recommended in symptomatic patients with met-Hgb levels >20%, and in asymptomatic patients with levels >30% [18, 23].

3.1. Follow Up. Methylene blue 1.5 mg/kg was administered intravenously, causing the patient's pulse oximetry to increase to 93% after 1-2 minutes and with immediate resolution of her cyanosis. Repeat co-oximetry demonstrated complete resolution of the met-Hgb. She was switched from primaquin-clindamycin to IV pentamidine to complete her therapy for PCP. While her met-Hgb never recurred, she did not survive her hospitalization. Supportive care was withdrawn after the development of severe MOSF. We suspect that methemoglobinemia may have played a role in her progression to MOSF, by converting a borderline hypoxemia into a profound deficiency in tissue oxygen delivery during her critical illness.

4. Conclusion

Many drugs routinely used in the ICU can cause methemoglobinemia, adding to deficient oxygen delivery in this vulnerable patient population. A high index of suspicion should be kept for methemoglobinemia in ICU patients. Clues to the presence of met-Hgb are cyanosis, chocolate brown blood, and dissociation between expected (from paO_2) and measured Hgb saturation, especially when pulse oximetry reads about 85%. Definitive diagnosis is made by sending an arterial blood sample for co-oximetry. Treatment is removal of the offending drug, with methylene blue administration if tissue hypoxia is critical.

References

[1] E. R. Jaffé, "Methemoglobin pathophysiology," *Progress in Clinical and Biological Research*, vol. 51, pp. 133–151, 1981.

[2] A. Mansouri and A. A. Lurie, "Concise review: methemoglobinemia," *The American Journal of Hematology*, vol. 42, no. 1, pp. 7–12, 1993.

[3] R. O. Wright, W. J. Lewander, and A. D. Woolf, "Methemoglobinemia: etiology, pharmacology, and clinical management," *Annals of Emergency Medicine*, vol. 34, no. 5, pp. 646–656, 1999.

[4] A. Mansouri, "Methemoglobin reduction under near physiological conditions," *Biochemical Medicine and Metabolic Biology*, vol. 42, no. 1, pp. 43–51, 1989.

[5] J. Ashurst and M. Wasson, "Methemoglobinemia: a systematic review of the pathophysiology, detection, and treatment," *Delaware Medical Journal*, vol. 83, no. 7, pp. 203–208, 2011.

[6] M. Whirl-Carrillo, E. M. McDonagh, J. M. Hebert et al., "Pharmacogenomics knowledge for personalized medicine," *Clinical Pharmacology & Therapeutics*, vol. 92, no. 4, pp. 414–417, 2012.

[7] E. C. Kennett, E. Ogawa, N. S. Agar, I. R. Godwin, W. A. Bubb, and P. W. Kuchel, "Investigation of methaemoglobin reduction by extracellular NADH in mammalian erythrocytes,"

International Journal of Biochemistry and Cell Biology, vol. 37, no. 7, pp. 1438–1445, 2005.

[8] T. L. Leunback, J. F. Pedersen, T. Trydal, P. Thorgaard, J. Helgestad, and S. Rosthøi, "Acute favism: methemoglobinemia may cause cyanosis and low pulse oximetry readings," *Pediatric Hematology-Oncology*. In press.

[9] M. Taleb, Z. Ashraf, S. Valavoor, and J. Tinkel, "Evaluation and management of acquired methemoglobinemia associated with topical benzocaine use," *American Journal of Cardiovascular Drugs*. In press.

[10] A. M. Mary and L. Bhupalam, "Metoclopramide-induced methemoglobinemia in an adult," *Journal of the Kentucky Medical Association*, vol. 98, no. 6, pp. 245–247, 2000.

[11] S. Chowdhary, B. Bukoye, A. M. Bhansali et al., "Risk of topical anesthetic-induced methemoglobinemia: a 10-year retrospective case-control study," *JAMA Internal Medicine*, vol. 173, no. 9, pp. 771–776, 2013.

[12] M. B. Sonbol, H. Yadav, R. Vaidya, V. Rana, and T. E. Witzig, "Methemoglobinemia and hemolysis in a patient with G6PD deficiency treated with rasburicase," *American Journal of Hematology*, vol. 88, no. 2, pp. 152–154, 2013.

[13] N. Ahmed, B. P. Hoy, and J. McInerney, "Methaemoglobinaemia due to mephedrone ('snow')," *BMJ Case Reports*, 2010.

[14] J. S. W. Chui, W. T. Poon, K. C. Chan, A. Y. W. Chan, and T. A. Buckley, "Nitrite-induced methaemoglobinaemia-aetiology, diagnosis and treatment," *Anaesthesia*, vol. 60, no. 5, pp. 496–500, 2005.

[15] J. A. Barclay, S. E. Ziemba, and R. B. Ibrahim, "Dapsone-induced methemoglobinemia: a primer for clinicians," *Annals of Pharmacotherapy*, vol. 45, no. 9, pp. 1103–1115, 2011.

[16] J. Canning and M. Levine, "Case files of the medical toxicology fellowship at banner good samaritan medical center in phoenix, AZ: methemoglobinemia following dapsone exposure," *Journal of Medical Toxicology*, vol. 7, no. 2, pp. 139–146, 2011.

[17] G. S. Kantor, "Primaquine-induced methemoglobinemia during treatment of *Pneumocystis carinii* pneumonia," *The New England Journal of Medicine*, vol. 327, no. 20, article 1461, 1992.

[18] S. M. Bradberry, "Occupational methaemoglobinaemia: mechanisms of production, features, diagnosis and management including the use of methylene blue," *Toxicological Reviews*, vol. 22, no. 1, pp. 13–27, 2003.

[19] E. R. Jaffe, "Methemoglobinemia in the differential diagnosis of cyanosis," *Hospital Practice*, vol. 20, no. 12, pp. 91–110, 1985.

[20] M. J. Percy, N. V. McFerran, and T. R. J. Lappin, "Disorders of oxidised haemoglobin," *Blood Reviews*, vol. 19, no. 2, pp. 61–68, 2005.

[21] J. E. Sinex, "Pulse oximetry: principles and limitations," *The American Journal of Emergency Medicine*, vol. 17, no. 1, pp. 59–66, 1999.

[22] J. B. Eisenkraft, "Pulse oximeter desaturation due to methemoglobinemia," *Anesthesiology*, vol. 68, no. 2, pp. 279–282, 1988.

[23] A. Skold, D. L. Cosco, and R. Klein, "Methemoglobinemia: pathogenesis, diagnosis, and management," *Southern Medical Journal*, vol. 104, no. 11, pp. 757–761, 2011.

[24] G. V. Baranoski, T. F. Chen, B. W. Kimmel, E. Miranda, and D. Yim, "On the noninvasive optical monitoring and differentiation of methemoglobinemia and sulfhemoglobinemia," *Journal of Biomedical Optics*, vol. 17, no. 9, Article ID 97005, 2012.

[25] O. W. van Assendelft, *Spectrophotometry of Haemoglobin Derivatives*, Charles C. Thomas, Springfield, IL, USA, 1970.

27

Combined Negative- and Positive-Pressure Ventilation for the Treatment of ARDS

Konstantinos Raymondos,[1] Jörg Ahrens,[2] and Ulrich Molitoris[3]

[1]*Anaesthesiology and Intensive Care Medicine, Hannover Medical School, 30625 Hannover, Germany*

[2]*Anaesthesiology and Intensive Care Medicine, Klinikum Links der Weser, 28277 Bremen, Germany*

[3]*Cardiothoracic, Transplantation and Vascular Surgery, Hannover Medical School, 30625 Hannover, Germany*

Correspondence should be addressed to Konstantinos Raymondos; raymondos@ards.eu

Academic Editor: Nicolas Nin

Objective. Tracheal intubation and positive-pressure ventilation as the current standard of care for the adult respiratory distress syndrome (ARDS) seem to have reached their limit in terms of a further relevant reduction of the still very high mortality. *Case Presentation.* A 75-year-old male patient developed ARDS after abscess drainage with deteriorating oxygenation, despite positive end-expiratory pressure (PEEP) values above 15 cm H_2O. We applied external negative-pressure ventilation with a chamber respirator using -33 cm H_2O at inspiration and -15 cm H_2O at expiration, combined with conventional pressure support using a PEEP of about 8 cm H_2O and a pressure support of 4–12 cm H_2O. Alveolar infiltrates disappeared rapidly and PaO_2/FiO_2 values surpassed 300 mmHg after the first application and 500 mmHg after the second. Negative-pressure ventilation was used for 6–18 hours/day over five days. Now, 13 years later, the patient is still alive and has a good quality of life. *Conclusion.* Using this or similar concepts, not only in intubated patients but also as a noninvasive approach in patients with ARDS, offers new options that may genuinely differ from the present therapeutic approaches and may, therefore, have the potential to decrease the present high mortality from ARDS.

1. Introduction

Continuous positive-pressure ventilation (CPPV) still represents the standard method of treating the adult respiratory distress syndrome (ARDS), despite the fact that it aggravates both lung injury and multisystem organ failure [1], with mortality from ARDS still as high as 50% [2, 3]. However, there are alternatives for the symptomatic treatment of ARDS. Decades ago, modified Emerson tank respirators were successfully used to treat ARDS with continuous negative pressure [4–6]. These patients had pneumonia and were neither intubated nor ventilated but breathed spontaneously surrounded by negative pressure [4–6]. According to observations of lung injury, it is not only spontaneous breathing under negative pressure that differs substantially from CPPV: this is certainly also the case for ventilation with negative pressure. Continuous external negative-pressure ventilation (CENPV) improves oxygenation under more physiological

conditions with lower transpulmonary, airway, and intra-abdominal pressures than with CPPV [7, 8].

Apart from these physiological studies, there are no reports on clinical experience with CENPV in ARDS or the combined use of negative- and positive-pressure ventilation.

2. Clinical Case

A 75-year-old male patient suffered from a peritonsillar abscess, which extended down to the hypopharynx. After anesthesia induction, the patient was intubated without any problems, and tonsillectomy and abscess drainage were performed. Following extubation, the peripheral oxygen saturation in the anesthesia recovery room decreased to 85% despite oxygen administration. Coarse bubbling and moist rales were auscultated over both lungs. Administration of intravenous furosemide administrations had no effect, and the initial chest X-ray revealed patchy bilateral infiltrates

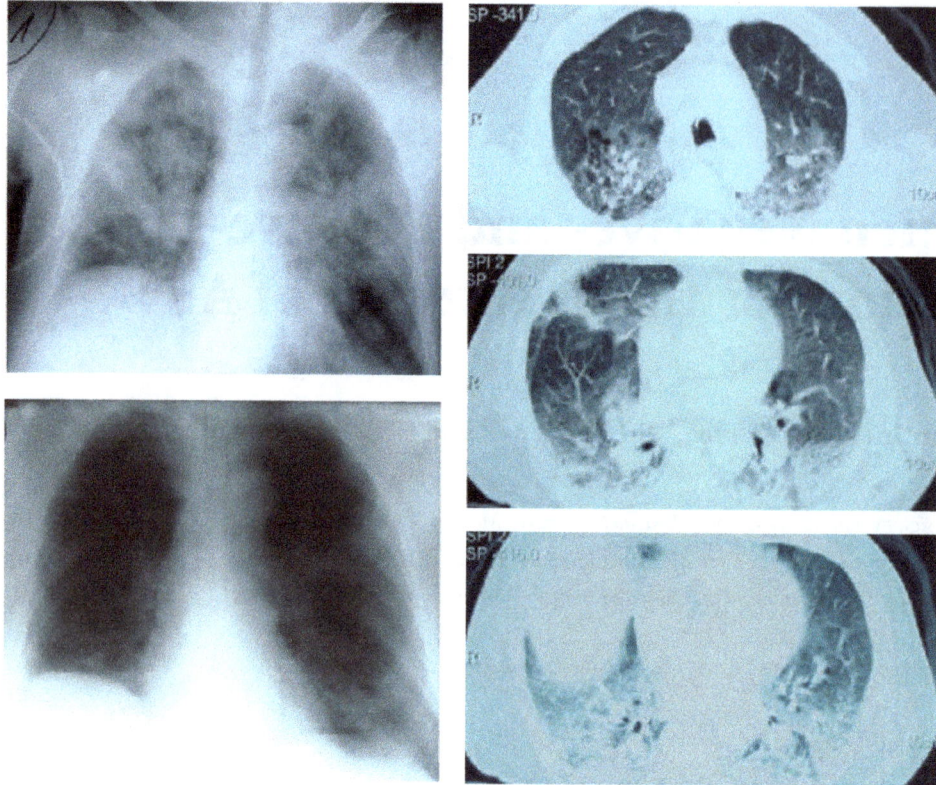

FIGURE 1: Chest X-rays and CT scan. Patchy bilateral infiltrates can be seen in the first chest X-ray made immediately postoperatively (top left). After three days of noninvasive ventilation and two days of invasive ventilation, the CT scan of the lungs was performed at a PEEP of 15 cm H_2O (right) showing bilateral dorsal infiltrates reaching from cranial (top right) to caudal lung regions (down right). The chest X-ray made after CENPV during the following day shows impressive regression of the infiltrates and pleural effusions (bottom left), corresponding to improved oxygenation.

but without enlarged heart (Figure 1). A cardiac etiology for the pulmonary edema was ruled out, also clinically, as a physical examination failed to reveal heart murmurs, jugular venous distension, or peripheral edema, and there was no sign of hemodynamic instability. The patient was ventilated noninvasively via a facemask with positive end-expiratory pressure (PEEP) of at least 5 cm H_2O and, from the second day, with a FiO_2 of 0.5. On the third day, respiratory insufficiency deteriorated and the patient was intubated. Two days later the patient was tracheostomized; CT scans of the lungs were performed at a PEEP level of 15 cm H_2O and showed bilateral patchy infiltrates and dorsal consolidation extending from cranial to caudal lung regions (Figure 1).

During the following day, the PaO_2/FiO_2 ratio again decreased below 200 mmHg, despite high PEEP values of not less than 15 cm H_2O (Figure 2) that were not sufficient to maintain lung volumes; even recruitment maneuvers using airway pressures up to 85 cm H_2O were unable to substantially improve oxygenation. In this situation, six days after the development of ARDS and three days after invasive CPPV, we decided to apply CENPV with the chamber respirator (Figure 3).

This device was constructed drawing on our clinical experience with a tank respirator that was built in our hospital in the early 1980s [7]. Gull-wing doors at both sides and one

at the head enabled rapid access to the intubated patient who was placed completely inside the chamber (Figure 3). Three air-sealing outlets at each side and two at the top enabled simple and rapid introduction of medical support devices; moreover, during their introduction (or when the doors were opened/closed), there was no need to disconnect any lines or connections.

After receiving permission from the patient's next of kin we started CENPV, applying chamber pressures of −33 cm H_2O at inspiration and −15 cm H_2O at expiration. We combined CENPV with conventional PEEP of about 8 cm H_2O and pressure support of 4–12 cm H_2O (Figure 2), applying tidal volumes of 6–8 mL/kg predicted bodyweight. For pressure support, we used the BIPAP assist mode of a conventional intensive care respirator (Evita 4, Dräger, Lübeck, Germany).

During the first application of the chamber ventilator (that lasted for 7 hours), the PaO_2/FiO_2 value increased from 236 to more than 300 mmHg (Figure 2), and alveolar infiltrates showed an impressive decrease. However, it was only during the second application time (after eight hours of CENPV) that the PaO_2/FiO_2 value increased to more than 500 mmHg (Figure 2), indicating significant recruitment of lung volume without the use of any recruitment maneuvers. Before opening the chamber respirator again, the PEEP

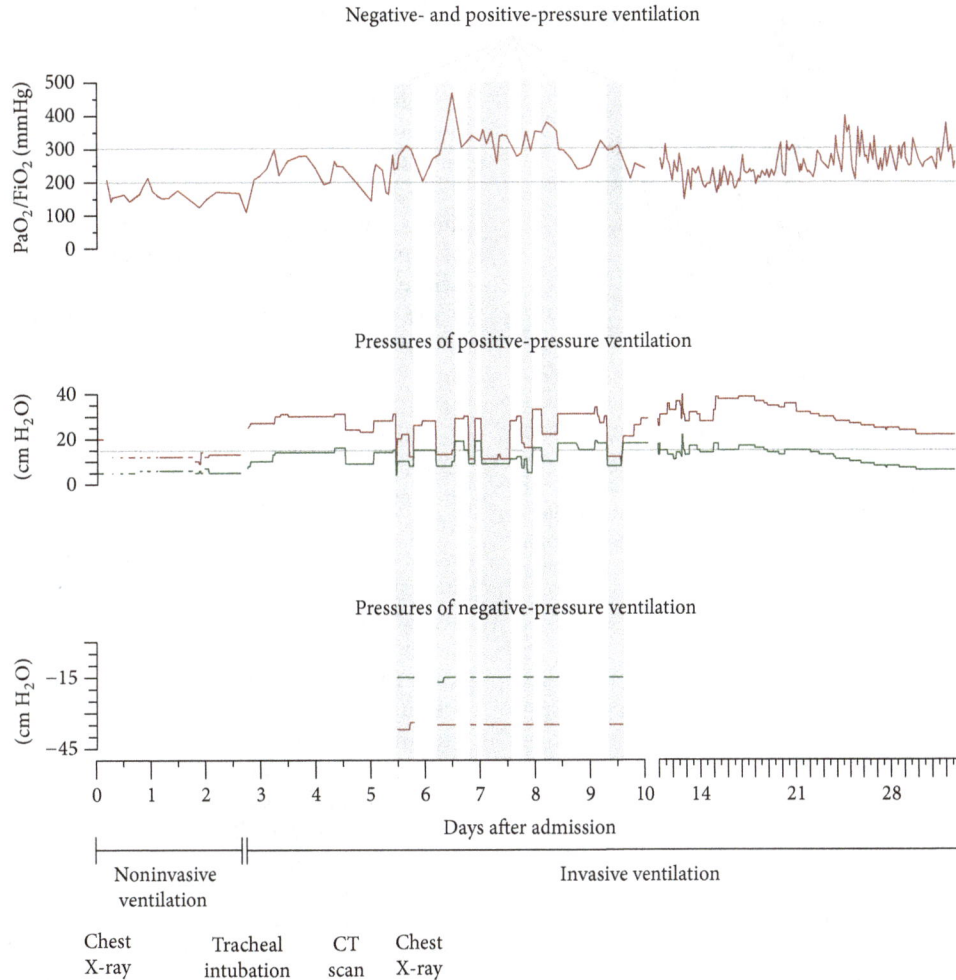

FIGURE 2: Course of gas exchange and ventilatory pressures. After three days of noninvasive positive-pressure ventilation, the patient was intubated and ventilated in a pressure-controlled mode. Three days later, negative-pressure ventilation was commenced in combination with conventional pressure support (gray columns). In both ventilatory modes, inspiratory pressures are shown as red and expiratory pressures as green lines. Ventilatory pressures represent inspiratory plateau pressures and positive end-expiratory pressures (PEEP) during conventional positive-pressure ventilation and maximum or minimum chamber pressures during negative-pressure ventilation.

level was elevated by at least 8 cm H_2O to compensate for the discontinuation of the end-expiratory negative chamber pressure (Figure 2).

During these first two applications of the chamber respirator, the patient was deeply sedated and CENPV was applied with a fixed setting without triggering the negative-pressure pump. During subsequent applications of CENPV, the patient's spontaneous breathing efforts triggered the external negative-pressure pump unit (Coppa, Biella, Italy) of the chamber ventilator via a thermistor that was fixed at the tracheal cannula. The resulting breaths triggered the pressure support function of the conventional respirator.

After applying CENPV for 5 days for 6–18 h/day, we decided to wean the tracheostomized patient from the ventilator and increased the PEEP to 19 cm H_2O before opening the chamber ventilator. Following cessation of CENPV, the patient breathed spontaneously at this high PEEP level with pressure support of only 4–8 cm H_2O (Figure 3). Most remarkably, he breathed slowly and very effectively, making

almost sole use of his diaphragm and only very marginal use of his accessory respiratory muscles. Subsequently, higher levels of pressure support became necessary and oxygenation deteriorated again, with PaO_2/FiO_2 values mainly between 200 and 300 mmHg (Figure 2). Three weeks after CENPV, the patient was successfully extubated and discharged to the normal ward.

Now, 13 years later, the patient is still alive and has a good quality of life, travelling extensively with his wife and enjoying his grandchildren, and one of his favorite and frequent activities is cycling.

3. Discussion

This patient probably developed ARDS due to the focus of infection that spread following abscess drainage; however, the definitive reason for the immediate postoperative development of lung injury remains unknown. Despite high pressure

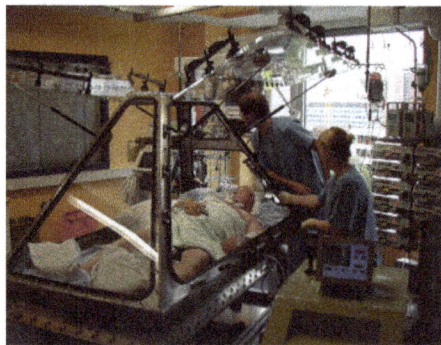

FIGURE 3: Patient with ARDS in the chamber respirator. CENPV has been discontinued and the chamber opened to enable better access for nursing procedures. The PEEP was elevated before opening the chamber to compensate for discontinuation of end-expiratory negative chamber pressure, and the patient is breathing spontaneously while receiving pressure support from the conventional ventilator. The separate pump unit (bottom right) was manufactured by Coppa S.r.l. (Biella, Italy) and was usually integrated into a tank respirator.

values, oxygenation could not be maintained using PEEP, and recruitment maneuvers proved unable to recruit lung volume. This not only reflects the severity of lung injury but also, in particular, indicates the limitations of conventional ventilator therapy in which only positive pressure is used.

In this situation, CENPV using the chamber respirator in combination with PEEP and pressure support was able to recruit and maintain lung volume, as indicated by persistently improved oxygenation over five days with PaO_2/FiO_2 values above 300 mmHg, associated with an impressive reduction of alveolar infiltrates. These effects may be caused by the different way in which ventilator pressures are applied, resulting in a much more effective means of distending the lungs and maintaining lung volumes, as the negative pressure acts across a broad surface of both the chest wall and abdomen. Therefore, in both surfactant-depleted rabbits and patients with ARDS, at matched end-expiratory and inspiratory lung volumes, applying lower transpulmonary pressures, CENPV presumably also resulted in better oxygenation as compared to CPPV [7, 8].

We decided to apply negative- and positive-pressure ventilation simultaneously, as we have found this combination to be highly effective in ventilating patients with ARDS. During CENPV, regional pleural pressure gradients probably exhibit a substantially different development compared with those in CPPV [7, 8]. Furthermore, transpulmonary pressures (TPP = alveolar pressure minus esophageal pressure), involved in both ventilator modes, should be cumulative when CENPV is combined with CPPV. We speculate that the distribution of ventilation is much more effective with this combination, resulting in alveolar recruitment, reduction of alveolar edema, and stabilization of recruited lung volume, even in severe cases of ARDS; we believe that these effects contributed to the favorable outcome in the present patient.

We observed similar effects in most of our other five patients with severe ARDS who were treated in the chamber respirator in 2002 and also in six additional patients with ARDS who were treated in a tank respirator after completing physiological studies [8]. In these (albeit limited number of) patients, no relevant adverse effects were observed that could be directly related to the combined use of negative- and positive-pressure ventilation. However, especially in patients with severe capillary leakage, external edema increased and decreased again under ambient air. In these latter patients, we limited this therapy to only several hours per day. Particularly in hypovolemic patients, we administered intravenous fluid before starting CENPV to avoid a pronounced decrease in blood pressure associated with low intrathoracic pressures and redistribution of intravascular volume. Finally, of all these patients, 50% survived their stay in the intensive care unit.

In line with this current standard of care, the patient described here was intubated and ventilated with CPPV; we then commenced CENPV as a rescue therapy in late-stage ARDS. Because we did not wish to risk applying CENPV in this patient (or other patients) without a tracheal tube during an early stage of lung injury, CENPV was applied only in intubated patients with severe ARDS. Generally, securing the airway with a tracheal tube is still deemed necessary when a patient with lung injury depends on high ventilatory pressures in conjunction with a high FiO_2 to maintain gas exchange. As in the presented case, noninvasive positive-pressure ventilation frequently fails in ARDS as a function of its severity and does not appear beneficial in severe ARDS [8]. We believe that CENPV has the potential to reduce this high failure rate, even in severe lung injury. Furthermore, after cessation of CENPV, our patient's breathing pattern with a low breathing frequency and high tidal volumes (making almost sole use of his diaphragm) may also indicate the potential of CENPV to reduce weaning failure. However, due to the paucity of data on this topic, randomized trials comparing noninvasive positive- and negative-pressure ventilation in patients with ARDS are needed to further support this hypothesis.

Devices far less clumsy than our self-made tank respirator or chamber respirator are now available. These include a much more practical Goretex suit that is effectively used with a highly efficient negative-pressure ventilator (Pegaso Vent, Dima S.r.l., Bologna, Italy). This device can be synchronized with spontaneous breathing and can be coupled to a conventional ventilator to optimally synchronize CENPV with CPPV.

Tracheal intubation and CPPV as the current standard of care for ARDS seem to have reached their limit in terms of a further relevant reduction of the still very high mortality rate [2, 3]. This unacceptably high mortality rate calls for alternative techniques that substantially differ from the present methods. CENPV might be worth considering as an alternative, as it has proven less injurious and resulted in better oxygenation in experimental lung injury [7] and also improved gas exchange in a physiologic study on patients with ARDS [8].

The present report is the first to demonstrate how both techniques can be successfully combined in an intubated patient with severe late-stage ARDS. We believe that this therapy made a substantial contribution to the patient's positive outcome and survival. The possibility of effectively applying this and similar concepts, not only in intubated but also in nonintubated patients with ARDS, offers new options that may genuinely differ from the present therapeutic approaches. Therefore, these options may have the potential to decrease the ongoing high mortality rate associated with ARDS.

Acknowledgments

The authors thank Dr. Ljiljana Verner, Professor Dr. Jörn Heine, and Professor Dr. Siegfried Piepenbrock for their support.

References

[1] V. M. Ranieri, F. Giunta, P. M. Suter, and A. S. Slutsky, "Mechanical ventilation as a mediator of multisystem organ failure in acute respiratory distress syndrome (multiple letters)," *The Journal of the American Medical Association*, vol. 284, no. 1, pp. 43–44, 2000.

[2] J. Villar, J. Blanco, J. M. Añón et al., "The ALIEN study: incidence and outcome of acute respiratory distress syndrome in the era of lung protective ventilation," *Intensive Care Medicine*, vol. 37, no. 12, pp. 1932–1941, 2011.

[3] A. W. Thille, D. Contou, C. Fragnoli, A. Cordoba-Izquierdo, F. Boissier, and C. Brun-Buisson, "Non-invasive ventilation for acute hypoxemic respiratory failure: intubation rate and risk factors," *Critical Care*, vol. 17, no. 6, article R269, 2013.

[4] S. K. Sanyal, R. Bernal, W. T. Hughes, and S. Feldman, "Continuous negative chest-wall pressure. Successful use for severe respiratory distress in an adult," *Journal of the American Medical Association*, vol. 236, no. 15, pp. 1727–1728, 1976.

[5] S. K. Sanyal, S. Turner, M. Ossi, and T. P. Coburn, "Continuous negative chest wall pressure therapy in management of severe hypoxemia due to aspiration pneumonitis: a case report," *Respiratory Care*, vol. 24, pp. 1022–1025, 1979.

[6] A. H. Morris and C. G. Elliott, "Adult respiratory distress syndrome: successful support with continuous negative extrathoracic pressure," *Critical Care Medicine*, vol. 13, no. 11, pp. 989–990, 1985.

[7] F. Grasso, D. Engelberts, E. Helm et al., "Negative-pressure ventilation: better oxygenation and less lung injury," *The American Journal of Respiratory and Critical Care Medicine*, vol. 177, no. 4, pp. 412–418, 2008.

[8] K. Raymondos, U. Molitoris, M. Capewell et al., "Negative-versus positive-pressure ventilation in intubated patients with acute respiratory distress syndrome," *Critical Care*, vol. 16, no. 2, article R37, 2012.

28

Fat Embolism Syndrome in Duchenne Muscular Dystrophy Patients: Early Recognition and Aggressive Therapy

Lee D. Murphy ⓘ,[1] Mouhammad Yabrodi,[1,2] and Riad Lutfi[1]

[1]*Division of Pediatric Critical Care Medicine, Department of Pediatrics, Indiana University School of Medicine, Indianapolis, IN, USA*
[2]*Division of Pediatric Cardiology, Department of Pediatrics, Indiana University School of Medicine, Indianapolis, IN, USA*

Correspondence should be addressed to Lee D. Murphy; ledmurph@iu.edu

Academic Editor: Chiara Lazzeri

We describe two pediatric patients with Duchenne muscular dystrophy that presented with acute neurologic deterioration and hypoxic respiratory failure requiring mechanical ventilation. These cases fulfill the clinical criteria for Fat Embolism Syndrome. Early recognition and aggressive supportive therapy with mechanical ventilation, right ventricular afterload reduction, and blood transfusion led to survival without any residual effects from the event. Fat Embolism Syndrome needs to be considered early in the course of patients with Duchenne muscular dystrophy who present with respiratory and neurological symptoms.

1. Introduction

Duchenne muscular dystrophy (DMD) is the most common inherited pediatric muscle disorder affecting approximately 1 in 3600 live male births [1]. Patients with DMD have a significant reduction in bone density due to chronic use of steroids, which results in increased incidence of long bone fractures and the potential development of Fat Embolism Syndrome (FES) [2]. When children with DMD present with altered mental status and respiratory compromise, the physician needs to consider FES in the differential diagnosis. We report two cases of pediatric patients with DMD that presented to the emergency department with altered mental status and respiratory compromise that were diagnosed with FES. Due to early recognition of the disease and aggressive supportive care with mechanical ventilation, right ventricular afterload reduction, and blood transfusion, both patients survived without any significant sequelae.

2. Case Report

2.1. Case 1. A 14-year-old male with DMD has been on daily oral steroid since 9 years of age. He weighed 53 kg (47th percentile) and was 147 cm tall (less than 3rd percentile). He became nonambulatory at 12 years of age. Forced vital capacity (FVC) was 2.37 L or 80% predicted. A polysomnogram was completed and revealed moderate obstructive sleep apnea. His echocardiogram (ECHO) was normal with cardiac magnetic resonance imaging (MRI) demonstrating normal left ventricular ejection fraction (LVEF). He participated in many school activities including wheelchair soccer.

He presented to the emergency department with confusion, tachycardia, tachypnea, and fever up to 39.2 degrees Celsius a few hours following soccer practice. During practice, he had been transferred from his wheelchair and his right leg had brushed the ground causing him to have to be placed on the ground until more help was obtained to put him back in his wheelchair. Brain computed tomography (CT) was negative for any acute intracranial process contributing to his current state. Chest computed tomography (CT) scan was negative for pulmonary embolism but showed patchy diffuse nodular airspace opacities seen scattered throughout both lung fields (Figure 1(a)). He had progressive acute hypoxic respiratory failure requiring mechanical ventilation. Shortly after intubation, he suffered cardiac arrest requiring 3 minutes of cardiopulmonary resuscitation (CPR) before return of spontaneous circulation. ECHOs were consistent with increased pulmonary vascular resistance including moderate right ventricle dysfunction and elevated pulmonary arterial pressure. Duplex ultrasound evaluation of lower extremities

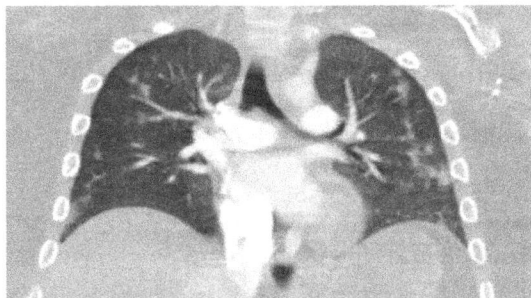

(a) Patchy diffuse nodular airspace opacities seen scattered throughout both lung fields

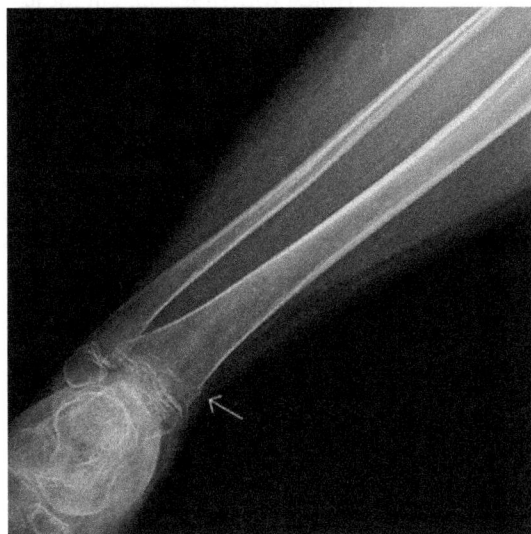

(b) Nondisplaced fracture at the distal right tibial metaphysis and fibular metaphysis

FIGURE 1

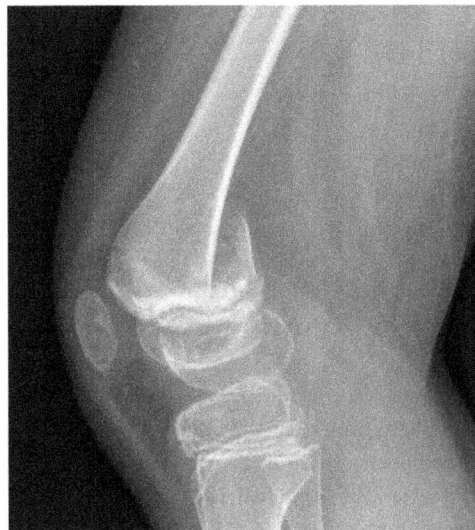

(a) Nondisplaced Salter-Harris type II fracture of the distal left femur

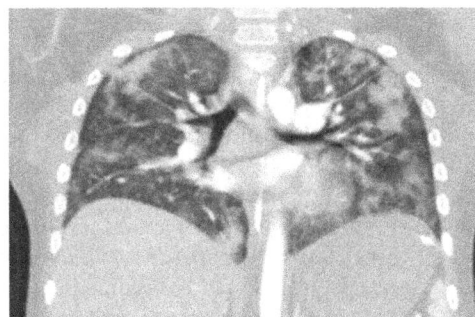

(b) Patchy diffuse nodular airspace opacities seen scattered throughout both lung fields

FIGURE 2

was without evidence of deep venous thrombosis bilaterally. X-rays of lower extremities revealed cortical step off at the proximal left femoral neck and nondisplaced fracture at the distal right tibial metaphysis and fibular metaphysis (Figure 1(b)). Ophthalmologic exam revealed Purtscher-like retinopathy. The patient was treated with 48 hours of antibiotics that were discontinued with negative blood, urine, and mini bronchoalveolar lavage (BAL) culture. The patient was treated with mechanical ventilation and right ventricular afterload reduction with milrinone and inhaled nitric oxide for pulmonary hypertension. These therapies were able to be weaned off, and the patient was able to be extubated on day five of admission. He was later transferred to the pediatric floor and later discharged home without any residual effects from the entire event.

2.2. Case 2. An 11-year-old male with DMD has been on daily oral steroid since 9 years of age. He weighed 30 kg (5.6th percentile) and he was 120 cm tall (less than 3rd percentile). He is able to ambulate without assistance. FVC was 1.5 L or 96% predicted. His ECHO was normal with cardiac MRI demonstrating normal LVEF.

He sustained a nondisplaced Salter-Harris type II fracture of the distal left femur (Figure 2(a)) from a fall that required surgical fixation and was able to be discharged home on the day of operation. He presented to the emergency department two days after his operation with seizure, tachycardia, tachypnea, and fever up to 38.6 degrees Celsius. He had progressive acute hypoxic respiratory failure requiring mechanical ventilation. Shortly after intubation, he developed pulmonary hemorrhage and anemia remedied with fresh frozen plasma, ventilator adjustments, and blood transfusion. A fast spin MRI of his head was negative. CT scan of his chest demonstrated bilateral patchy infiltrates; no pulmonary embolism was identified (Figure 2(b)). ECHO revealed mildly elevated tricuspid regurgitation velocities representing increased right ventricular and pulmonary artery pressures. He was placed on broad spectrum antibiotics for 72 hours but blood, urine, and mini BAL remained negative. Mechanical ventilation was able to be weaned and the patient was extubated on day five of admission. He was later transferred to the pediatric floor and later discharged home without any residual effects from the entire event.

Table 1: Gurd's criteria to diagnose fat embolism syndrome.

	CASE 1	CASE 2
MAJOR CRITERIA		
Petechial Rash	Yes	No
Respiratory Insufficiency	Yes	Yes
Cerebral Involvement	Yes	Yes
MINOR CRITERIA		
Tachycardia	Yes	Yes
Pyrexia	Yes	Yes
Retinal changes: fat or petechiae	Yes	No
Jaundice	No	No
Renal: anuria/oliguria or lipiduria	No	No
Sudden fall in hemoglobin concentration	Yes	Yes
Sudden Thrombocytopenia	No	No
High erythrocyte sedimentation Rate	Yes	Yes
Fat macroglobulinemia	No	N/A

3. Discussion

The diagnosis of FES is made up of a group of nondescript symptoms that could represent a multitude of diagnoses [3, 4]. Many cases go unnoticed and therefore the true incidence of FES is unknown [5]. The pathophysiology is thought to be a result of fat droplets released from bone marrow, most commonly after traumatic fractures or orthopedic procedures [4]. Small fat droplets are released into the venous circulation. These droplets can either become lodged in the pulmonary circulation or pass into the systemic circulation and lodge in the cerebral vasculature causing microinfarcts [6]. In DMD patients, FES is increasingly becoming a well-recognized complication as patients with this condition are prone to falls and minor trauma, leading to fractures due to the use of chronic corticosteroids and prolonged immobility [1].

Clinical presentation can range from asymptomatic to cardiac arrest from right ventricular heart failure. Typically, the onset of symptoms happens within the first 12–24 hours after trauma, although some cases may occur as late as 36–72 hours [5, 6]. There are no standardized, prospectively validated diagnostic criteria for FES. The diagnosis is made by recognizing the characteristic clinical syndrome in the context of supportive imaging and a predisposing insult. Given the absence of a gold-standard diagnostic test, a number of authors have proposed clinical diagnostic criteria. The most frequently cited, despite low sensitivity and specificity, are Gurd's criteria (Table 1). Gurd's criteria have been adapted over the years to include the following variations: 1 major with 4 minor or 2 major and 2 minor are the most commonly used definition to diagnose FES [7]. Major criteria include respiratory failure, neurologic changes, and a petechial rash [6, 7].

The lungs are usually the most affected organs with rapidly progressing tachypnea and hypoxemia as the primary clinical symptoms [3, 6]. Chest X-ray shows a diffuse bilateral infiltrate that is hard to differentiate from pediatric acute respiratory distress syndrome. Chest computed tomography

(CT) does not add much to a regular chest x-ray in terms of diagnosis; however, it is usually done to rule out pulmonary embolism. Alveolar hemorrhage can be also seen in FES [8].

The brain is the second most affected organ. Neurological symptoms are extremely variable between irritability, anxiety, agitation, confusion, delirium, convulsions and coma, and hypertonia. Cerebral CT scan is usually negative. MRI with DWI is a more specific diagnostic modality [6, 9].

Skin petechiae represent the third most important sign for clinical diagnosis. These tiny lesions (1-2 mm) are, in fact, small hemorrhages caused by the rupture of skin capillaries. The time elapsed from trauma to petechial onset varies with their location but the typical pattern is found in the axillary and high presternal region, in lateral surfaces of the neck, and in eye conjunctiva [5].

In addition to lungs, brain, skin, and conjunctivas, there are minor criteria that include tachycardia, fever, retinal changes, anuria or oliguria, sudden hematocrit and/or platelets drop, and positive fat on sputum [3]. Some patients will develop acute pulmonary hypertension and subsequent acute right heart failure and cardiovascular collapse. Using right ventricular afterload reduction with milrinone and/or inhaled nitric oxide may be beneficial in this setting [10, 11].

A recent systematic review specifically looking at the few published case reports about Fat Embolism Syndrome in children with Duchenne muscular dystrophy found that 7 out of the 16 (44%) children died [12]. In our paper, we report two cases of FES with favorable outcomes. Early recognition and aggressive supportive treatment are key elements for good outcomes in this fragile population. Anticipating potential complications such as anemia, thrombocytopenia, right ventricular failure, or acute kidney injury is another key of the management.

4. Conclusion

Our report highlights the need of high index of suspicion for FES in the DMD population and the need for aggressive supportive therapy when these children present with acute altered mental status and respiratory distress.

References

[1] K. Bushby, R. Finkel, D. J. Birnkrant et al., "Diagnosis and management of Duchenne muscular dystrophy, part 1: diagnosis, and pharmacological and psychosocial management," *The Lancet Neurology*, vol. 9, no. 1, pp. 77–93, 2010.

[2] V. H. Morgenroth, L. P. Hache, and P. R. Clemens, "Insights into bone health in Duchenne muscular dystrophy," *BoneKEy Reports*, vol. 1, 2012.

[3] A. R. Gurd and R. I. Wilson, "The fat embolism syndrome," *The Journal of Bone & Joint Surgery*, vol. 56B, no. 3, pp. 408–416, 1974.

[4] L. C. McAdam, A. Rastogi, K. MacLeod, and W. Douglas Biggar, "Fat Embolism Syndrome following minor trauma in Duchenne

muscular dystrophy," *Neuromuscular Disorders*, vol. 22, no. 12, pp. 1035–1039, 2012.

[5] N. Shaikh, "Emergency management of fat embolism syndrome," *Journal of Emergencies, Trauma, and Shock*, vol. 2, no. 1, pp. 29–33, 2009.

[6] S. Akhtar, "Fat Embolism," *Anesthesiology Clinics*, vol. 27, no. 3, pp. 533–550, 2009.

[7] A. R. Gurd, "Fat embolism: an aid to diagnosis," *The Journal of Bone & Joint Surgery (British Volume)*, vol. 52, no. 4, pp. 732–737, 1970.

[8] S. K. Dash, A. Bansal, B. S. Wankhade, and R. Sharma, "Alveolar hemorrhage in a case of fat embolism syndrome: A case report with short systemic review," *Lung India*, vol. 30, no. 2, pp. 151–154, 2013.

[9] P. M. Parizel, H. E. Demey, G. Veeckmans et al., "Early diagnosis of cerebral fat embolism syndrome by diffusion-weighted MRI (starfield pattern)," *Stroke*, vol. 32, no. 12, pp. 2942–2944, 2001.

[10] E. Brotfain, L. Koyfman, R. Kutz et al., "Use of Early Inhaled Nitric Oxide Therapy in Fat Embolism Syndrome to Prevent Right Heart Failure," *Case Reports in Critical Care*, vol. 2014, pp. 1–4, 2014.

[11] A. Amigoni, P. Corner, F. Zanella, and A. Pettenazzo, "Successful use of inhaled nitric oxide in a child with fat embolism syndrome," *Journal of Trauma*, vol. 68, no. 3, pp. E80–E82, 2010.

[12] D. Feder, M. E. Koch, B. Palmieri, F. L. A. Fonseca, and A. A. D. S. Carvalho, "Fat embolism after fractures in duchenne muscular dystrophy: An underdiagnosed complication? A systematic review," *Therapeutics and Clinical Risk Management*, vol. 13, pp. 1357–1361, 2017.

29

Effect of Hemoadsorption for Cytokine Removal in Pneumococcal and Meningococcal Sepsis

Francesca Leonardis ⓘ,[1] Viviana De Angelis,[1] Francesca Frisardi,[1]
Chiara Pietrafitta,[1] Ivano Riva,[2] Tino Martino Valetti,[2] Valentina Broletti,[2]
Gianmariano Marchesi,[2] Lorenza Menato,[3] Roberto Nani,[3] Franco Marson,[3]
Mirca Fabbris,[3] Luca Cabrini,[4] Sergio Colombo,[4] Alberto Zangrillo,[4]
Carlo Coniglio,[5] Giovanni Gordini,[5] Lucia Stalteri,[6] Giovanni Giuliani,[6]
Vittorio Dalmastri,[6] and Gaetano La Manna ⓘ[6]

[1]*Intensive Care Unit, Fondazione Policlinico Tor Vergata, Viale Oxford 81, 00133 Roma RM, Italy*
[2]*Intensive Care Unit 3, Department of Anesthesia and Intensive Care, ASST Papa Giovanni XXIII, Piazza OMS 1, 24127 Bergamo BG, Italy*
[3]*Intensive Care Unit, Azienda ULSS 2 Marca Trevigiana, Presidio Ospedaliero di Treviso, Piazzale dell'Ospedale 1, 31100 Treviso TV, Italy*
[4]*Anesthesia and Intensive Care Unit, IRCSS San Raffaele, Via Olgettina 60, 20132 Milano MI, Italy*
[5]*Resuscitation and Territorial Emergency Unit, Maggiore Hospital, Largo Nigrisoli 2, 40133 Bologna BO, Italy*
[6]*Nephrology, Dialysis and Transplantation Unit, Azienda Ospedaliera-Universitaria di Bologna, Via Massarenti 9, 40138 Bologna BO, Italy*

Correspondence should be addressed to Francesca Leonardis; francesca.leonardis@uniroma2.it

Academic Editor: Zsolt Molnár

Bacterial meningitis and septicemia are invasive bacterial diseases, representing a significant cause of morbidity and mortality worldwide. Both conditions are characterized by an impressive inflammatory response, resulting rapidly in cerebral edema, infarction, hydrocephalus, and septic shock with multiple organ failure. Despite advances in critical care, outcome and prognosis remain critical. Available adjunctive treatments to control the inflammatory response have shown encouraging results in the evolution of patients with sepsis and systemic inflammation, but meningococcal or pneumococcal infection has not been investigated. We herein report five patients with similar critical pathological conditions, characterized by pneumococcal or meningococcal sepsis and treated with hemoadsorption for cytokine removal. All patients showed a progressive stabilization in hemodynamics along with a rapid and marked reduction of catecholamine dosages, a stabilization in metabolic disorders, and less-than-expected loss of extremities. Therapy proved to be safe and well tolerated. From this first experience, extracorporeal cytokine removal seems to be a valid and safe therapy in the management of meningococcal and pneumococcal diseases and may contribute to the patient stabilization and prevention of severe sequelae. Further studies are required to confirm efficacy in a larger context.

1. Introduction

Bacterial meningitis and septicemia are invasive bacterial diseases affecting, respectively, the central nervous system (CNS) and the blood, representing a significant cause of morbidity and mortality worldwide [1, 2] with rising risk of poor outcome in case of combination of these diseases.

Reported in-hospital mortality range is between 24% [3] and 41% [4] and the most frequent causes of death are systemic complications in the elderly (>50 years of age) and cerebral complications in the younger patients (<2 years of age) [5].

Neisseria meningitidis (Gram-negative bacteria) and *Streptococcus pneumoniae* (Gram-positive bacteria) are the leading causative pathogens of invasive bacterial disease, with the latter being responsible for two-thirds of the reported cases in Western Europe and the US [5].

Once these bacteria have entered the bloodstream through the nasopharynx mucosa, they may survive and proliferate thanks to their polysaccharide capsule, provoking an immune and inflammatory reaction, which may rapidly lead to fulminant septic shock [6]. Then these bacteria may also invade the blood-brain barrier, causing bacterial meningitis and provoking an immanent inflammatory reaction in the CNS. This inflammation contributes to neuronal injury and involves the subarachnoid space, the meninges, and the brain parenchymal vessels. A hallmark of the inflammatory response associated with the infection is the excessive production of cytokines, chemokines, and other inflammatory mediators [6–9] with sometimes fulminant, devastating courses. This can lead to an uncontrolled, overwhelming reaction of the body's host response against itself leading to cerebral edema, infarction, hydrocephalus, and septic shock with multiple organ failure [10, 11].

Despite advances in critical care and early administration of antibiotics and corticosteroids, invasive bacterial diseases still represent a major challenge to physicians. Bacterial meningitis, if treated successfully, presents a high burden of sequelae so that approximately half of the survivors exhibit neurological sequelae [11]. Septicemia may be a dramatic fulminant consequence of bacterial meningitis or may be present on its own, increasing the high mortality rate of these patients [6–11].

A common dramatic feature is the occurrence of disseminated intravascular coagulation (DIC) [12], characterized by extensive activation of the coagulation system, amplified by inhibition of anticoagulant pathways, and often associated with the rapid onset of hypotension, acute adrenal hemorrhage, and multiorgan failure, leading to poor outcome [11, 12].

Despite the necessity of early recognition of symptoms and the prompt administration of antibiotics treatment, new adjunctive therapies are on their way. Inhibition of leukocyte recruitment or pattern recognition receptors, adjuvant erythropoietin/corticosteroid/complex vitamin B treatments, radical scavenging, and therapeutic hypothermia, have been described extensively elsewhere [8–10]. Since pneumococcal and meningococcal PAMPs act proinflammatorily provoking the generation of proinflammatory cytokines and chemokines, inhibition of these would seem a reasonable approach. Previous attempts to fight sepsis or the systemic inflammatory response syndrome (SIRS) by removing a single, specific cytokine have not been able to demonstrate an improvement in outcome. This brings up the question as to whether a broad, rather than specific, approach to remove the multitude of cytokines and other factors at fault in the disease may be more promising. In this context, extracorporeal blood purification therapies with the potential ability to alter the host inflammatory response through broad-spectrum, nonselective removal of inflammatory mediators have come into focus. A new hemoadsorption device, Cytosorb (Cytosorbents Corp, USA), intended as adjunctive treatment for patients with elevated cytokine levels in the setting of SIRS, sepsis, and septic shock has shown encouraging results in

the evolution of these critical patients [13–18], but clinical cases are not available for meningococcal or pneumococcal infections.

Therefore, the aim of this case series is to report our clinical experience about the use of hemoadsorption for cytokine removal in that kind of patients.

2. Clinical Cases

We herein present five patients with pneumococcal or meningococcal sepsis early treated with Cytosorb for cytokine removal as adjunctive therapy.

Patient characteristics, treatments, clinical parameters, and patient outcome are presented in Table 1.

All the Cytosorb treatments were performed continuously until a hemodynamic, metabolic, and inflammatory improvement was observed, in combination with continuous renal replacement therapy (CRRT). Blood flows were set among 100 and 180 ml/min, according to the hemodynamic response of the patient, while dialysis doses were in the range of 30 and 35 ml/kg/h. A citrate-based protocol was used in all the patients.

2.1. Case 1. Case 1 is a 40-year-old male, presenting with general malaise, arthralgia in his extremities, facial cyanosis, and fever (39°C). In the medical history, a post-traumatic splenectomy was reported. Empirical antibiotic therapy started with ceftriaxone (2 g every 12h) and vancomycin (500 mg every 6h). After several bacteriological analysis, secondary sepsis caused by meningitis from *Streptococcus pneumoniae* was diagnosed. The patient was transferred to the intensive care unit (ICU) where his clinical status rapidly deteriorated, showing a severe hemodynamic instability with need for vasopressor support (norepinephrine 0.4 μg/kg/min), persistent hypotension, and a pronounced inflammatory state with C-reactive protein (CRP) at 176.3 mg/l and procalcitonin (PCT) at 485.88 ng/ml. The patient also exhibited metabolic abnormalities, with lactate levels of 7.8 mmol/l, and severe coagulative disorders.

In face of a persistent anuria, continuous renal replacement therapy (CRRT), hemodiafiltration mode (CVVHDF, Prismaflex, M150, Baxter, USA) was started, together with Cytosorb cartridge, for a total of 68 hours (start of treatment <24h after ICU admission).

A general improvement was obtained already during the first treatment. PCT could be reduced to 6 ng/ml at the end of the treatments. Similarly, CRP also dropped to 136.41 mg/l during the course of the treatments. On the metabolic level, the patient showed a marked improvement in lactate acidosis, with lactate levels decreasing to 1.9 mmol/dl. From a hemodynamic point of view, a MAP stabilization could be achieved paralleled with a reduction in the need for norepinephrine. The patient could be stopped from CRRT after 12 days with a recovery of diuresis. The course for norepinephrine demand during Cytosorb treatment is presented in Figure 1, whereas the course of lactate and PCT is shown in Figure 2.

The patient was still hospitalized after 2 months, however in an alert, collaborative, tracheotomised, spontaneously breathing state, waiting for transfer to a rehabilitation facility.

TABLE 1: Patient characteristics, treatments, clinical parameters, and patient outcome. M: male, F: female, Cat-free: catecholamine-free, CRRT: continuous renal replacement therapy, SOFA: Sequential Organ Failure Assessment, and PELOD: Paediatric Logistic Organ Dysfunction (*only case 4).

Case number	1	2	3	4*	5
Sex	M	F	M	M	F
Age	40	66	40	14	36
Diagnosis	Pneumococcal Sepsis	Pneumococcal Sepsis	Meningococcal Sepsis (Serotype C)	Meningococcal Sepsis (Serotype C)	Meningococcal Sepsis (Serotype C)
Antibiotics	Ceftriaxone/ Vancomycin	Ceftriaxone/ Levofloxacin	Meropenem/ Amikacin/ Ceftriaxone	Dexamethasone/ Ceftriaxone	Levofloxacin / Ceftriaxone
Cytosorb treatments (n)	4	1	3	2	4
Cytosorb treatment time (h)	68	24	72	32	96
Delay (h)	<24	<15	15	11	8
SOFA Score/*PELOD Score Admission	13	17	18	22	12
SOFA Score/*PELOD Score Post treatment	10	20	16	13	8
Cat-free (days)	6	3	5	3	4
CRRT (days)	12	10	12	4	5
Ventilation (days)	20	53	10	4	5
ICU stay (days)	49	53	17	6	7
Amputation need	Yes/Phalange	Yes/Limbs	Yes/Phalanges	No	Yes/Toe
ICU mortality	No	Yes	No	No	No
28-day survival	Yes	Yes	Yes	Yes	Yes
Hospital mortality	No	Yes	No	No	No

2.2. Case 2. Case 2 is a 66-year-old female, presenting with general illness, fever (40°C), and hypotension. Prior medical history included beta-blocker therapy for tachyarrhythmia, appendectomy, colon cancer, and splenectomy for colonic metastases. On admission, she exhibited skin ischemic lesions with rapid deterioration to whole body cyanosis and metabolic and lactic acidosis. Empirical antibiotic therapy started with ceftriaxone (2 g every 12h) and levofloxacin (500 mg every 12h). After 24h, blood cultures confirmed the diagnosis of sepsis from *Streptococcus pneumoniae* paralleled with severe purpura fulminans. Empirical antibiotic therapy continued for 11 and 7 days, respectively, with adjustments due to renal function changes. In the further course, she became oligoanuric, severely hypotonic with hemodynamic instability (epinephrine 0.4 μg/kg/min), and thrombocytopenic, presenting severe bleeding.

A CVVHDF treatment (Multifiltrate, AV1000, Fresenius Medical Care, Germany) was started in combination with one 24-hour session of Cytosorb hemoadsorption immediately after the ICU admission.

This combined treatment resulted in a clear and progressive hemodynamic stabilization accompanied by a marked reduction of epinephrine to 0.1 μg/kg/min (Figure 1) and a reduction of CRP, from 17.5 mg/dl to 13 mg/dl. Initially diuresis started to work again; however this went back to anuria in the first 12 hours (probably due to sepsis-associated tubular

necrosis) and fully recovered later on day 10. Lactacidemia, elevated at the admission (15 mmol/l), decreased until 4 in the first 24h. At the same time, PCT decreased from 18.35 ng/ml to 2 ng/ml after 6 days (Figure 2).

Subsequent to this first acute event, the patient showed a recrudescence of the septic state. Blood cultures were positive for *Enterobacter aerogenes*, which colonise the body through the injured intestine wall, resulting from purpura fulminans. Because of her severe injuries at the extremities, the patient needed amputations and 2 months later, the reoccurrence of the second septic episode caused the death of the patient.

2.3. Case 3. Case 3 is a 47-year-old male showing fever (38°C), asthenia, and lumbar pain with signs of diffuse petechiae. In the further course, he became severely hypovolemic and tachycardic, showing also metabolic acidosis (lactate 12 mmol/l). Blood cultures were taken and empirical antibiotic therapy was started with meropenem (2 g every 8h) and amikacin (1 g every 24h). Diagnoses confirmed by blood cultures were septic shock secondary to *Neisseria meningitidis* infection (Serotype C) and antibiotic therapy was replaced with ceftriaxone (2 g every 12h). After transfer to the ICU, norepinephrine infusion was started at 0.2 μg/kg/min and rapidly increased to 0.5 μg/kg/min, in combination with epinephrine infusion at 0.2 μg/kg/min. Inflammation was controlled with PCT, which was extremely elevated, 121.7

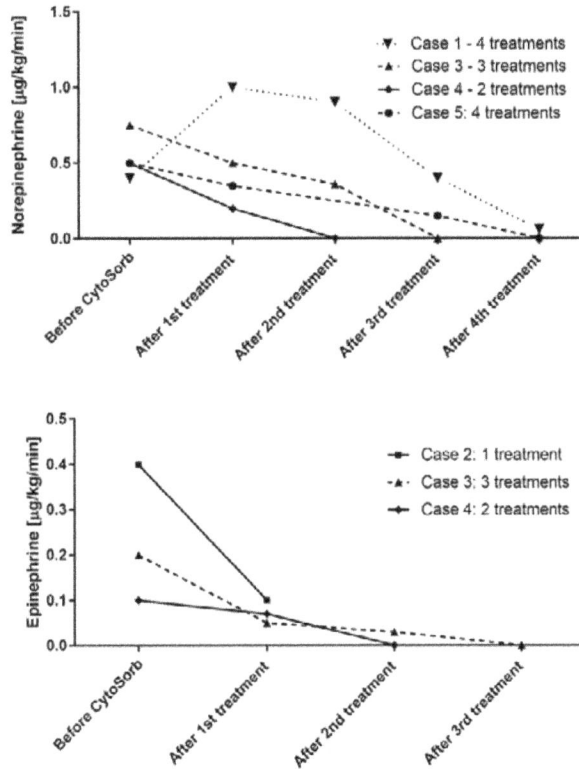

FIGURE 1: Course of norepinephrine and epinephrine demand during Cytosorb treatment in all treated patients. Values are shown at the beginning of the treatment and after every treatment until the end.

ng/ml. In the following hours, a worsening of general conditions of the patient was reported, with extension of petechiae and severe bleeding from the insertion points of the catheters and severe hypotension with the increase of norepinephrine up to 0.75 μg/kg/min. In face of a persistent condition of oligoanuria, it was necessary starting a hemofiltration treatment (CVVH, Prismaflex, M150, Baxter, USA) and Cytosorb was additionally installed into the CVVH circuit the next day (start of treatment: 15h after ICU admission).

Within the course of 72-hour Cytosorb treatments, the patient witnessed a hemodynamic improvement with norepinephrine and epinephrine being tapered off after the third session (Figure 1) as well as a stabilization of lactate values and inflammation, with PCT decreased until 16.52 ng/ml (Figure 2).

The patient also showed an attenuation of disseminated intravascular coagulopathy, a demarcation of skin necrosis areas, and a recovery of vital functions. The patient could be extubated 10 days and weaned from CVVH 12 days after the ICU admission. He was transferred to rehabilitation medicine after 23 days from the recovery, waiting for plastic surgeon consultant for the amputation of some phalanges.

2.4. Case 4. Case 4 is a young male, presenting with fever (40°C), vomiting, pain in the lower limbs, and petechiae in extension with suspected disseminated intravascular coagulopathy and septic shock. He exhibited hemodynamic instability and metabolic acidosis (lactate 13 mmol/l). The patient was immediately transferred to ICU and

pharmacological therapy with dexamethasone (10 mg every 6h) and immunoglobulins were immediately started. Diagnosis was septic shock secondary to *Neisseria meningitidis* infection (serotype C), confirmed by labs, and maxillary sinusitis was set as the probable cause of infection. Antibiotic therapy was then modified to ceftriaxone (2 g every 12h). The patient developed acute kidney injury and CRRT, hemodialysis mode, was started (CVVHD, Multifiltrate, AV1000S, Fresenius Medical Care, Germany).

Hemodynamic instability was observed with a median arterial pressure of 75 mmHg, necessitating administration of epinephrine at 0.1 μg/kg/min and norepinephrine at 0.5 μg/kg/min. In the following hours diuresis partially recovered; however the general critical condition did not improve and therefore Cytosorb was performed for a total of 32 hours in combination with CRRT (start of treatment: 11h after ICU admission). Three hours after start of Cytosorb, norepinephrine could be reduced to 0.2 μg/kg/min and epinephrine to 0.07 μg/kg/min. After the second treatment, norepinephrine and epinephrine infusion were stopped (Figure 1) and there was no more need for renal support. During the hemoadsorption treatment, we further noticed a clear stabilization of lactic acidosis from initially 13 to 1.78 mmol/l and a total recovery of diuresis. The course of lactate and PCT is shown in Figure 2.

The patient could be extubated 1 day after the cessation of Cytosorb treatment and transferred to paediatrics two days later in good medical condition without severe consequences or amputation need.

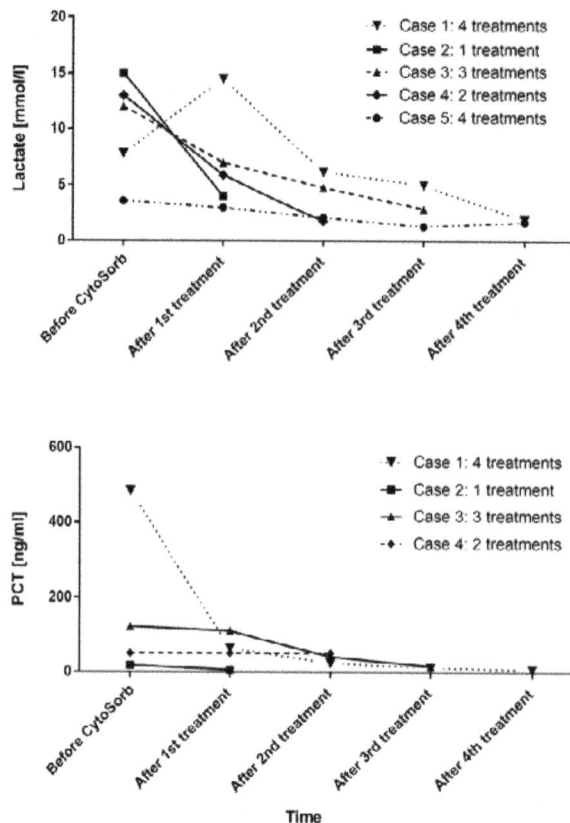

FIGURE 2: Course of lactate and PCT during Cytosorb treatment in all treated patients. PCT is not presented for Case 5 because it has not been measured with routine. Values are shown at the beginning of the treatment and after every treatment until the end.

2.5. Case 5. Case 5 is a 36-year-old female, showing a persistent fever, severe polymyalgia, and diffuse petechiae in expansion to the limbs and arms. Antibiotic therapy was started with levofloxacin (750 mg every 24h) and ceftriaxone (2 g every 12h). The patient was immediately transferred to ICU with a suspected diagnosis of sepsis secondary to meningitis. The patient presented hypotension, requiring the administration of norepinephrine at 0.5 μg/kg/min and dobutamine in the next day. Lab tests confirmed the diagnosis of bacterial meningitis infection caused by *Neisseria meningitidis* (Serotype C) and underlined a condition of thrombocytopenia, acute renal failure, and inflammation, initially monitored with CRP (17.5 mg/l). Lactate level was at 3.6 mmol/l. Immediately after the ICU admission, a CVVHDF treatment (Prismaflex, Oxiris, Baxter, USA) was started in combination with Cytosorb (start of treatment: 8h after ICU admission).

Within the course of hemoadsorption treatments, performed for a total of 96 hours, a hemodynamic stabilization was observed, associated with a reduction in need of inotrope drugs. Indeed, dobutamine could be stopped after 48h and norepinephrine after 78h. The course of norepinephrine is shown in Figure 1. The patient showed a stabilization lactate level, reduced at 1.7 mmol/l, as presented in Figure 2. Moreover, the inflammatory status was also monitored during Cytosorb treatment dosing IL-6 levels (Figure 3), directly adsorbed by the sorbent. After 12h of hemoperfusion, IL-6

values were 4.326 ng/ml and decreased dramatically during the course of treatments until 60.1 ng/ml after 60h and 35 ng/ml after 72h. Petechiae and skin lesions were stable already after the first day of treatment. A complete recovery of renal function and diuresis was observed after 9 days from the admission and the patient could be transferred to medicine after 7 days. The patient was followed by dermatologists and vascular surgeons for the outcome of the septic embolism complication, evaluating the possible amputation of one toe.

3. Discussion

Morbidity and mortality for bacterial meningitis and sepsis remain high [1–4]. The risk factors for a poor outcome, besides other medical conditions, include systemic compromise and a low level of consciousness. Importantly, outcome largely depends on rapid initiation of an effective empiric treatment [5–9]. Despite the necessity of early recognition of symptoms and the prompt administration of antibiotics, new adjunctive extracorporeal therapies [8, 9] focused on the control of the inflammatory response caused by pneumococcal and meningococcal bacteria would seem a reasonable approach [13–18].

These case reports appear to be among the first published applications of Cytosorb as an adjunctive treatment in the management of meningococcal and pneumococcal sepsis.

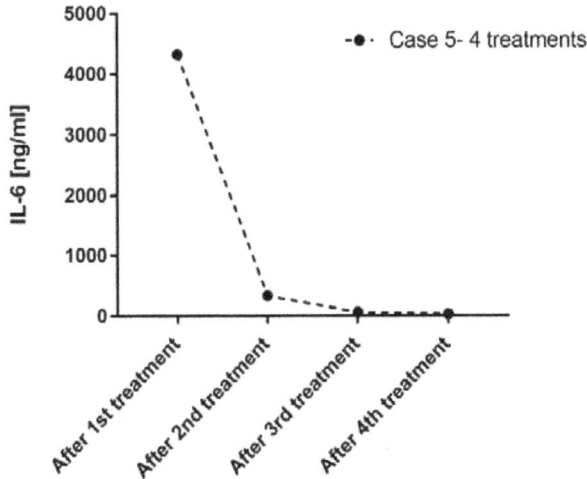

FIGURE 3: Course of IL-6 during Cytosorb treatment in Case 5. Values are shown after the first Cytosorb treatment, and then after every 24h until the end.

The combined treatment of CRRT and Cytosorb was well tolerated in all patients.

The main results to be drawn from our experiences are predominantly a progressive and clear stabilization in hemodynamics along with a rapid and marked reduction of catecholamine dosages (Figure 1). Moreover, we consistently recorded a stabilization in metabolic disorders as seen by a decrease in lactate levels (Figure 2). Except for one patient, dying after 2 months from a secondary septic episode, all patients survived. All the patients showed also a stabilization within normal range of coagulation parameters, showing an attenuation of the embolic septic status. Importantly, despite commonly occurring coagulation disorders leading to amputations, we noticed only minor loss of extremities in three patients (some phalanges and one toe) or even no need for an amputation in one patient.

Two of our patients had undergone splenectomy, one with a post-traumatic background and the other by elective surgery due to colonic metastases. While the first patient survived, the latter died. Importantly, hyposplenic patients are at high risk for overwhelming sepsis caused by pneumococcal bacteria [3].

The patients described herein have all been treated early between 8 and 24 hours after initial diagnosis. A prospective study performed on two ICUs over a period of 6 years in patients with acute community-acquired bacterial meningitis could show that the overall severity of the disease within 24 hours of admission may be the major indicator of adverse in-hospital clinical outcome [10].

A recently published case series underlined the more pronounced effects of Cytosorb treatment in septic shock patients when therapy was started within 24 hours of sepsis diagnosis. On the other hand, a delay in the start of therapy was associated with a poor response in terms of reduction of catecholamine demand and survival [13].

As underlined in literature [13–18], we performed each hemoadsorption treatment for 24 hours, except in two patients (cases 1 and 4) in which we changed the entire extracorporeal circuit after approximately 12 hours due to the severe coagulative disorders of the patients at the beginning. The continuation of the treatment was decided in function of the patient clinical improvement. In particular, the therapy was continued until catecholamine demand was stopped (cases 3, 4, and 5) or drastically decreased from the beginning of the treatment (cases 1 and 2) and an important reduction in lactate levels was observed (in all cases, lactate levels normalized around the reference limit value).

Overall, an improvement in hemodynamics seems to be one of the consistent key clinical benefits seen with this therapy, also confirmed in preclinical studies and published evidences [13–18].

Regarding the inflammatory response in these patients, pneumococcal and meningococcal compounds are extremely aggressive because of their polysaccharide capsule, letting them to escape from phagocytosis in blood and once recognized by specified receptors, they trigger an expression of inflammatory cytokines, chemokines, and reactive oxygen species [6]. Their excessive and uncontrolled action might have harmful effects and once they become systemic, sepsis with multiple organ failure might occur. Cutting off these high peak-plasma levels of several inflammatory mediators would be desirable [6–9].

Although cytokine levels were not recorded, except in one patient (Figure 3) which showed an impressive reduction of IL-6, as these types of measurements are not routine in all institutions, cytokine reduction may be at the background of the hemodynamic and metabolic improvements in all patients [13–18].

The inflammatory response modulation might have a benefit effect also on the coagulation status because it has been found that cytokines influence both procoagulant and anticoagulant pathways [6]. Therefore, their control might contribute to the recovery of homeostasis, in addition to the action on microcirculation, leading to an improvement in blood perfusion through blocked vessels [13–18].

All patients were empirically treated with broad-spectrum antibiotics and steroids without change in dosage.

4. Conclusion

To our knowledge, this is the first report on the successful use of hemoadsorption for cytokine removal therapy in a set of patients with meningococcal and pneumococcal sepsis. Effects associated with its application included a rapid and clear stabilization in hemodynamics along with a reduction in catecholamine dosages, a decrease in lactate as well as a less-than-expected loss of extremities. Therapy proved to be safe and well tolerated. After these promising initial data, a solid proof of efficiency is needed for the implementation in a larger context.

References

[1] D. van de Beek, M. C. Brouwer, G. E. Thwaites, and A. R. Tunkel, "Advances in treatment of bacterial meningitis," *The Lancet*, vol. 380, no. 9854, pp. 1693–1702, 2012.

[2] D. van de Beek, J. de Gans, A. R. Tunkel, and E. F. M. Wijdicks, "Community-acquired bacterial meningitis in adults," *The New England Journal of Medicine*, vol. 354, no. 1, pp. 44–53, 2006.

[3] S. Kastenbauer and H.-W. Pfister, "Pneumococcal meningitis in adults: Spectrum of complications and prognostic factors in a series of 87 cases," *Brain*, vol. 126, no. 5, pp. 1015–1025, 2003.

[4] R. Muralidharan, F. J. Mateen, and A. A. Rabinstein, "Outcome of fulminant bacterial meningitis in adult patients," *European Journal of Neurology*, vol. 21, no. 3, pp. 447–453, 2014.

[5] M. C. Brouwer, A. R. Tunkel, and D. van de Beek, "Epidemiology, diagnosis, and antimicrobial treatment of acute bacterial meningitis," *Clinical Microbiology Reviews*, vol. 23, no. 3, pp. 467–492, 2010.

[6] N. Pathan, S. N. Faust, and M. Levin, "Pathophysiology of meningococcal meningitis and septicaemia," *Archives of Disease in Childhood*, vol. 88, no. 7, pp. 601–607, 2003.

[7] D. van de Beek, J. de Gans, L. Spanjaard, M. Weisfelt, J. B. Reitsma, and M. Vermeulen, "Clinical features and prognostic factors in adults with bacterial meningitis," *The New England Journal of Medicine*, vol. 351, no. 18, pp. 1849–1859, 2004.

[8] R. Nau, M. Djukic, A. Spreer, and H. Eiffert, "Bacterial meningitis: New therapeutic approaches," *Expert Review of Anti-infective Therapy*, vol. 11, no. 10, pp. 1079–1095, 2013.

[9] T. Barichello, A. Collodel, J. S. Generoso et al., "Targets for adjunctive therapy in pneumococcal meningitis," *Journal of Neuroimmunology*, vol. 278, pp. 262–270, 2015.

[10] J. M. Flores-Cordero, R. Amaya-Villar, M. D. Rincón-Ferrari et al., "Acute community-acquired bacterial meningitis in adults admitted to the intensive care unit: Clinical manifestations, management and prognostic factors," *Intensive Care Medicine*, vol. 29, no. 11, pp. 1967–1973, 2003.

[11] M. Hoogman, D. van de Beek, M. Weisfelt, J. de Gans, and B. Schmand, "Cognitive outcome in adults after bacterial meningitis," *Journal of Neurology, Neurosurgery & Psychiatry*, vol. 78, no. 10, pp. 1092–1096, 2007.

[12] J. Thachil, "Disseminated Intravascular Coagulation: A Practical Approach," *Anesthesiology*, vol. 125, no. 1, pp. 230–236, 2016.

[13] K. Kogelmann, D. Jarczak, M. Scheller, and M. Drüner, "Hemoadsorption by CytoSorb in septic patients: A case series," *Critical Care*, vol. 21, no. 1, p. 74, 2017.

[14] K. Träger, C. Skrabal, and G. Fischer, "Hemoadsorption treatment of patients with acute infective endocarditis during surgery with cardiopulmonary bypass—A case series," *The International Journal of Artificial Organs*, vol. 40, no. 5, pp. 240–249, 2017.

[15] K. Träger, D. Fritzler, G. Fischer et al., "Treatment of post-cardiopulmonary bypass SIRS by hemoadsorption: A case series," *The International Journal of Artificial Organs*, vol. 39, no. 3, pp. 141–146, 2016.

[16] Z.-Y. Peng, M. J. Carter, and J. A. Kellum, "Effects of hemoadsorption on cytokine removal and short-term survival in septic rats," *Critical Care Medicine*, vol. 36, no. 5, pp. 1573–1577, 2008.

[17] B. Hinz, O. Jauch, T. Noky, S. Friesecke, P. Abel, and R. Kaiser, "CytoSorb, a novel therapeutic approach for patients with septic shock: a case report," *The International Journal of Artificial Organs*, vol. 38, no. 8, pp. 461–464, 2015.

[18] S. Friesecke, S.-S. Stecher, S. Gross, S. B. Felix, and A. Nierhaus, "Extracorporeal cytokine elimination as rescue therapy in refractory septic shock: a prospective single-center study," *The International Journal of Artificial Organs*, vol. 20, no. 3, pp. 252–259, 2017.

30

Fatal Heat Stroke in a Schizophrenic Patient

María Jesús Gómez Ramos,[1] Francisco Miguel González Valverde,[2] Carmen Sánchez Álvarez,[1] Lisa Ortin Katnich,[1] and Francisco Pastor Quirante[3]

[1] *Department of ICU, Reina Sofía General University Hospital, University of Murcia, 30.003 Murcia, Spain*
[2] *Department of Surgery, Reina Sofía General University Hospital, University of Murcia, 30.003 Murcia, Spain*
[3] *Department of Pathology, Reina Sofía General University Hospital, University of Murcia, 30.003 Murcia, Spain*

Correspondence should be addressed to F. Miguel González Valverde, migova@terra.es

Academic Editors: M. Egi, A. Grippo, H. Kern, and J. Starkopf

Objective. The case of a patient who developed a fatal post-exertional heat stroke is reported. *Case Report.* A 20-year-old man with a history of morbid obesity, hypertension, and schizophrenia was admitted to our intensive care unit because of multiorgan failure due to severe heat stroke. He had been working under the sun. Treatment included aggressive body cooling but, in spite of the best supportive care, the patient succumbed in a few hours. We concluded that the adverse event was possibly associated with his obesity and the use of antipsychotics. Histological evaluation revealed lesions consistent with severe hyperthermia and shock. *Conclusions.* Heat stroke is an uncommon clinical entity characterized by systemic heat and loss of the body's normal mechanisms for dealing with heat stress, such as sweating and temperature control. When heat stroke is diagnosed early and supportive care begins promptly the prognosis is optimal but it becomes a life-threatening disease when treatment is delayed. Lack of physical acclimatization and the use of certain medications that interfere with salt and water balance can impair thermoregulation under conditions of high environmental temperature. Health professionals must be adequately prepared to prevent, recognise, and treat them urgently.

1. Introduction

Heat stroke (HS) is a potentially life-threatening disease characterized by an extreme elevation of core body temperature and neurologic disorders resulting in delirium, convulsion, or coma [1]. It is usually the result of exposure to high environmental temperature and strenuous exercise. Although treatable and preventable, a substantial number of people die from extreme heat in Europe each year.

The most frequent cause of death directly attributable to heat is HS but heat conditions are known to aggravate chronic disorders and leads to increased all-cause mortality, specially circulatory and respiratory mortality. So, the reported incidence of heat-related mortality is imprecise and grossly underdiagnosed in specific risk groups as the elderly, those with chronic medical diseases or morbid obesity, and the socially isolated [2].

2. Case Report

In late May 2008, a man aged 20 years was working in a field in Murcia (south-eastern Spain) for 4 hours in 30°C heat. He had a history of arterial hypertension, morbid obesity, and schizophrenia. His medications included risperidone 6 mg, biperiden hydrochloride, and enalapril 20 mg daily. At 4 pm he complained of dizziness and headache. After about 10 minutes he came running out in a highly agitated state and suddenly collapsed. The patient stayed under direct sunlight during approximately 2 hours until emergencies arrived and found him moaning and unresponsive (Glasgow Coma Scale 7: E2, V2, M3), with eye deviation, and breathless. His skin felt very hot and dry, blood pressure was 80/25 mmHg, pulse rate 176 bpm, and his axillary temperature—which underestimates core temperature—39.6°C. The patient was given intravenous fluids, intubated, rapidly cooled, and transported to our hospital, 50 minutes away.

On arrival to the ICU the patient was deeply sedated and still hypotensive (50/20 mm Hg). At this time his rectal temperature was 41.8°C. Electrocardiogram revealed sinus tachycardia with diffuse subendocardial lesion in ST; serum levels of myocardial markers were remarkably high and diffuse hypokinesis was observed on the echocardiogram. Chest X-ray was compatible with an early pulmonary edema. The cerebral CT scan did not reveal any pathology and, to exclude an infectious origin, a lumbar puncture was performed yielding normal cerebrospinal fluid.

Laboratory results revealed severe acidosis (pH 7.11, PCO2 70 mmHg, HCO3 17) and abnormal serum levels: creatinine (2.6 mg/dL) as well as blood urea nitrogen (BUN: 30 mg/dL) were elevated indicating the beginning of renal failure. Sodium was 138 mmol/L, potassium 4.6 mmol/L and chloride 115 mmol/L. Haematology analysis presented low platelet count (41.000) and severe alteration of coagulation levels (prothrombin time 13%, partial thromboplastin time >200 sec, INR 737, and fibrinogen 70). Hematocrit was 52.9%, hemoglobin 189 g/L, and leukocyte count 28400 (58% neutrophils and 12% band cells).

During the first hours, temperature control methods were continued with intravenous cold fluid infusion, vitamin K, sodium bicarbonate 1 molar, platelet, and fresh frozen plasma therapy. Conventional external cooling devices such as cooling blankets, cold compresses, and fans, warm water sprayed, and a gastric irrigation with cold water did not lead to any significant decrease in body temperature.

One hour of intensive care later, core body temperature was 39°C. The patient started bleeding by venous access and gastrointestinal tube. Because of subsequent deterioration of the patient's condition and insufficient temperature control, use of vasopressors (noradrenaline) and hemodynamic monitoring with pulmonary artery catheter was required. Despite aggressive therapy, multiorgan dysfunction syndrome with anuria and disseminated intravascular coagulopathy developed and the patient died 9 hours after his access to ICU.

In the autopsy, severe superficial skin burns with epidermal loss were observed on groin, neck, trunk, axillae, and other non-exposure areas (Figure 1). The lungs, the larynx, and the high respiratory airways were heavily congested and hemorrhagic (Figure 2). Histological study also revealed moderate brain edema, necrosis of the renal tubules, subendocardial necrosis (Figure 3), numerous petechial haemorrhages, and generalized visceral congestion. The underlying cause of death was heat stroke.

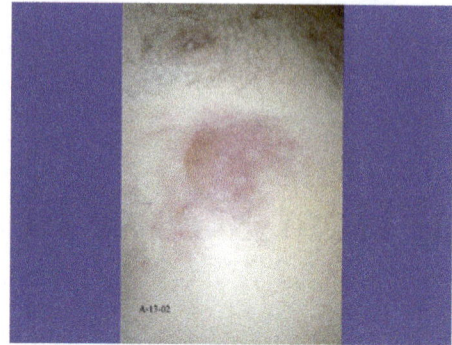

FIGURE 1: Superficial burn blisters with epidermal loss on non-exposure areas.

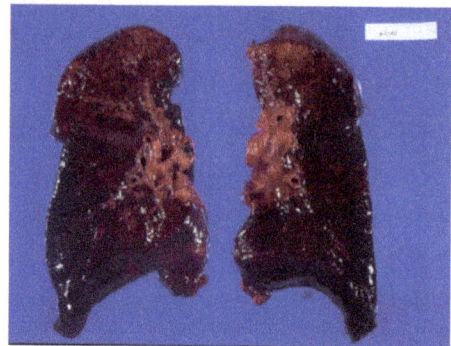

FIGURE 2: The lungs were heavily congested and hemorrhagic.

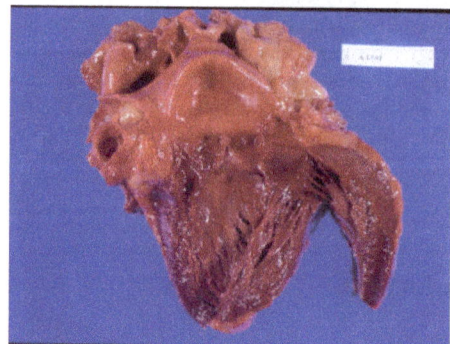

FIGURE 3: Heart specimen showing acute subendocardial-myocardial infarction.

3. Discussion

The incidence of heat-related disorders is higher during the summer but it can also occur in moderate conditions, depending on environmental factors, age, and the use of several drugs (Table 1). The continuum of classic heat-related illnesses includes mild disease (heat edema, rash, cramps, syncope), heat exhaustion, and the most severe form, heat stroke. The last two situations are commonly treated in critical care units because of the highest risk of morbid-mortality. Clinically HS is distinguished from heat exhaustion by disturbances of the central nervous system, usually prolonged unconsciousness and coma often preceded by confusion, delirium, ataxia, or convulsions [3, 4].

Although HS has been classically documented as a medical condition, a universally accepted definition is lacking because its pathophysiology is not fully understood. It must be considered in anyone who presents with hyperthermia (exceeding 40°C) and altered mental status. Despite adequate hypothermia or other care-therapy, permanent neurological damage occurs in approximately 20% of patients and the mortality rate may be as high as 10 to 80% [1, 4–6].

TABLE 1: Conditons contributing to the risk of heat illness.

	Risk factors	Mechanism
Physical conditions	Prolonged exertion	
	Fever	
	Dehydration	
Medications	Drugs of abuse: amphetamines, heroine, cocaine, LSD, ethanol.	Increase endogenous heat production
	Anticholinergic: tricyclic antidepressants, antispasmodics and phenothiazides.	Disrupt hypothalamic function and reduce sweating
	Beta-adrenergic and Calcium channel blockers	Inhibit the compensatory increase in cardiac output
	Diuretics	Produce a relative state of dehydration that affects central thermoregulation and sweating
	Others: antiparkinsonian agents, antihistamines	
Chronic illness	Cardiac conditions	
	Cystic fibrosis	
	Extensive skin disease	
	Hyperthyroidism	
	Psychiatric conditions	
Older age		

TABLE 2

Characteristic	Classic	Exertional
Health condition	Predisposing factors	Healthy
Age	Elderly	Younger
Conditions	High environmental temp	Occurs sporadically
Sweating	Usually absent	Present
Activity	Sedentary	Strenuous
Disseminated intravascular coagulation	Mild	Marked
Acute renal failure	<5% patients	25–30% patients
Lactic acidosis	Rare	Common
Hyperuricemia	Moderate	Severe
Hypocalcemia	Rare	Common
Hypoglycaemia	Rare	Common
Hypokalemia	Rare	Common
Rhabdomyolysis	Rare	Common
CPK	Mildly elevated	Marked elevated
Mechanism	Poor dissipation of environmental heat	Excessive endogenous heat production

Information from [3, 8].

Hyperpyrexia and neurologic dysfunction are necessary but not sufficient to diagnose HS. Associated clinical manifestations such as extreme fatigue and flu-like symptoms; hot dry skin or heavy perspiration; nausea; vomiting; diarrhea; disorientation; dizziness; uncoordinated movements; reddened face are frequently observed (Table 2). Clinical signs of dehydration and salt depletion are almost always present in the form of tachycardia, hypotension, and diaphoresis. Potential complications related to severe HS are acute renal failure, disseminated intravascular coagulation, rhabdomyolysis, acute respiratory distress syndrome, acid-base disorders, and electrolyte disturbances [4, 7, 8]. Above 42.4°C, thermal damage becomes critical, oxidative phosphorylation becomes uncoupled, proteins denature inducing changes in

TABLE 3: Heat illness.

	Edema	Cramps	Tetany	Syncope	Exhaustion	Stroke
Symptoms	Minimal clinical significance but important interstitial fluid accumulation	Cramps	Cramps, carpopedal spasm, and perioral and distal paresthesias	Nausea, sighing, yawning, restlessness, and orthostatic syncope	Flulike	Flulike
Central nervous system symptoms	NO	NO	NO	NO	NO	Present
Temperature	<41°C	<41°C	<41°C	<41°C	<41°C	>41°C
Sweating	Present	Present	Present	Present	Present	Absent
Mechanism	Unacclimatisation, peripheral vasodilatation	Unacclimatisation and negative sodium balance	Unacclimatisation and severe negative sodium balance	Unacclimatisation, dehydration and inadequate cardiac output	Excess sweating in a hot humid environment causing volume depletion	Heat production exceeds dissipation
Treatment	Periodic exercise, elevation of the legs, or diuretic medication	Oral sodium replacement	Oral or parenteral sodium replacement	Placing supine position, and replacing water deficit	Cool area to rest, placing supine position and replacing water deficit	Emergency treatment

the membrane fluidity, and enzyme systems are affected [4]. HS resembles sepsis in many aspects, and endotoxemia and cytokines may be implicated in its pathogenesis [1, 9, 10].

Two forms of HS are recognized (Table 3): classic (no exertional), usually occurring in elderly persons with chronic illnesses, children, the obese, and those receiving medications such as diuretics, antipsychotics, antihypertensives, and antidepressants; exertional HS, more common in physically active individuals who develop a strenuous and exceptional exercise [3, 6, 8–10].

In our case the patient was a morbidly obese subject that intook antipsychotics and antihypertensives, practising a strenuous activity at sunshine, and accompanied by inadequate fluid intake. Clinical manifestation was sudden and concurrent with exertional type but he had no sweating and hypoglycaemia, presenting several characteristics of the classic type. Certain drugs may induce or worsen heat-related illnesses. Drugs with anticholinergic effects can inhibit sweating and reduce heat elimination. Neuroleptics and tranquillizers, such as phenothiazines, have combined anticholinergic and central thermoregulatory effects. The set point of the temperature regulation centre can be elevated by the antidopaminergic effect of antipsychotics, such as phenothiazines and thioxanthenes [11–13].

The diagnosis of HS is suspected in the presence of a markedly elevated temperature and changes in mental status following heat exposure. Medical work-up include chest X-ray, electrocardiogram, and lab work with a complete blood count, electrolytes, BUN and creatinine, liver enzymes, creatine kinase, prothrombin time and partial thromboplastin time, arterial blood gasses, and urinalysis. The differential diagnosis includes hyperthyroid storm, pheochromocytoma, central nervous system injury, infection, anticholinergic poisoning, drug ingestion, and neuroleptic malignant syndrome [3].

In autopsy, edema of the brain, leptomeninges, petechial haemorrhages, and neuronal degeneration may be observed. The cardiovascular system may show right heart dilatation, pericardial effusion, edema, degeneration, and necrosis of myocardial fibres. Pulmonary infarction and high airways submucosal haemorrhages have also been described. The kidneys are enlarged with numerous petechial haemorrhages as well as the gastrointestinal submucosa. The liver may be congestive but structural injuries are infrequently found. Skin scalds with different depth degree on non-exposure areas and rigid and contracted muscles with necrosis of fibres are possible [14–16].

Assuming that HS is an acute life threatening emergency, the prognosis can be greatly improved if the symptoms are recognised early and emergency measures are instituted promptly. The prognosis is poorest when treatment is delayed >2 hours [10, 17, 18]. Early management should include the use of cold water or watersoaked towels, support of organ-system function, fluid resuscitation and electrolyte replacement if possible, and immediate transfer to a hospital. Aggressive cooling measures should be continued until the core temperature reaches 39°C. There is controversy regarding which cooling techniques are most effective. A combination of cold-water immersion and evaporative methods (spraying the body with atomised 15°C water and warmed air) is the best option for treatment [19, 20]. Other methods include ice packs placed over the axilla, groin, and neck. Disadvantages include peripheral vasoconstriction that retard heat loss; induced shivering, resulting in increased internal heat generation. If shivering does occur, medications as meperidine and diazepam can inhibit it; extreme discomfort to patients and medical attendants; difficulty in monitoring and resuscitating vital signs of patient [8, 20]. Internal methods for cooling as cold water irrigation to the stomach or rectum may be used but only in addition to external cooling methods [20]. Peritoneal lavage and cardiopulmonary bypass in severe cases have been advocated but their clinic efficacy is debated.

The use of pharmacological agents as antipyretics or steroids is not helpful in the treatment of HS. The hypothalamic setpoint is not elevated as it is in fever so that aspirin and acetaminophen are ineffective; furthermore aspirin is contraindicated for its effect on platelets and clotting [1, 4, 8]. Supportive cares are necessary and respiratory, neurologic, and cardiac status must be specially monitored [21]. In a comatose patient, a cuffed endotracheal tube should be placed to protect the airway as respiratory assistance is indicated. Invariably a venous access to replace fluids is required even if the patient is not hypotensive. Furthermore hemodynamic monitoring with pulmonary artery catheter may be indicated. This technique helps us for fluidotherapy management and vasopressors drugs if hypotension is not controlled well. Other aspects of monitoring include urine output measurement as indicator of acute renal failure.

Due to the risk and the prognosis, the best treatment is prevention. It requires awareness of risk factors and appropriate hydration.

4. Conclusions

Heat stroke is a true medical emergency requiring immediate admission to an intensive care unit. Early recognition and management with aggressive measures to lower the body temperature with other supportive therapies can substantially reduce the mortality. Emergency departments and public health agencies should be adequately prepared to prevent, suspect, and manage heat-related illnesses, especially during heat waves.

Abbreviations

HS: Heat stroke
pm: Post meridiem
bpm: Beats per minute.

References

[1] A. Bouchama and J. P. Knochel, "Medical progress: heat stroke," *The New England Journal of Medicine*, vol. 346, no. 25, pp. 1978–1988, 2002.

[2] G. M. Varghese, G. John, K. Thomas, O. C. Abraham, and D. Mathai, "Predictors of multi-organ dysfunction in heatstroke," *Emergency Medicine Journal*, vol. 22, no. 3, pp. 185–187, 2005.

[3] M. W. Barrow and K. A. Clark, "Heat-related illnesses," *American Family Physician*, vol. 58, no. 3, pp. 749–756, 1998.

[4] T. A. Waters, "Heat illness: tips for recognition and treatment," *Cleveland Clinic Journal of Medicine*, vol. 68, no. 8, pp. 685–687, 2001.

[5] Centers for Disease Control, "Heat-related illness and deaths—United States, 1994-1995," *Morbidity and Mortality Weekly Report (MMWR)*, vol. 44, pp. 465–468.

[6] J. E. Dematte, K. O'Mara, J. Buescher et al., "Near-fatal heat stroke during the 1995 heat wave in Chicago," *Annals of Internal Medicine*, vol. 129, no. 3, pp. 173–181, 1998.

[7] A. S. Howe and B. P. Boden, "Heat-related illness in athletes," *American Journal of Sports Medicine*, vol. 35, no. 8, pp. 1384–1395, 2007.

[8] R. Khosla and K. K. Guntupalli, "Heat-related illnesses," *Critical Care Clinics*, vol. 15, no. 2, pp. 251–262, 1999.

[9] K. C. Lu, J. Y. Wang, S. H. Lin, P. Chu, and Y. F. Lin, "Role of circulating cytokines and chemokines in exertional heatstroke," *Critical Care Medicine*, vol. 32, no. 2, pp. 399–403, 2004.

[10] H. Grogan and P. M. Hopkins, "Heat stroke: implications for critical care and anaesthesia," *British Journal of Anaesthesia*, vol. 88, no. 5, pp. 700–707, 2002.

[11] J. S. S. Kwok and T. Y. K. Chan, "Recurrent heat-related illnesses during antipsychotic treatment," *Annals of Pharmacotherapy*, vol. 39, no. 11, pp. 1940–1942, 2005.

[12] K. Martin-Latry, M. P. Goumy, P. Latry et al., "Psychotropic drugs use and risk of heat-related hospitalisation," *European Psychiatry*, vol. 22, no. 6, pp. 335–338, 2007.

[13] T. H. Reilly and M. A. Kirk, "Atypical antipsychotics and newer antidepressants," *Emergency Medicine Clinics of North America*, vol. 25, no. 2, pp. 477–497, 2007.

[14] J. P. Knochel, W. R. Beisel, E. G. Herndon, E. S. Gerard, and K. G. Barry, "The renal, cardiovascular, hematologic and serum electrolyte abnormalities of heat stroke," *The American Journal of Medicine*, vol. 30, no. 2, pp. 299–309, 1961.

[15] M. Rav-Acha, E. Hadad, Y. Epstein, Y. Heled, and D. S. Moran, "Fatal exertional heart stroke: a case series," *American Journal of the Medical Sciences*, vol. 328, no. 2, pp. 84–87, 2004.

[16] K. Niizato, K. Tsuchiya, K. Oshima et al., "An autopsied case of schizophrenic patient who died from heat stroke," *No To Shinkei*, vol. 58, no. 5, pp. 418–424, 2006.

[17] J. L. Glazer, "Management of heatstroke and heat exhaustion," *American Family Physician*, vol. 71, no. 11, pp. 2133–2140, 2005.

[18] T. P. Yeo, "Heat stroke: a comprehensive review," *AACN Clinical Issues*, vol. 15, no. 2, pp. 280–293, 2004.

[19] J. S. Weiner and M. Khogali, "A physiological body-cooling unit for treatment of heat stroke," *The Lancet*, vol. 1, no. 8167, pp. 507–509, 1980.

[20] T. L. Lee-Chiong and J. T. Stitt, "Heatstroke and other heat-related illnesses: the maladies of summer," *Postgraduate Medicine*, vol. 98, no. 1, pp. 26–36, 1995.

[21] S. H. Chen, F. M. Chang, H. K. Chang, W. C. Chen, K. F. Huang, and M. T. Lin, "Human umbilical cord blood-derived CD34+ cells cause attenuation of multiorgan dysfunction during experimental heatstroke," *Shock*, vol. 27, no. 6, pp. 663–671, 2007.

31

Bilateral Cerebrovascular Stroke as an Initial Presenting Symptom of Moyamoya Disease

Ester Ilyayeva ⓘ**, Khaled Nada** ⓘ**, Roxane Farahi Far, Kamal Albright,
Manmeet Kaur Gujral, and Menachem Gold**

Lincoln Medical and Mental Health Center, 234 E 149Th St., Bronx, NY 10451, USA

Correspondence should be addressed to Ester Ilyayeva; ilyayeve1@nychhc.org

Academic Editor: Kurt Lenz

Moyamoya disease is a rare condition affecting the circle of Willis and its branching arteries. While the pathogenesis is unclear, it causes progressive occlusion of multiple cerebral vessels leading to severe strokes. We report a case of a 47-year-old Hispanic woman with HTN presented with altered mental status and bilateral upper and lower extremity weakness with dystonic-like upper extremity movement. Serial brain CTs and angiography were performed which showed massive frontal and parietal cerebral infarcts with radiological evidence of moyamoya disease.

1. Introduction

Bilateral cerebroocclusive events occurring simultaneously are extremely rare and are often due to an alternative underlying etiology. Moyamoya is a rare progressive cerebrovascular disease that presents as a hemorrhagic or ischemic event in adults. Moyamoya is a chronic cerebral vasculopathy first described in 1957 by Takeuchi and Shimizu. It is characterized by chronic worsening occlusion of the arteries of the circle of Willis leading to the development of abnormal collateral vessels. The term "moyamoya" refers to the appearance of the collateral vessels that resemble a "puff of smoke" in Japanese. While computed tomography (CT), MRI-angiography, or ultrasonography may be used as diagnostic tools, the gold standard for visualizing the collateral circulation network characteristic of moyamoya disease is conventional angiography. Here we present a patient with bilateral infarction of the ACA and left MCA with a network of collateral vessels consistent with moyamoya disease.

2. Case Presentation

A 47-year-old female with a past medical history of hypertension presented to the emergency department at Lincoln Hospital, Bronx, New York, with altered mental status. As per the patient's daughter, she was found confused in the bathroom, with last well known time eight hours prior to her presentation. Upon examination in the emergency department, she appeared altered, nonverbal, but responsive to painful stimuli, involuntarily opening and closing her eyes, and able to protect her airway. The patient was afebrile, tachycardic to 130 with a blood pressure of 140/90. Neurological exam was remarkable for left gaze preference, spasticity of all extremities, bilateral lower extremity hyperreflexia, occasional myoclonus, and positive Babinski sign bilaterally. She was also noted to be moving all extremities purposelessly. All labs were normal including complete blood count, basic metabolic panel, creatinine kinase, and troponin. Serum levels of salicylate, acetaminophen, carbamazepine, lithium, valproic acid, and alcohol were negative, and urine toxicology screen was also negative for any illicit drugs. EKG showed normal sinus rhythm.

Initial brain CT was negative for hemorrhage or any infarcts [Figure 1]. A few hours later, the patient became more lethargic, unable to protect her airway, and, given the high risk for aspiration, she was intubated and admitted to the medical ICU. Lumbar puncture was done and CSF analysis was negative for bacterial meningitis, as well as CMV, HSV

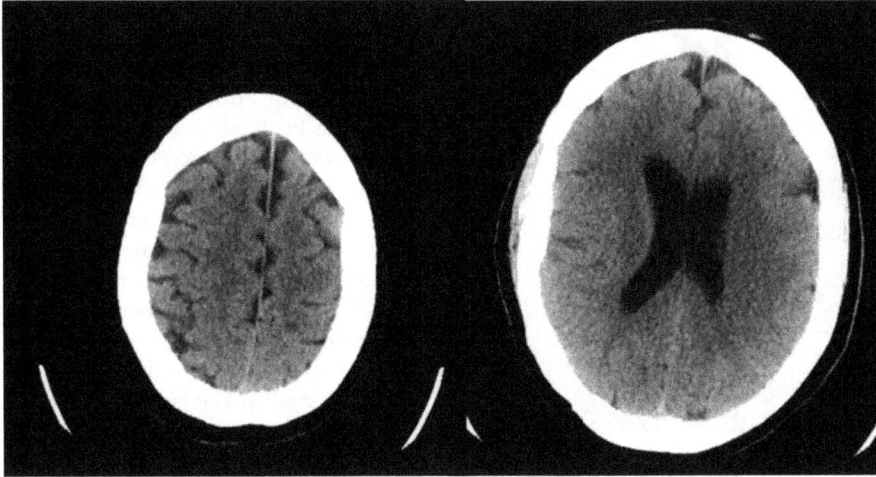

FIGURE 1: Brain CT on presentation.

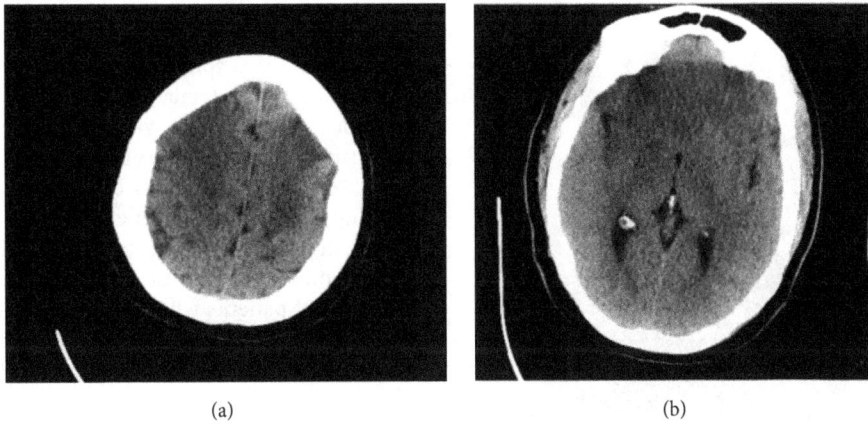

(a)

(b)

FIGURE 2: Axial CT images demonstrating bilateral large areas of hypoattenuation consistent with acute MCA and ACA infarcts.

PCR, toxoplasma, west Nile virus, and oligoclonal bands. She had a repeat CT the next day that demonstrated large areas of low attenuation in both cerebral hemispheres consistent with acute ACA and MCA infarcts [Figures 2(a) and 2(b)]. In view of the patient's presentation and absence of classical stroke risk factors, CT angiography and vasculitis work-up were sent including ANA, c-ANCA, p-ANCA, ESR, CRP, antiphospholipid antibodies, Factor V Leiden, prothrombin gene mutation, protein C, protein S, cryoglobulins, and complement C3 and C4 levels. Results of the vasculitis workup were negative, excluding vasculitis as a cause for her presentation.

Brain CT angiography was remarkable for acute bilateral ACA and large right MCA territory infarcts. The intracranial segments of the ICA were diffusely decreased in caliber; there was a complete occlusion of the right MCA from its origin and at least moderate stenosis of the M1 and M2 segments of the left MCA. ACAs were patent but diffusely decreased in caliber, and prominent lenticulostriate vessels were noted in the basal ganglia bilaterally [Figures 3 and 4]. Repeat brain CT the next day showed worsening edema with mass effect

on the lateral ventricle and midline shift; thus neurosurgery was consulted and the patient had a left hemicraniectomy. However, mental status remained poor; the patient had a tracheostomy and percutaneous endoscopic gastrostomy and was transferred to a long-term acute care facility.

3. Discussion

Acute cerebrovascular events typically present as a constellation of unilateral neurological deficits coinciding to the appropriate unilateral ischemic event. Simultaneous bilateral cerebrovascular infarction is relatively rare [1]. Bilateral ACA territory infarction can be due to vasospasm that occurs as a complication of subarachnoid hemorrhage [2]. Rarer causes of bilateral cerebrovascular infarction can include rupture of an aneurysm of the ACA, thrombus of the precommunicating part of the ACA with an agenesis of the contralateral part [3], or the result of an anomalous unilateral cerebral artery that can mimic a space-occupying lesion [1]. Although transient ischemic attacks (TIAs) and cerebrovascular accidents (CVAs) can typically present with

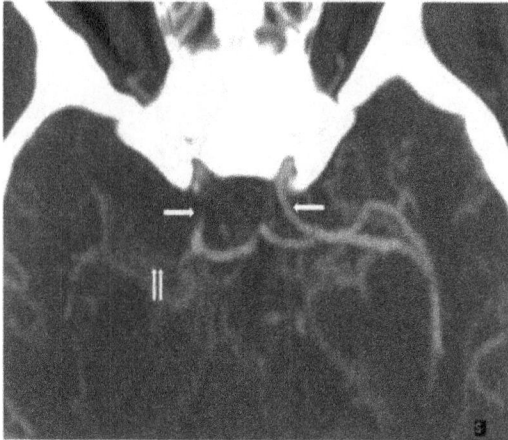

FIGURE 3: Maximum intensity projection (MIP) axial image of the CT angiogram demonstrates severe stenosis of the internal carotid arteries (single arrows) and occlusion of the Rt, MCA (double arrows).

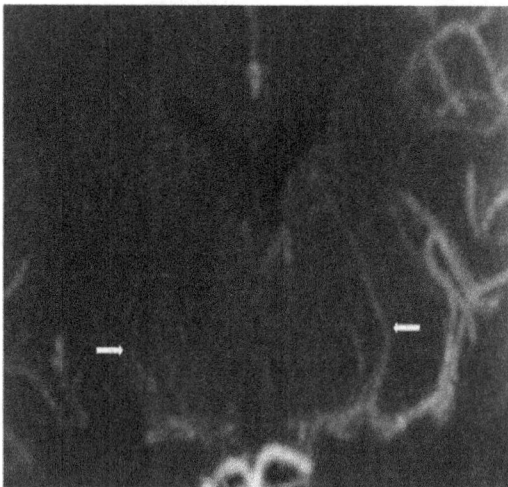

FIGURE 4: Coronal MIP demonstrates prominent lenticulostriate collaterals in the basal ganglia (arrows).

bilateral symptoms as in moyamoya disease, they are not typical. Moyamoya disease in adults commonly presents as either hemorrhagic or ischemic events with ischemic events as the most common presentation in children and adults [4]. Moyamoya disease tends to have a bimodal age distribution affecting children at around 10 years of age and adults aged 30-40 years [5]. In addition to TIA and CVA's, patients with moyamoya disease can present with seizures, headaches, and cognitive impairment. Patients also have a tendency to develop repeated TIAs when they are hyperventilating possibly due to vasodilation of normal vessels and subsequent hypoperfusion in a vulnerable area via steal phenomenon [5]. It is imperative to rule out similar cerebrovascular lesions such as meningitis, brain tumors, TBIs, autoimmune diseases, etc. Diagnosis of moyamoya is a challenge itself due to the rarity of the disease and inclusion criteria as outlined by the

research committee on spontaneous occlusion of the circle of Willis (moyamoya disease). The challenge is evident in the acute setting with an initial presentation of symptoms not typical for stroke, as the distribution of neurological deficit was bilateral. An angiogram is recommended at this stage to evaluate intracranial stenosis for possible neurointervention, though it is still controversial. In the SAMM-PRIS trial, patients with recent TIA/CVA with intracranial arterial stenosis were questioned if they would benefit with percutaneous transluminal angioplasty and stenting (PTAS) in addition to aggressive medical therapy. Those with PTAS were associated with an increased risk of recurrent stroke when compared to medical therapy alone [6]. Surgical bypass or intracranial angioplasty may offer additional treatment options for moyamoya in the future, though its current efficacy in clinical practice is limited [7].

4. Conclusion

Moyamoya disease is a rare clinical syndrome that requires a high index of suspicion to detect. This case presentation outlines an atypical bilateral presentation for an evolving ischemic stroke, with moyamoya disease as the most likely diagnosis. Our findings suggest that, in addition to vasculitis, toxic, and infectious etiologies, moyamoya ischemic pathology should be considered as the cause for a patient to present with altered mental status, sudden onset bilateral upper motor neurological exam findings, and aphasia. We propose that patients with similar presentations be evaluated with an early angiography for evaluation for possible neurointervention, though evidence is currently thin.

References

[1] B. F. Menezes, B. Cheserem, J. Kandasamy, and D. O'Brien, "Acute bilateral anterior circulation stroke due to anomalous cerebral vasculature: A case report," *Journal of Medical Case Reports*, vol. 2, no. 1, 2008.

[2] G. Orlandi, P. Moretti, C. Fioretti, M. Puglioli, P. Collavoli, and L. Murri, "Bilateral medial frontal infarction in a case of azygous anterior cerebral artery stenosis," *Italian Journal of Neurological Sciences*, vol. 19, no. 2, pp. 106–108, 1998.

[3] F. Borggreve, P. P. De Deyn, P. Mariën, P. Cras, and R. A. Dierckx, "Bilateral infarction in the anterior cerebral artery vascular territory due to an unusual anomaly of the circle of willis," *Stroke*, vol. 25, no. 6, pp. 1279–1281, 1994.

[4] P. H. Janda, J. G. Bellew, and V. Veerappan, "Moyamoya disease: case report and literature review," *The Journal of the American Osteopathic Association*, vol. 109, no. 10, pp. 547–553, 2009.

[5] J. S. Kim, "Moyamoya disease: Epidemiology, clinical features, and diagnosis," *Journal of Stroke*, vol. 18, no. 1, pp. 2–11, 2016.

[6] Stenting and Aggressive Medical Management for Preventing Recurrent Stroke in Intracranial Stenosis Trial Investigators,

"Mechanisms of stroke after intracranial angioplasty and stenting in the SAMMPRIS trial," *Neurosurgery*, vol. 72, no. 5, pp. 777–795, 2013.

[7] R. Shastri, N. Chaudhary, A. Pandey, C. Roark, B. Thompson, and J. Gemmete, "E-048 moya moya syndrome: evaluation and treatment in patients with inflammatory conditions causing a puff of smoke," *Journal of NeuroInterventional Surgery*, vol. 7, pp. A63–A64, 2015.

32

Meningococcemia Presenting as a Myocardial Infarction

Daniel Lachant and David Trawick

Division of Pulmonary and Critical Care Medicine, University of Rochester Medical Center, 601 Elmwood Avenue, Rochester, NY 14624, USA

Correspondence should be addressed to Daniel Lachant; daniel_lachant@urmc.rochester.edu

Academic Editor: Chiara Lazzeri

Neisseria meningitidis is an encapsulated gram negative diplococcus that colonizes the nasopharynx and is transmitted by aerosol or secretions with the majority of cases occurring in infants and adolescents. Meningococcemia carries a high mortality which is in part due to myocarditis. Early recognition and prompt use of antibiotics improve morbidity and mortality. We report a 55-year-old male presenting to the emergency department with chest pain, shortness of breath, and electrocardiogram changes suggestive of ST elevation MI who developed cardiogenic shock and multisystem organ failure from *N. meningitidis*. We present this case to highlight the unique presentation of meningococcemia, the association with myocardial dysfunction, and the importance of early recognition and prompt use of antibiotics.

1. Introduction

Neisseria meningitidis is an encapsulated gram negative diplococcus that normally colonizes the nasopharynx of humans and is transmitted by aerosol or secretions [1]. The annual incidence of meningococcal infections is estimated at 1,500–3,000 cases per year in the United States, typically occurring in the late winter and early spring [1]. Although infants and adolescents account for the majority of cases, adults over thirty comprise up to 30% of infections [1, 2]. Risk factors for infection acquisition include terminal complement deficiency, immune deficiencies, crowded living spaces [1], eculizumab [3], and asplenia [4]. Mortality ranges from 9% to as high as 40% in meningococcemia [1]. Myocarditis has been associated with meningococcemia in both children and adults and is associated with increased mortality [5, 6]. We report a unique case of meningococcemia presenting as chest pain and ST elevations on ECG mimicking an acute anterior myocardial infarction without any preceding infectious symptoms in a 55-year-old male.

2. Case

A 55-year-old male with history of smoking and substance abuse presented to the emergency department (ED) with acute onset worsening chest pain and shortness of breath of 18-hour duration. He had no complaints of subjective fever, cough, sputum production, sweats, neck pain, or headache. On presentation, his core temperature by Foley catheter was 35.7°C, blood pressure 110/80 mmHg, respiratory rate 28 breaths per minute, heart rate 134 beats per minute, and hemoglobin saturation on 100% oxygen 95%. He was noted to be anxious and to have cool mottled skin; the remainder of his exam was benign. His initial ECGs performed by EMS and in the emergency department, respectively, demonstrated atrial fibrillation with a rapid rate and ST elevation in V1–V3 (Figure 1). The Myocardial Infarction Team was called as there was concern that the patient was experiencing an acute anterior ST elevation myocardial infarction. He was taken for emergent rescue percutaneous intervention before his initial blood work came back. The left heart catheterization revealed no obstructing lesion, no dissection, and an ejection fraction of 20%; his echo from one year previously demonstrated a normal ejection fraction. A concomitant right heart catheterization (RHC) revealed a right atrial pressure of 15 mmHg, a pulmonary artery occlusion pressure of 28 mmHg, systemic vascular resistance of 1172 dynes/sec/cm^5, and a cardiac index of 2.68 liters per minute per meter squared. The pulmonary artery catheter was not left in and his hemodynamic parameters were not trended.

(a)

(b)

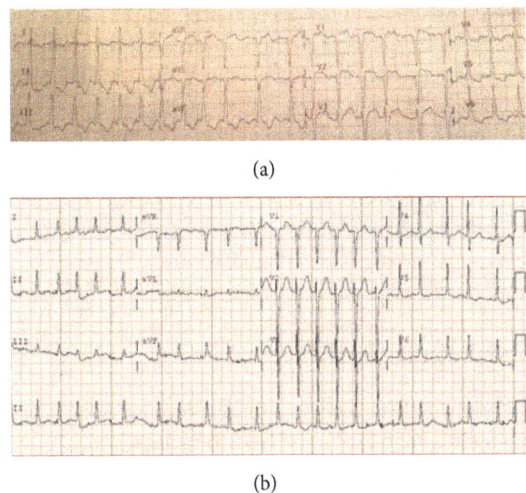

FIGURE 1: (a) Electrocardiogram from EMS showing ST elevation in V1–V3 with ST depressions in V4–V6, I, II, II, and AVF in the setting of chest pain. (b) Electrocardiogram 3 days later with resolution of ST changes.

During the catheterization the initial labs drawn in the ED returned. The arterial blood gas was 7.21/34/161, serum lactate 6.6 millimoles/L, troponin <0.01 ng/mL (it was not trended but on day 2 it was 1.26 ng/mL), bicarbonate 14 millimoles/L, creatinine 2.17 mg/dL, INR 2.4, aPTT 52.5, fibrinogen 103 mg/deciliter, white blood cell count 7,900/μL (with 14% bands), hemoglobin level 12.1 g/dL, and platelets count 17,000/microliter.

There was now concern for severe sepsis of unknown etiology, and vancomycin, piperacillin-tazobactam, and azithromycin were initiated 3 hours after admission. Five hours after the antibiotic administration, the patient developed refractory hypotension despite fluid resuscitation. Vasopressors were initiated including norepinephrine (peaking at 70 mcg/min within 12 hours of starting), vasopressin 0.04 units/min was started after norepinephrine reached 30 mcg/min (this is the dosing used at our institution, and it is not titrated), and hydrocortisone 50 mg was given every 6 hours. He subsequently developed respiratory failure shortly after vasopressors were started and was intubated. A CT chest/abdomen/pelvis showed possible multifocal pneumonia versus pulmonary edema. A gram stain of his sputum after antibiotics initiation revealed a few gram negative diplococci and gram positive cocci. Sixteen hours after presentation, his echocardiogram now showed global biventricular systolic dysfunction with an ejection fraction of 18% and cardiac index calculated to be 1.32. The patient developed persistent metabolic acidosis requiring high bicarbonate and calcium infusions. Following consultation with nephrology, the MICU team initiated continuous venovenous hemodialysis to better address the evolving acute renal failure, hypocalcemia, and metabolic acidosis.

Within 24 hours after admission one blood culture turned positive for gram negative diplococci eventually identified as *Neisseria meningitidis* Group A. High dose ceftriaxone was added and continued for 10 days. An LP was never performed

due to his coagulopathy and hemodynamic instability. CT and MRI of his head did not show evidence of infection or bleed. Vasopressors were weaned off in 4 days and steroids were stopped 6 days after presentation, respectively.

By day 11, a repeat echocardiogram revealed that his ejection fraction had improved to 42% and a month later it went back to 55%. After his critical illness resolved he returned and remained in normal sinus rhythm. The areas of mottling on admission were demarcated at both hands and all of his toes developing gangrene ultimately requiring left transmetatarsal amputation, left transradial amputation, and partial right hand amputation. After working with physical therapy he is able to ambulate and requires assistance with activities of daily living. His renal function never recovered and he remains on dialysis.

3. Discussion

This is a unique case of a 55-year-old male with an intact immune system with meningococcemia without meningitis who presented after 24 hours of chest pain in the absence of an infectious prodrome and was noted to have an ECG strongly suggestive of an acute anteroseptal myocardial infarction. The chest pain and ECG changes were likely from myocarditis leading to congestive heart failure and cardiogenic shock as his coronary angiogram at the time was normal. In previous reports detailing meningococcemia with associated ST segment elevation the patients presented with an infectious prodrome which was absent in our patient [7–9]. However, similar to our patient, the previous cases also had elevated troponins, decreased left ventricular function on echocardiogram, developed shock requiring vasopressor and/or inotropic support, and angiograms which revealed normal coronary arteries without obstructing lesions [8, 9].

The causes of the ECG changes associated with meningococcemia are not known but are probably multifactorial, and some authors postulate transmural ischemia [7]. The incidence of myocardial ischemia is increased in acute meningococcemia in pediatric patients and correlates with myocardial dysfunction. Early recognition of myocardial injury allows for myocardial support and early replacement therapy with PC, AIII, factor VIII, or fibrinogen that might improve outcome in acute meningococcemia in children [6]. Myocarditis probably plays a role as autopsy series suggests associated rates of 27–57% in children and as high as 85% in adults [5]. Acute myocarditis, in general, may present with chest pain, ECG changes, and elevated serum markers, all of which were seen in our case [10] and may trigger coronary spasm mimicking myocardial infarction [11].

Septic shock, in general, is characterized by peripheral vasodilatation and hypotension. Sepsis-associated myocardial dysfunction has been known for years but is not always readily evident due to the concomitant elevated cardiac index [12]. However, the cardiovascular response to meningococcemia may be fundamentally different than what is seen with other forms of gram negative sepsis. Monsalve and colleagues retrospectively reviewed the hemodynamic data of patients admitted to their ICU with shock from *Neisseria meningitidis*;

hemodynamic data of 19 of them were obtained within the first 6 hours [13]. These were compared to 20 patients admitted with shock from other gram negative organisms who underwent similar hemodynamic monitoring. Before volume expansion, the *Neisseria* group had a cardiac index of 2.3 $\pm$ 0.07 L/min^2 and systemic vascular resistance of 1338 $\pm$ 205 dynes/sec/cm^5 versus 3.5 $\pm$ 0.6 L/min^2 and 826 $\pm$ 207 dynes/sec/cm^5, respectively. The hemodynamic data from the *Neisseria* group in this study is very similar to what we found on right heart catheterization in our patient and further underscores why our case first appeared to be a cardiogenic rather than septic event. After the RHC the pulmonary artery catheter was removed and we were unable to trend further hemodynamic numbers as his shock progressed and improved.

The cardiac dysfunction occurs earlier compared to other gram negative bacteremia and typically precedes manifestations of shock [13]. In our patient, the RHC demonstrated a low cardiac index and high systemic vascular resistance during a time when the patient was normotensive despite a concomitant metabolic profile suggesting a metabolic acidosis with acute kidney injury and a complete blood count demonstrating a significant bandemia.

Previous studies have shown that TNFα and interleukin 1β contribute to myocardial dysfunction in sepsis [14]. However, in meningococcal sepsis, interleukin 6 appears to play more significant role than the one that has previously been ascribed to it [15]. Furthermore, there appears to be a significant relationship between interleukin 6 levels and disease severity in meningococcal disease and the levels often remain elevated for up to 48 hours after disease presentation which could explain the persistence noted in cardiac dysfunction following the onset of sepsis [16–19].

From our case and review of the literature, we believe the hypotension in meningococcal-induced shock is due, at least initially, to cardiogenic rather than distributive factors. The initial hemodynamic support measures may require more attention focused on inotropic support rather than vasopressors as the latter could theoretically contribute to vascular ischemia and subsequent gangrenous necrosis often seen in severe meningococcemia. In suspected cases of shock caused by meningococcemia, consideration should be given to using a pulmonary artery catheter to help elucidate cardiogenic versus distributive shock and help guide decisions regarding inotropic versus vasopressor therapy. In some cases, intra-aortic balloon pumps have been used successfully as an initial support measure [20]. Whether more aggressive use of inotropic support in our patient would have prevented or ameliorated his vascular complications is not known.

In conclusion we present this case of meningococcemia with a unique presentation of chest pain, ST elevation on ECG, and cardiogenic shock and without neurologic involvement or any preceding infectious symptoms. Prompt recognition and early use of antibiotics are the mainstay of treatment for this rapidly progressive infection given its high morbidity and mortality. Furthermore, as the initial hypotension in meningococcemia may be more cardiogenic than distributive, invasive hemodynamic monitoring with a pulmonary artery catheter may better guide hemodynamic management. In retrospect, the combination of mottled skin and low cardiac output with elevated right sided pressures could serve as a clue to possible meningococcal etiology if other lab data suggests infection. As the incidence of adults with meningococcemia presenting without neurologic involvement is extremely low, physicians are not typically thinking about this as a cause of cardiogenic shock especially in the presence of ST segment elevation.

Authors' Contribution

The authors of this paper originally prepared all materials. They also have read and approved the paper.

References

[1] N. E. Rosenstein, B. A. Perkins, D. S. Stephens, T. Popovic, and J. M. Hughes, "Meninggococcal disease," *The New England Journal of Medicine*, vol. 344, no. 18, pp. 1378–1388, 2001.

[2] N. E. Rosenstein, B. A. Perkins, D. S. Stephens et al., "The changing epidemiology of meningococcal disease in the United States, 1992–1996," *Journal of Infectious Diseases*, vol. 180, no. 6, pp. 1894–1901, 1999.

[3] J. N. George and C. M. Nester, "Syndromes of thrombotic microangiopathy," *The New England Journal of Medicine*, vol. 371, no. 7, pp. 654–666, 2014.

[4] L. G. Rubin and W. Schaffner, "Care of the asplenic patient," *The New England Journal of Medicine*, vol. 371, no. 4, pp. 349–356, 2014.

[5] N. S. Garcia, J. S. Castelo, V. Ramos, G. S. Rezende, and F. E. Pereira, "Frequency of myocarditis in cases of fatal meningococcal infection in children: observations on 31 cases studied at autopsy," *Revista da Sociedade Brasileira de Medicina Tropical*, vol. 32, no. 5, pp. 517–522, 1999.

[6] M. Razminia, Y. Salem, M. Elbzour, D. Teves, H. Deshmukh, and S. Khosla, "Importance of early diagnosis and therapy of acute meningococcal myocarditis: a case report with review of literature," *American Journal of Therapeutics*, vol. 12, no. 3, pp. 269–271, 2005.

[7] O. Gach, P. Lancellotti, and L. A. Pierard, "Acute ST-segment elevation in neisseria meningitis," *Acta Cardiologica*, vol. 56, no. 5, pp. 327–329, 2001.

[8] G. S. Filippatos, D. Kardara, E. Sioras et al., "Acute myocardial infarction with normal coronary arteries during septic shock from *Neisseria meningitidis*," *Intensive Care Medicine*, vol. 26, no. 2, article 252, 2000.

[9] G. Briassoulis, P. Kalabalikis, V. Thanopoulos, and T. Hatzis, "Non-Q wave acute myocardial infarction in acute meningococcemia in a 10-year-old girl," *Pediatric Emergency Care*, vol. 16, no. 1, pp. 33–38, 2000.

[10] Z. I. Bitar, M. Swede, and K. Almerri, "ST elevation without myocardial infarction," *BMJ Case Reports*, 2014.

[11] A. Kumar, R. Bagur, P. Béliveau et al., "Acute myocarditis triggering coronary spasm and mimicking acute myocardial

infarction," *World Journal of Cardiology*, vol. 6, no. 9, pp. 1045–1048, 2014.

[12] S. Price, P. B. Anning, J. A. Mitchell, and T. W. Evans, "Myocardial dysfunction in sepsis: mechanisms and therapeutic implications," *European Heart Journal*, vol. 20, no. 10, pp. 715–724, 1999.

[13] F. Monsalve, L. Rucabado, A. Salvador, J. Bonastre, J. Cuñat, and M. Ruano, "Myocardial depression in septic shock caused by meningococcal infection," *Critical Care Medicine*, vol. 12, no. 12, pp. 1021–1023, 1984.

[14] A. Kumar, V. Thota, L. Dee, J. Olson, E. Uretz, and J. E. Parrillo, "Tumor necrosis factor α and interleukin 1β are responsible for in vitro myocardial cell depression induced by human septic shock serum," *Journal of Experimental Medicine*, vol. 183, no. 3, pp. 949–958, 1996.

[15] N. Pathan, C. A. Hemingway, A. A. Alizadeh et al., "Role of interleukin 6 in myocardial dysfunction of meningococcal septic shock," *The Lancet*, vol. 363, no. 9404, pp. 203–209, 2004.

[16] B. Gardlund, J. Sjolin, A. Nilsson, M. Roll, C.-J. Wickerts, and B. Wretlind, "Plasma levels of cytokines in primary septic shock in humans: correlation with disease severity," *Journal of Infectious Diseases*, vol. 172, no. 1, pp. 296–301, 1995.

[17] J. A. Hazelzet, I. M. Risseeuw-Appel, R. F. Kornelisse et al., "Age-related differences in outcome and severity of DIC in children with septic shock and purpura," *Thrombosis and Haemostasis*, vol. 76, no. 6, pp. 932–938, 1996.

[18] J. A. Hazelzet, E. van der Voort, J. Lindemans, P. G. J. ter Heerdt, and H. J. Neijens, "Relation between cytokines and routine laboratory data in children with septic shock and purpura," *Intensive Care Medicine*, vol. 20, no. 5, pp. 371–374, 1994.

[19] M. van Deuren, J. van der Ven-Jongekrijg, A. K. M. Bartelink, R. Van Dalen, R. W. Sauerwein, and J. W. M. Van der Meer, "Correlation between proinflammatory cytokines and antiinflammatory mediators and the severity of disease in meningococcal infections," *Journal of Infectious Diseases*, vol. 172, no. 2, pp. 433–439, 1995.

[20] Y.-H. Chiu, C.-K. How, C.-H. Chern, L.-M. Wang, and C.-I. Huang, "Cardiac rescue with intra-aortic balloon counterpulsation in refractory shock due to acute meningococcemia," *The American Journal of Emergency Medicine*, vol. 25, no. 2, pp. 253–254, 2007.

33

Use of Hemadsorption in a Case of Pediatric Toxic Shock Syndrome

Andrea Berkes,[1] **Edit Szikszay,**[1] **János Kappelmayer,**[2] **Adrienne Kerényi,**[2] **Tamás Szabó,**[1] **László Ujhelyi,**[3] **Krisztina Bari,**[4] **György Balla,**[1,5] **and József Balla**[3]

[1]*Department of Pediatrics, University of Debrecen, Debrecen 4012, Hungary*
[2]*Institute of Laboratory Medicine, University of Debrecen, Debrecen 4012, Hungary*
[3]*Department of Medicine, Faculty of Medicine, University of Debrecen, Debrecen 4012, Hungary*
[4]*Fresenius Medical Care, NephroCare University of Debrecen, Debrecen 4012, Hungary*
[5]*HAS-UD Vascular Biology and Myocardial Pathophysiology Research Group, Hungarian Academy of Sciences,*
 Debrecen 4012, Hungary

Correspondence should be addressed to József Balla; balla@belklinika.com

Academic Editor: Mehmet Doganay

Background. Toxic shock syndrome is a potentially fatal toxin-mediated disease. The role of toxins in this clinical entity made us hypothesize that extracorporeal blood purification with CytoSorb® could play a beneficial role in the clinical management of toxic shock syndrome. This case report describes the successful treatment of toxic shock syndrome using a combination of renal replacement therapy and hemadsorption in a pediatric patient. *Case Presentation.* A 5-year-old girl with Down's syndrome presented with an inflamed area surrounding an insect bite, signs of systemic inflammation, and multiple organ failure. As previous attempts of immune modulation therapy were unsuccessful, renal replacement therapy was supplemented by the cytokine absorber CytoSorb. Treatment using this combination was associated with a rapid and significant stabilization in the hemodynamic situation and a decrease in inflammatory mediators within hours after the initiation of therapy. The application of CytoSorb therapy was simple and safe. *Conclusion.* The use of extracorporeal blood purification with CytoSorb proved potentially beneficial by removing toxins and inflammatory mediators in this case and could therefore play a role in the clinical management of toxic shock syndrome. Whether CytoSorb has the potential to even positively influence mortality in patients with toxic shock syndrome still needs to be confirmed.

1. Introduction

Toxic shock syndrome (TSS) is a potentially fatal toxin-mediated disease caused by infection from *Staphylococcus aureus* or Group A Streptococcus (GAS). This multisystem disorder is the consequence of an uncontrolled systemic inflammatory response syndrome caused by bacterial super-antigens that broadly activate T-cells and lead to hypercytokinemia and hyperinflammation [1]. Consequently, the excessive release of various cytokines, leukotrienes, and prostaglandins, causing a "cytokine storm," leads to the generation of the symptoms of this syndrome. The goal of therapy in TSS is to eradicate infection, mitigate the overwhelming inflammatory response, and prevent complications.

Therefore, the fatal role of toxins in this disease entity made us hypothesize that extracorporeal blood purification with a novel sorbent, CytoSorb, might be capable of removing toxins, cytokines, and other inflammatory mediators and could play a beneficial role in the clinical management of TSS. This case report describes the successful treatment of toxic shock syndrome using CytoSorb in a five-year-old girl with Down's syndrome. Consent on publishing has been gathered from the patients' legal parents.

2. Case Report

A 5-year-old girl with Down's syndrome presented with an erythematous, indurated area on her right leg surrounding an insect bite noticed two days prior to admission. Oral cefaclor therapy was started for suspected systemic infection by *S. pyogenes* or *S. aureus/epidermidis* the day before admission by the GP. Despite antibiotics, the erythema continued to migrate proximally towards the inguinal region. On arrival at the emergency department, the conscious patient presented with diarrhea but stable vital signs: breathing rate 26 breaths/min, heart rate 110 beats/min, and blood pressure 98/57 mmHg. Blood examination revealed leukocytosis (15.44 G/L), neutrophilia (84.8%, absolute or 13.1 G/L), mild anemia (Hb 107 g/L, Hct 32%), a normal platelet count (238 G/L), and an elevated CRP (260.98 mg/L).

During the first two hours her status deteriorated so rapidly that she needed to be transferred to the intensive care unit. Capillary blood gas analysis revealed a severe uncompensated metabolic acidosis: pH 6.77, pCO_2 37.6 mmHg, HCO_3 5.2 mmol/L, and lactate 7 mmol/L. Septic shock was diagnosed and three intravenous fluid boluses (20 mL/kg) and oxygen therapy were started. Blood cultures were taken and the antibiotic therapy augmented by parenteral clindamycin and vancomycin. Due to an unsatisfactory cardiovascular response to fluid resuscitation, dopamine was started at 5 μg/kg/min and then increased to 10 μg/kg/min. Low ventricular contractility on ultrasonography required additional dobutamine at 5 μg/kg/min while clinical signs of decreased systemic vascular resistance necessitated noradrenaline at 0.1 μg/kg/min which had to be increased up to 0.5 μg/kg/min later. Due to pronounced cardiovascular instability and suspected adrenal gland insufficiency, hydrocortisone was prescribed at 2 mg/kg/12 hours.

Considering the well-known immunodeficiency of patients with Down's syndrome, an antimycotic agent (fluconazole) was administered preventively, and intravenous immunoglobulin therapy (1 g/kg) for septic shock due to *S. pyogenes* or *S. aureus* was given on the day of admission and the following day. Fresh frozen plasma (15 mL/kg) and low molecular weight heparin (enoxaparin 6 mg/kg) were administered for laboratory signs of disseminated intravascular coagulation (DIC). Deep vein thrombosis of the right lower extremity was ruled out by Doppler ultrasonography. Chest X-ray revealed increased perihilar lung markings.

Eight hours after admission to the ICU an altered state of consciousness, hypercapnia, tachydyspnoe, and increasing oxygen needs required intubation and pressure controlled SIMV at PIP 17 cm H_2O, PEEP 5 cm H_2O, respiratory rate 25/min, and FiO_2 0.4.

Based on the Surviving Sepsis Campaign guidelines multiorgan failure was diagnosed. The patient had cardiovascular instability requiring complex vasoactive therapy (dopamine, dobutamine, noradrenaline, and milrinone); DIC indicated deteriorating liver function, poor lung function on ventilatory support alluding to Acute Respiratory Distress Syndrome (ARDS), and deteriorating kidney function. Microbiological examinations were inconclusive as to the causative pathogen.

During the first 48 hours of therapy diffuse erythroderma with purpura and petechiae appeared, while the right leg became livid, and bullae appeared in places subjected

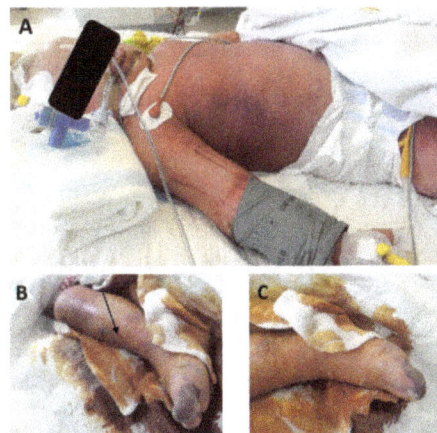

FIGURE 1: Diffuse erythroderma, purpura, and petechiae with severe generalized edema (A). Erythroderma, livid swelling, confluent bullae, and diffuse desquamation of the right leg (B, C). Arrow indicates site of the initial insect bite.

to external pressure (Figure 1). Periodic pediatric surgery consultation excluded necrotizing fasciitis. The clinical picture now matched that of TSS. While skin lesions improved gradually and necrotic areas recovered fully under local conservative therapy from day seven onwards, new bullous eruptions continued to appear.

In an attempt to modulate the dysregulated immune response, plasma exchange therapy was performed without complications. Despite an increasing urine output during the first 24 hours from 0.4 to 5.4 ml/kg/hour her fluid balance remained positive. Thereafter, diuresis declined and the patient became anuric by hour 56 such that continuous venovenous hemodialysis was started. Thrombocytopenia, anemia, and hypoproteinemia were supported by blood products and an augmentation of the low neutrophil levels by granulocyte-colony stimulating factor tried on days four and five.

As previous attempts of immune modulation therapy were unsuccessful, renal replacement therapy was supplemented by the cytokine absorber CytoSorb (Cytosorbents Corp., Monmouth Junction, NJ, USA). CVVHD was performed with multiFiltrate (Fresenius Medical Care) machine, using a AV400S polysulfone dialyzer. Blood flow (Qb) of 40 mL/min could be achieved; dialysis fluid (MultiBic) flow (Qd) of 800 mL/hour was maintained, with an ultrafiltration rate of 100 mL/hour. Because of hepatic failure with DIC, regional citrate anticoagulation was used during the whole course of CRRT without any remarkable complication. As a result of a 72-hour uneventful course of the CVVHD-CytoSorb therapy, cardiovascular stability improved on lower vasopressor doses; FiO_2 decreased from 0.95 to 0.4, airway pressures PIP/PEEP from 27/10 to 24/8 cm H_2O, and respiratory rate from 25 to 15/min, respectively. In addition, levels of important laboratory parameters decreased (Table 1) as did plasma concentrations of proinflammatory and immunomodulatory cytokines (Figure 2). This attenuation of the inflammatory response correlated with the clinical improvement. The need for platelets decreased

TABLE 1: Laboratory parameters during the course of multiple immune-modulatory therapies including CVVHD + CytoSorb.

Time from admission	pH	Lactate [mmol/L]	CRP [mg/L]	PCT [μg/L]	WBC [10^3/μL]	Platelets [10^3/μL]	BUN [mmol/L]	Creatinine [μmol/L]	ALT [U/L]	AST [U/L]	LDH [U/L]
0	6,42	8.6	178.7	218.4	14.97	204	10.5	196	38	21	344
6 hr					Start of hydrocortisone, IVIG						
15 hr	7.35	4.4	114	95.07	8.67	67	11.1	134	—	—	—
42 hr	7.37	3.9	105.1	32.85	7.72	34	17.3	147	—	—	—
63 hr	7.39	3.6	113.5	20.54	8.15	12	24.3	210	—	—	—
67 hr					Start of plasma exchange therapy						
69 hr	7.39	4.2	87.46	19.02	6.96	21	26.4	223	270	150	887
78 hr					Start of CVVHD-CytoSorb						
91 hr	7.41	1.9	50.5	4.06	1.91	5	18.8	163	214	101	554
133 hr	7.47	1.5	87.46	3.33	4.31	5	12.8	98	274	146	676
150 hr					End of CVVHD-CytoSorb						
212 hr	7.39	0.7	76.01	2.8	3.78	20	7.6	78	78	94	587

CRP: C-reactive protein, PCT: procalcitonin, WBC: white blood cell, BUN: blood urea nitrogen, ALT: alanine aminotransferase, AST: aspartate aminotransferase, LDH: lactate dehydrogenase, IVIG: intravenous immune globulin, and CVVHD: continuous venovenous hemodialysis. Normal values of laboratory results provided by the examiner institution: lactate: 0,5–2,2 mmol/L, CRP: <2,2 mg/L, PCT: 0,5 μg/L, WBC: 4,5–11,5 G/L, platelets: 150–500 G/L, BUN: 1,8–6,4 mmol/L, creatinine: 18–53 mmol/L, ALT: <40 U/L, AST: <40 U/L, and LDH: <340 U/L.

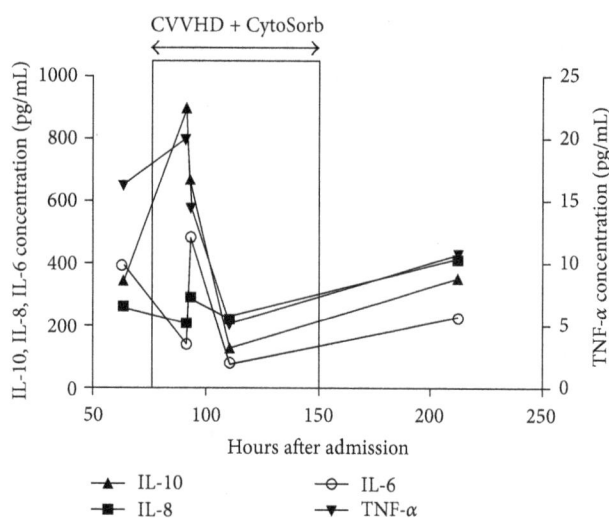

FIGURE 2: Course of proinflammatory and immunomodulatory cytokines before, during, and after combined CVVHD + CytoSorb treatment.

dramatically 48 hours after CytoSorb therapy and the diffuse erythroderma, purpura, and petechiae started to fade. CVVHD was continued for a further 8 days due to pronounced fluid overload, reaching normal rates of diuresis on day 17, three days after successful extubation and termination of the initial empiric antibiotic combination therapy. After six days of total parenteral nutrition the patient was switched to enteral feeding.

On day 20, her condition deteriorated again with tachypnea and desaturation together with elevated levels of CRP, PCT. This time, blood cultures revealed a staphylococcal infection; however, sepsis did not develop during the targeted

antibiotic therapy. After 25 days the patient left the intensive care unit although her right ankle was still swollen.

The reappearance of fever accompanied by mildly elevated inflammatory laboratory parameters gave rise to the thought of deep tissue infection. MRI could not rule out an osteomyelitis of the os naviculare. The patient remained afebrile while the inflammation of the ankle became smaller under local conservative therapy. Complex physiotherapy tried to counteract muscle wasting and decreased tone. The girl was discharged home after 42 days where she recovered completely.

3. Discussion

In the present case report, we treated a 5-year-old girl with Down's syndrome who developed toxic shock syndrome and multiple organ failure after an insect bite, using a combination of CVVHD and hemadsorption. Treatment was associated with a rapid and significant stabilization of the hemodynamic situation accompanied by declining catecholamine dosage, improved respiratory status, and a decrease in inflammatory mediators within hours after initiation of therapy. Moreover, the need for platelets decreased dramatically and the diffuse erythroderma, purpura, and petechiae vanished.

These findings are in line with two published case reports on the use of CytoSorb in patients with toxic shock syndrome showing the potential role of this therapy in stabilizing hemodynamics, decreasing vasopressor requirements, improving lactate clearance, and reducing erythema as short term effects [2, 3].

The clinical picture in our case was ambiguous. The cutaneous lesion, as probable origin of the disease, suggested *Streptococcus pyogenes* as the causative agent, while the generalized erythroderma was typical for *Staphylococcus* infection.

As bacteria from neither blood cultures nor skin and mucosal lesions were isolated, the microbiological background of our case remains unknown. Interestingly, a study that set out to quantify the ability of the CytoSorb polymer to adsorb a broad selection of inflammatory pathogen-associated molecular pattern molecules (PAMPs), damage-associated molecular pattern molecules (DAMPs), and cytokines from whole blood in a single compartment in vitro recirculation system provided that substantial quantities of a broad spectrum of DAMPS, PAMPS, and cytokines (i.e., S100A8, complement C5a, procalcitonin, HMGB-1, MIP1-α, IL-6, IFN-γ, TNF-α, Staph enterotoxin TSST-1, and aflatoxin B1) were removed [4]. Therefore, direct removal of streptococci toxins may potentially have played a role in the current case. These results might be of particular interest in a case such as the one presented herein, where the pathological origin is not clear but the diagnosis of TSS was established.

One of the striking features of systemic TSS is the speed of excess cytokine and toxin production. Our patient had been treated with multiple immune-modulatory therapies (i.e., hydrocortisone, IVIG, and plasma exchange therapy) achieving only moderate reductions in the laboratory parameters that characterize systemic inflammation. However, from the start of CVVHD/CytoSorb initiation, plasma levels of inflammatory mediators such as IL-6, IL-10, IFN-γ, CRP, and PCT but also of metabolic parameters (i.e., lactate) started to decrease rapidly. This attenuation of the inflammatory response correlated well with the clinical improvement of the patient.

Previous studies have shown that inflammatory mediators can be removed from the circulation with different blood purification techniques such as plasma exchange, high-volume and very high-volume hemofiltration, and a number of hybrid therapies encompassing high-permeability hemofiltration, super high-flux hemofiltration, hemadsorption or coupled filtration, and adsorption [5]. These therapeutic modalities have been associated with lower mortality in patients with sepsis [6, 7]. Whether CytoSorb has the potential to positively influence mortality in TSS patients needs to be confirmed in randomized, controlled trials.

However, despite the fact that most experience with CytoSorb in the clinical setting to date is still limited to case reports, the first multicenter randomized controlled study using treatment with CytoSorb hemadsorption in septic patients with acute lung injury showed that application of the device over a 7-day treatment period was safe and effectively decreased the blood concentration levels of several key cytokines [8–11]. From this perspective, further studies to elucidate the potential clinical impact of this new therapy option are urgently warranted.

4. Conclusion

The use of extracorporeal blood purification with a novel sorbent, CytoSorb, proved potentially beneficial by removing toxins, cytokines, and other inflammatory mediators in this case of toxic shock syndrome in a pediatric patient and could therefore play a future role in the clinical management of toxic shock syndrome. Whether CytoSorb has the potential to even positively influence mortality in patients with toxic shock syndrome needs to be confirmed in randomized, controlled trials.

Abbreviations

TSS: Toxic shock syndrome
GAS: Group A Streptococcus
Hb: Hemoglobin
Hct: Hematocrit
CRP: C-reactive protein
DIC: Disseminated intravascular coagulation
PIP: Peak inspiratory pressure
PEEP: Positive end-expiratory pressure
PCT: Procalcitonin
WBC: White blood cell
IVIG: Intravenous immune globulin
CVVHD: Continuous venovenous hemodialysis.

References

[1] A. S. DeVries, L. Lesher, P. M. Schlievert et al., "Staphylococcal toxic shock syndrome 2000-2006: Epidemiology, clinical features, and molecular characteristics," *PLoS ONE*, vol. 6, no. 8, Article ID e22997, 2011.

[2] N. Lees, A. Rosenberg, A. Hurtado-Doce et al., "Combination of ECMO and cytokine adsorption therapy for severe sepsis with cardiogenic shock and ARDS due to Panton–Valentine leukocidin—positive Staphylococcus aureus pneumonia and H1N1," *Journal of Artificial Organs*, vol. 19, no. 4, pp. 399–402, 2016.

[3] G. W. van der Linde and A. F. Grootendorst, "First case of toxic shock treated with haemoadsorption by CytoSorb® in the Netherlands," *Netherlands Journal of Critical Care*, vol. 24, pp. 27–29, 2016.

[4] M. Gruda, "In vitro adsorption of a broad spectrum of inflammatory mediators with CytoSorb® hemoadsorbent polymer beads," *Critical Care*, vol. 20, p. 194, 2016.

[5] P. M. Honore, R. Jacobs, O. Joannes-Boyau et al., "Newly designed CRRT membranes for sepsis and SIRS-a pragmatic approach for bedside intensivists summarizing the more recent advances: A systematic structured review," *ASAIO Journal*, vol. 59, no. 2, pp. 99–106, 2013.

[6] M. Joannidis, "Continuous renal replacement therapy in sepsis and multisystem organ failure," *Seminars in Dialysis*, vol. 22, no. 2, pp. 160–164, 2009.

[7] F. Zhou, Z. Peng, R. Murugan, and J. A. Kellum, "Blood purification and mortality in sepsis: A meta-analysis of randomized trials," *Critical Care Medicine*, vol. 41, no. 9, pp. 2209–2220, 2013.

[8] D. Schädler, C. Porzelius, A. Jörres et al., "A multicenter randomized controlled study of an extracorporeal cytokine hemoadsorption device in septic patients," *Critical Care*, vol. 17, p. 62, 2013.

[9] K. Kogelmann, D. Jarczak, M. Scheller, and M. Drüner, "Hemoadsorption by CytoSorb in septic patients: a case series," *Critical Care*, vol. 21, no. 1, 2017.

[10] C. G. Cirstoveanu, I. Barascu, and S. Mc Kenzie Stancu, "Hemadsorption with Adult CytoSorb® in a Low Weight Pediatric Case," *Case Reports in Critical Care*, vol. 2017, Article ID 6987167, pp. 1–5, 2017.

[11] S. David, K. Thamm, B. M. Schmidt, C. S. Falk, and J. T. Kielstein, "Effect of extracorporeal cytokine removal on vascular barrier function in a septic shock patient," *Journal of Intensive Care*, vol. 5, no. 12, 2017.

34

A Curious Case of Acute Respiratory Failure: Is It Antisynthetase Syndrome?

Gurveen Malhotra,[1] Nitya Ramreddy,[2] Serafin Chua,[3] Mira Iliescu,[4] and Tanjeev Kaur[1]

[1] *University of Illinois at Chicago, Chicago, IL 60612, USA*
[2] *Internal Medicine, Mount Sinai Hospital, Chicago, IL 60608, USA*
[3] *Rheumatology, Mount Sinai Hospital, Chicago, IL 60608, USA*
[4] *Pulmonary & Critical Care Medicine, Mount Sinai Hospital, Chicago, IL 60608, USA*

Correspondence should be addressed to Gurveen Malhotra; gurveen22@gmail.com

Academic Editor: Chiara Lazzeri

Antisynthetase (AS) syndrome is a major subgroup of inflammatory myopathies seen in a minority of patients with dermatomyositis and polymyositis. Although it is usually associated with elevated creatine phosphokinase level, some patients may have amyopathic dermatomyositis (ADM) like presentation with predominant skin involvement. Interstitial lung disease (ILD) is the main pulmonary manifestation and may be severe thereby determining the prognosis. It may rarely present with a very aggressive course resulting in acute respiratory distress syndrome (ARDS). We report a case of a 43-year-old male who presented with nonresolving pneumonia who was eventually diagnosed to have ADM through a skin biopsy without any muscle weakness. ADM may be associated with rapidly progressive course of interstitial lung disease (ADM-ILD) which is associated with high mortality. Differentiation between ADM-ILD and AS syndrome may be difficult in the absence of positive serology and clinical presentation may help in clinching the diagnosis.

1. Introduction

Antisynthetase (AS) syndrome is a rare disease entity with predominant interstitial lung disease associated with the presence of anti-Jo-1 antibodies. It may pose a diagnostic challenge and needs early aggressive immunosuppression for better outcomes.

2. Case Presentation

A 43-year-old male without any past medical history presented with progressive dyspnea, fever, and nonproductive cough for 1 month. He denied orthopnea, paroxysmal nocturnal dyspnea, hemoptysis, or weight loss. There was no history of recent travel, sick contacts, or prolonged immobilization. He had no history of cigarette smoking, second-hand smoking, or alcohol or illicit drug use.

He was afebrile and hemodynamically stable on presentation. He had mild periorbital edema with erythema on supraorbital areas but no heliotrope rash. He also had erythematous patchy scaly lesions on bilateral elbows and metacarpophalangeal joints with periungual erythema without distinct Gottron papules. Breath sounds were decreased on the right base with crackles and scattered rhonchi. There was no gallop rhythm or jugular venous distention. Mildly tender metacarpophalangeal and proximal interphalangeal joints without synovitis were noted bilaterally. Muscle strength was normal and equal bilaterally in all four extremities. Initial blood work showed aspartate transaminase 94 U/L, alanine transaminase 70 U/L, and no leucocytosis.

He later developed a fever and chest X-ray (Figure 1) was done which revealed bilateral lower and right middle lobe infiltrates. Respiratory panel, blood culture, sputum culture, fungal culture, *Legionella* antigen, *Histoplasma* antigen, QuantiFERON Gold, hepatitis panel, and HIV test were all negative. A computed tomography scan of the chest (Figure 2) showed patchy subpleural bilateral opacities more prominent in the bases with subtle reticulonodular opacities

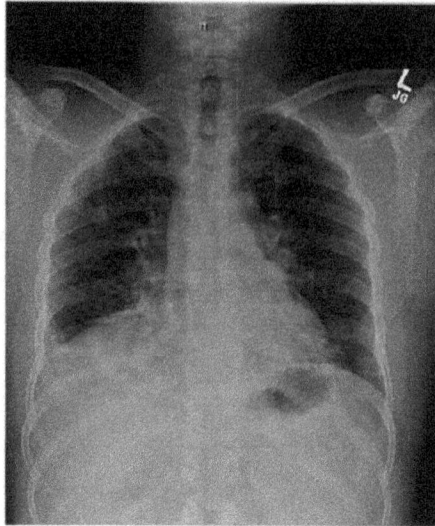

FIGURE 1: Chest X-ray showing bibasilar and right middle lobe infiltrate on presentation.

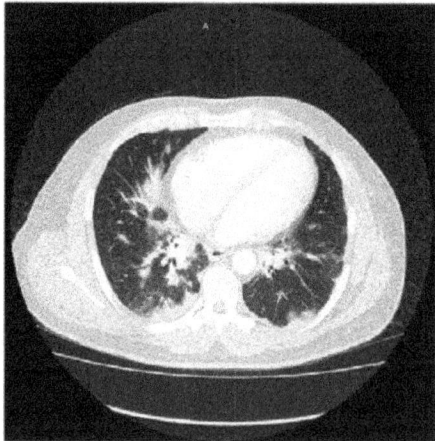

FIGURE 2: CT chest revealing bilateral basilar fibrosis along with reticulonodular and subpleural wedge shaped opacities.

in both lungs along with traction bronchiectasis. No significant pleural effusion, pneumothorax, or lymphadenopathy was seen. He was recently treated for pneumonia at another hospital and was thus empirically started on antibiotics for treatment of suspected health care associated pneumonia. Bronchoscopy with transbronchial biopsy revealed chronic inflammation and fibrosis. Autoimmune workup including anti-cyclic citrullinated peptide, anti-nuclear antibody, double-stranded DNA antibody, anti-proteinase 3, anti-myeloperoxidase, Scl-70, anti-smooth muscle, anti-Jo-1 antibody, and cryoglobulin was unremarkable. Aldolase was elevated at 13.7 (normal < 8.1 U/L), C-reactive protein was 10.4 (normal 0–8 mg/L), creatine phosphokinase was 351 (normal 30–223 IU/L), and rheumatoid factor was 71 (normal < 14 IU/mL). Skin biopsy of lesions over metacarpophalangeal joints revealed mild epidermal acanthosis and papillomatosis with perivascular inflammation suggestive of dermatomyositis (Figure 3).

Pulse dose of intravenous methylprednisolone 1000 mg was given for 3 days. Video assisted thoracoscopic lung biopsy could not be performed because of his worsening respiratory status. The clinical picture with the presence of ILD, fever, and arthritis in the setting of ADM suggested a diagnosis of AS syndrome and immunosuppression with cyclophosphamide was initiated. Although he was initially placed on noninvasive ventilation, his condition eventually deteriorated requiring intubation and mechanical ventilation for hypoxemic respiratory failure. Repeat chest X-ray showed findings consistent with acute respiratory distress syndrome (ARDS) and he was placed on RotoProne bed. Repeat creatine kinase level was minimally elevated at 292 IU/L and urinalysis revealed red blood cell casts. He subsequently developed acute kidney injury with metabolic acidosis requiring hemodialysis. He eventually went into shock requiring vasopressor support and progressed to multiorgan failure. His condition continued to deteriorate leading to refractory shock with no improvement

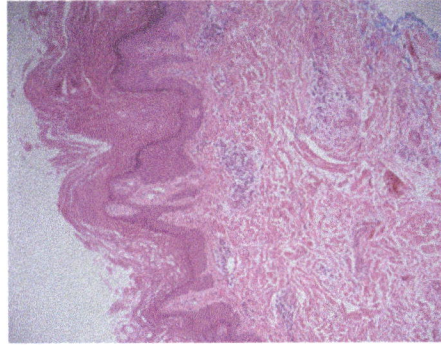

FIGURE 3: Skin biopsy shows acanthosis and papillomatosis with focal dermal perivascular lymphocytic infiltrate (10x).

in the overall status; the family decided not to resuscitate in the event of a cardiac arrest and he unfortunately died.

3. Discussion

Inflammatory myopathies are a diverse group of autoimmune disorders with polymyositis, dermatomyositis, and inclusion body myositis as the major entities. Skin disease may precede the development of myopathy while in others the disease only affects the skin, ADM.

A major subgroup of inflammatory myopathies are AS syndrome characterized by ILD, chronic polyarthritis, Raynaud's phenomenon, fever, and "mechanics" hands [1]. Diagnosis is confirmed by the presence of anti-tRNA synthetase autoantibodies with anti-Jo-1 antibody being the most common [2]. Other less commonly tested antibodies include anti-PL-7 (anti-threonyl), anti-PL-12 (anti-alanyl), and antityrosyl tRS antibody which are found in only 2–5% of the cases [3]. The true incidence of AS syndrome is unknown; however, the annual incidence of inflammatory myopathies ranges between 2 and 10 cases per million per year [4] and antisynthetase antibodies are found in 25–40% of them [5]. Interestingly, AS syndrome is very infrequently seen in ADM [6].

Lung involvement is rare in ADM with nonspecific interstitial pneumonia being the most common pattern [6] and associated with poor prognosis [7, 8]. Other presentations may include diffuse alveolar damage, usual interstitial pneumonia, cryptogenic organizing pneumonia, and ARDS [9]. Although data on ILD in ADM is not very clear, two different forms have been established: acute and chronic [10]. The acute subtype is more prevalent in the amyopathic type as compared to the classic dermatomyositis and associated with much higher mortality. Acute ILD rapidly deteriorates into respiratory failure which is the leading cause of death in these patients. The presence of traction bronchiectasis may help in differentiating rapidly deteriorating subtype from the chronic form and hence determining the prognosis [11]. The acute form of ILD is also associated with a high mortality of up to 67% when compared to the chronic form [8].

There is no current established treatment but the mainstay of therapy has been high dose steroids and immunosuppressive agents like cyclophosphamide and cyclosporine

[2, 12]. In resistant cases, tacrolimus [13], intravenous immunoglobulin, and rituximab have shown benefit [14].

Kidney injury is infrequent in ADM. Rhabdomyolysis and myoglobulinuria leading to acute tubular necrosis are the most common cause while glomerulonephritis is less frequently seen [15]. The major glomerulopathies are membranous nephritis, membranoproliferative glomerulonephritis, and diffuse proliferative glomerulonephritis. The serological tests for various vasculitides as well as the viral hepatitis were all negative. Our patient could not get a kidney biopsy because of his hemodynamically unstable condition.

It is therefore a challenge to diagnose AS syndrome in the absence of confirmatory serological tests, and, in such a scenario, ADM-ILD should be considered. Diagnosis can be made in similar situations after ruling out various connective tissue diseases as the primary etiology. The clinical scenario presented by the authors here emphasizes the need for physicians to become familiar with this clinical entity of AS syndrome since early diagnosis and treatment usually lead to better outcomes. A delay in the diagnosis as in our patient may result in severe complications and a poor prognosis despite aggressive treatment. Further, management may be difficult and requires corticosteroids and immunosuppression in either situation. Both AS syndrome and ILD can rapidly deteriorate into acute respiratory failure which may prove fatal.

Competing Interests

The authors declare that they have no competing interests.

References

[1] C. Marguerie, C. C. Bunn, H. L. C. Beynon et al., "Polymyositis, pulmonary fibrosis and autoantibodies to aminoacyl-tRNA synthetase enzymes," *Quarterly Journal of Medicine*, vol. 77, no. 282, pp. 1019–1038, 1990.

[2] J. Solomon, J. J. Swigris, and K. K. Brown, "Myositis-related interstitial lung disease and antisynthetase syndrome," *Jornal Brasileiro de Pneumologia*, vol. 37, no. 1, pp. 100–109, 2011.

[3] M. Hirakata, "Autoantibodies to aminoacyl-tRNA synthetases," *Internal Medicine*, vol. 44, no. 6, pp. 527–528, 2005.

[4] C. V. Oddis, C. G. Conte, V. D. Steen, and T. A. Medsger Jr., "Incidence of polymyositis-dermatomyositis: a 20-year study of

hospital diagnosed cases in Allegheny County, PA 1963–1982," *Journal of Rheumatology*, vol. 17, no. 10, pp. 1329–1334, 1990.

[5] L. A. Love, R. L. Leff, D. D. Fraser et al., "A new approach to the classification of idiopathic inflammatory myopathy: myositis-specific autoantibodies define useful homogeneous patient groups," *Medicine*, vol. 70, no. 6, pp. 360–374, 1991.

[6] V. Cottin, F. Thivolet-Béjui, M. Reynaud-Gaubert et al., "Interstitial lung disease in amyopathic dermatomyositis, dermatomyositis and polymyositis," *European Respiratory Journal*, vol. 22, no. 2, pp. 245–250, 2003.

[7] N. Sakamoto, H. Mukae, T. Fujii et al., "Nonspecific interstitial pneumonia with poor prognosis associated with amyopathic dermatomyositis," *Internal Medicine*, vol. 43, no. 9, pp. 838–842, 2004.

[8] A. Sauty, T. Rochat, O. D. Schoch et al., "Pulmonary fibrosis with predominant CD8 lymphocytic alveolitis and anti-Jo-1 antibodies," *European Respiratory Journal*, vol. 10, no. 12, pp. 2907–2912, 1997.

[9] T. Suda, T. Fujisawa, N. Enomoto et al., "Interstitial lung diseases associated with amyopathic dermatomyositis," *European Respiratory Journal*, vol. 28, no. 5, pp. 1005–1012, 2006.

[10] H. Mukae, H. Ishimoto, N. Sakamoto et al., "Clinical differences between interstitial lung disease associated with clinically amyopathic dermatomyositis and classic dermatomyositis," *Chest*, vol. 136, no. 5, pp. 1341–1347, 2009.

[11] G. Ideura, M. Hanaoka, T. Koizumi et al., "Interstitial lung disease associated with amyopathic dermatomyositis: review of 18 cases," *Respiratory Medicine*, vol. 101, no. 7, pp. 1406–1411, 2007.

[12] E. Miyazaki, M. Ando, T. Muramatsu et al., "Early assessment of rapidly progressive interstitial pneumonia associated with amyopathic dermatomyositis," *Clinical Rheumatology*, vol. 26, no. 3, pp. 436–439, 2007.

[13] A. L. Rigby, M. Plit, and A. R. Glanville, "Tacrolimus rescue therapy for severe respiratory failure in the anti-synthetase syndrome," *Respirology Case Reports*, vol. 2, no. 2, pp. 70–72, 2014.

[14] I. Marie, S. Dominique, A. Janvresse, H. Levesque, and J.-F. Menard, "Rituximab therapy for refractory interstitial lung disease related to antisynthetase syndrome," *Respiratory Medicine*, vol. 106, no. 4, pp. 581–587, 2012.

[15] T. H. Yen, P. C. Lai, C. C. Chen, S. Hsueh, and J. Y. Huang, "Renal involvement in patients with polymyositis and dermatomyositis," *International Journal of Clinical Practice*, vol. 59, no. 2, pp. 188–193, 2005.

35

A Case of Waterhouse-Friderichsen Syndrome Resulting from an Invasive Pneumococcal Infection in a Patient with a Hypoplastic Spleen

Kazumasa Emori, Nobuhiro Takeuchi, and Junichi Soneda

Department of Cardiovascular Surgery, Kobe Tokusyukai Hospital, 1-3-10 Kamitakamaru, Tarumi-ku, Kobe-shi, Hyogo 655-0017, Japan

Correspondence should be addressed to Kazumasa Emori; soofog09@yahoo.co.jp

Academic Editor: Zsolt Molnar

A 50-year-old male was brought to our emergency department by ambulance with complaints of pain and numbness in both legs. At arrival, purple spots were evident on his neck and face. Examination of the vital sign indicated septic shock. Laboratory data and blood gas analysis revealed disseminated intravascular coagulation, multiple organ failure, and metabolic acidosis. Peripheral blood smears revealed Howell-Jolly bodies, indicating decreased splenic function. A rapid urinary pneumococcal antigen test was also found to be positive. After admission to the intensive care unit, extensive treatment, including polymyxin-B direct hemoperfusion and administration of methylprednisolone and broad spectrum antibiotics was immediately initiated. Despite of our efforts to save his life, the patient died six hours after the arrival. The following day, blood cultures revealed the presence of *Streptococcus pneumoniae*. An autopsy revealed a hypoplastic spleen and a bilateral adrenal hemorrhage, indicating acute adrenal insufficiency caused by sepsis. Finally, the patient was diagnosed with Waterhouse-Friderichsen syndrome. Although severe infection may be seen in the splenectomized patients, it should be noted that patients with a hypoplastic spleen may have acute severe infections. We, therefore, report a case of Waterhouse-Friderichsen syndrome resulting from an invasive pneumococcal infection in a patient with a hypoplastic spleen.

1. Background

Waterhouse-Friderichsen syndrome (WFS) is an emergency condition, characterized by fever, cyanosis, bruises, and/or shock [1]. WFS is reported to occur in splenectomized patients, and in patients with congenital asplenia or decreased splenic function [2–5]. Here, we report a rare case of WFS, presenting with purpura fulminans, resulting from an invasive pneumococcal infection.

2. Case Presentation

A 50-year-old male was brought to our hospital by ambulance with complaints of pain and numbness in both legs. According to his wife, he presented with a high-grade fever (39.0°C), pain in both legs, vomiting, and diarrhea on the preceding day. His past medical history also included duodenal ulcer,

which was treated by conservative therapy. He was previously diagnosed with fatty liver and an idiopathic leukopenia. According to his wife, the patient had undergone dental treatment three months before. The patient was employed as a system engineer. He had a habit of having 100 cc of whisky and smoking 20 cigarettes daily. Upon arrival, the patient was alert and repeatedly complained of severe pain and numbness in his legs. Furthermore, cyanosis of the whole body was evident, and purple spots were apparent on the patient's neck and face. Examination of the vital signs showed the following results; blood pressure, 85/64 mmHg; heart rate, 113 beats/min; body temperature, 38.2°C; and percutaneous oxygen saturation could not be measured because of apparent peripheral circulatory disturbance. Septic shock was suspected based on the clinical symptoms. An arterial blood gas analysis revealed hypoxemia and metabolic acidosis (pH = 7.280, pO$_2$ = 57.0 mmHg,

(a)

(b)

(c)

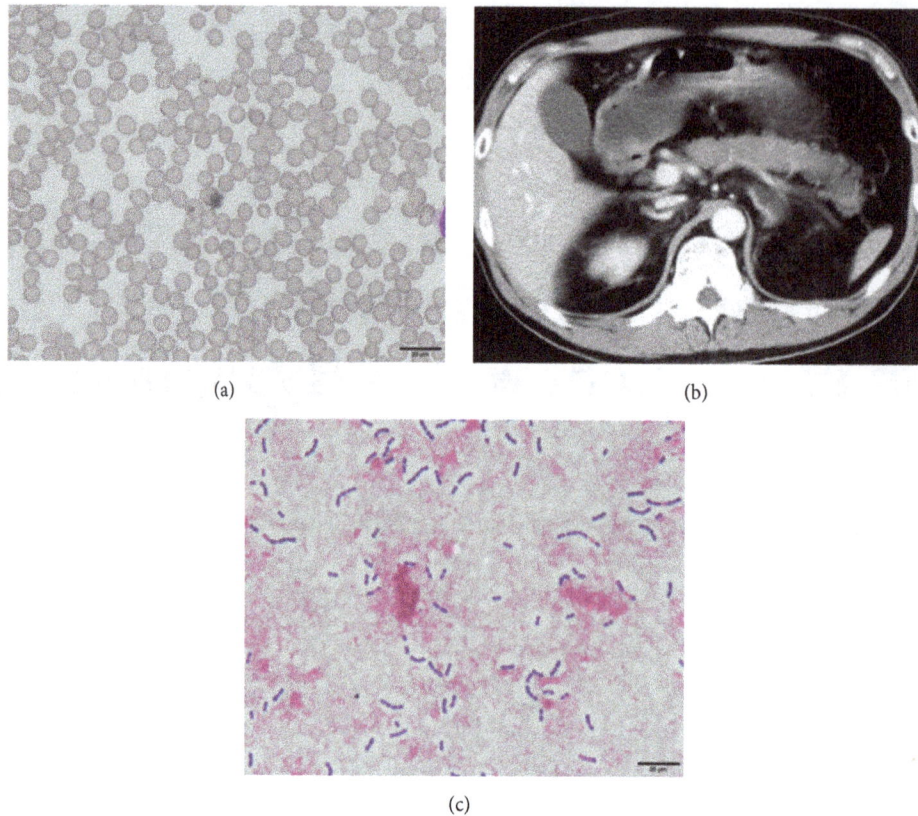

FIGURE 1: Peripheral blood smear, CT, and blood culture. (a) Peripheral blood smear revealed Howell-Jolly bodies. (b) Contrast CT demonstrated a hypoplastic spleen and retrospective fat tissue stranding around the left adrenal gland. (c) A blood culture revealed streptococci with capsules.

HCO_3^- = 9.2 mmol/L, BE = −15.8 mmol/L). Blood examination revealed leukopenia (3,310 cells/μL), moderately elevated levels of liver enzymes (aspartate aminotransferase 111 IU/L and alanine transaminase 61 IU/L), renal dysfunction (serum creatinine 4.43 mg/dL and blood urea nitrogen 30.3 mg/dL), and coagulation dysfunction (prothrombin time 26%, international normalized ratio 2.42, fibrinogen 37 mg/dL, fibrin and fibrinogen degradation product 86 μg/mL, D-dimer 28 μg/mL, and antithrombin III 58%), and remarkably elevated procalcitonin levels (>100 ng/mL). A peripheral blood analysis revealed Howell-Jolly bodies (Figure 1(a)), indicating decreased splenic function, and a rapid urinary pneumococcal antigen test was also positive. In the emergency department, he was immediately intubated and respiratory management was initiated. At the time of intubation, the pharyngeal mucosa was remarkably reddish and spotted. According to the Japanese Association for Acute Medicine, the disseminated intravascular coagulation (DIC) score was 8; therefore, his condition decisively satisfied the DIC criteria. Contrast computed tomography (CT) did not reveal abscess formation, but a small-sized spleen was noted (Figure 1(b)). Based on the findings of the blood examination along with the clinical symptoms, his condition was compatible with purpura fulminans, and the patient was supposedly in the state of sepsis-associated multiple organ failure as well as acute respiratory distress syndrome (ARDS). Immediately

after admitting to the intensive care unit (ICU), a dialysis catheter was inserted to initiate hemodialysis, including continuous hemodiafiltration (CHDF) and polymyxin-B direct hemoperfusion (PMX-DHP). Considerable extracellular fluid along with the transfusion of red blood cells and fresh frozen plasma was administered. Concurrent broad spectrum antibiotics, including imipenem/cilastacin, clindamycin, and piperacillin, were administered. Sivelestat sodium hydrate was initiated for the treatment of ARDS, and 1000 mg of methylprednisolone was administered for the treatment of septic shock. Four hours after the initiation of CHDF and PMX-DHP, his blood pressure suddenly decreased resulting in cardiac arrest. The administration of several doses of adrenaline, as well as chest compressions, restored his heartbeat. However, several minutes after cardiac restoration, cardiac arrest was repeated three to four times. Eventually, he passed away six hours upon arrival. The following day, blood culture results revealed the presence of *Streptococcus* (Figure 1(c)). An autopsy was performed under the consent of his family. Gloss examination of the entire body revealed purple spots across the face, neck, and chest (Figure 2(a)). The autopsy also revealed splenic hypoplasia, with the organ weighting 20 g (Figure 2(b)). Microscopic analysis of the spleen disclosed striking neutrophil infiltration (Figure 2(c)), providing the evidence of sepsis and the analysis of the adrenal glands showed hemorrhage in all layers of the cortex

(a)

(b)

(c)

(d)

(e)

(f)

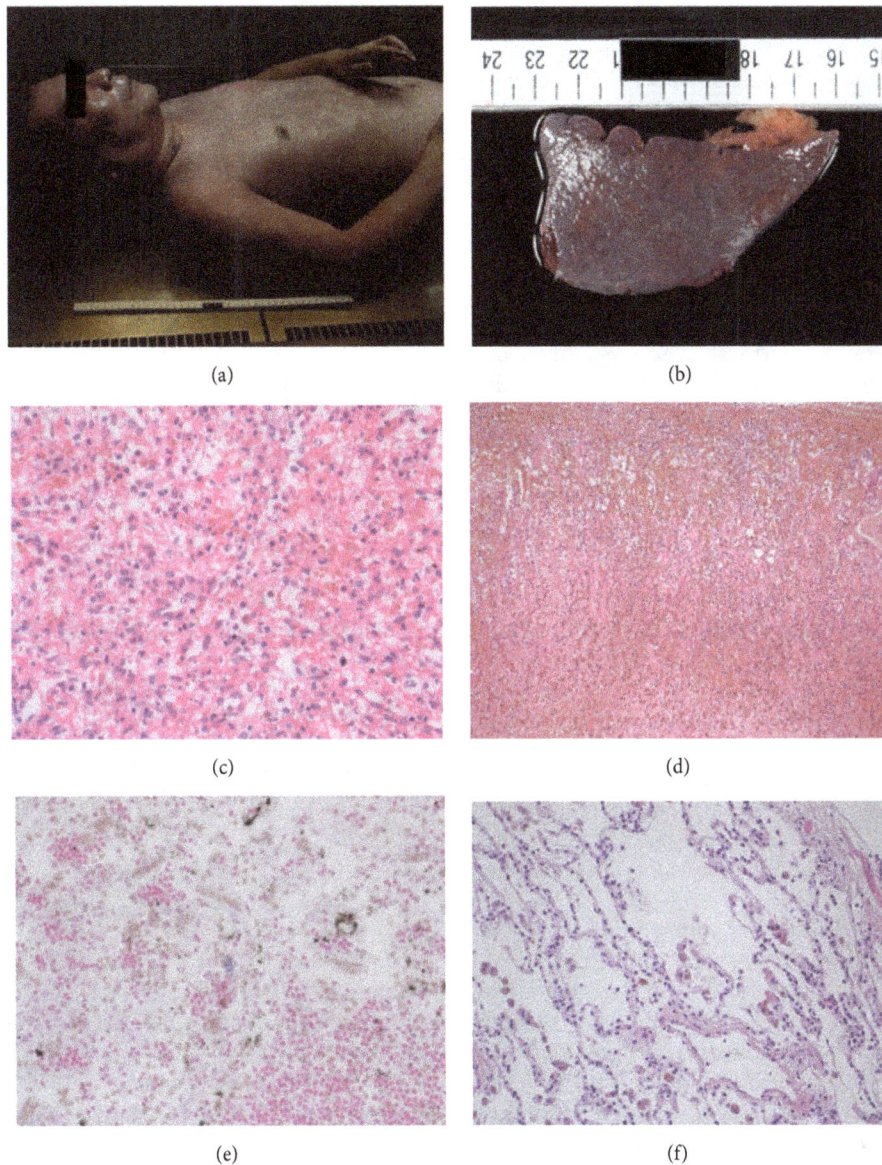

FIGURE 2: Autopsy analysis. (a) Gross inspection of the entire body revealed purpura fulminans in the face, neck, and chest. (b) Macroscopic analysis of the spleen. The spleen weighted 20 g, with a size of 7.5 × 4.0 × 1.8 cm. (c) Microscopic analysis of the spleen revealed striking neutrophil infiltration. This finding was compatible with acute splenitis, showing evidence of sepsis. (d) Microscopic analysis of the adrenal glands demonstrated hemorrhage in all the layers of the cortex and medulla. Hemosiderin dispositions are apparent. (e, f) Microscopic analysis of the tonsils (e) and lungs (f) revealed streptococci (gram staining).

and medulla (Figure 2(d)). Gram staining of the tonsil and lungs provided evidence of streptococcal infection (Figures 2(e) and 2(f)). Thus, the presence of *Streptococcus* in his lungs and tonsils along with bilateral adrenal hemorrhage revealed that the autopsy was consistent with WFS.

3. Discussion

It is well- known that splenectomized patients are likely to contract severe infection, which may be fatal; this condition is known as overwhelming post splenectomy infection (OPSI) syndrome [6]. On the other hand, it is less well known that patients with a hypoplastic splenic or decreased splenic

function are vulnerable to bacterial infections [7]. The spleen plays a vital role in controlling infections, including bacterial phagocytosis, antigen presentation, antigen production, and production of bacterial opsonin. If spleen function is decreased, it is also known that severe infections can be caused by polysacharide-encapsulated bacteria. In this patient, an enhanced-CT scan demonstrated the small size of the spleen. In general, splenic dysfunction may not only be a result of splenic hypoplasia but also liver cirrhosis, portal hypertension, ulcerative colitis, amyloidosis, sarcoidosis, and collagen diseases. It was revealed at the initial interview that the patient previously had been notified about his decreased peripheral blood cell count resulting from splenic hypoplasia, but no preventative measures had been taken.

Howell-Jolly bodies are seen along with a markedly decreased splenic function. Some reports show that counting Howell-Jolly bodies are a simple and useful measure for assessing splenic function [8] and, in our case, the sample of peripheral blood cells shows the inclusion of Howell-Jolly bodies. Based on this finding along with the evidence provided by the enhanced-CT scan revealing a hypoplastic spleen, the patient was considered to have a decreased splenic function.

Purpura fulminans is a critical syndrome, involving intravascular thrombosis and hemorrhagic infarction of the skin, which rapidly progresses, and is accompanied by vascular collapse or DIC [9]. It is characterized by small vessel thrombosis, leading to tissue necrosis, and is associated with a high mortality rate of approximately 43% [10]. The condition sometimes requires aggressive surgical treatment, including limb amputation, to prevent further dissemination of toxins or to save patients afflicted by purpura fulminans [10]. In our case, with the rapidly worsening condition, surgical treatment was not feasible.

WFS is an emergency condition, characterized by fever, cyanosis, bruises, and/or shock [1]. Even if it is treated, patients with WFS usually die within 24 h after presentation of the syndrome [2]. On autopsy, our case was compatible with the diagnosis of WFS. It is challenging to properly diagnose WFS during the treatment of patients with septic shock and it is supposed that many patients with WFS pass away when left undiagnosed.

Hence, till late, WFS has been considered a post-mortem diagnosis; however, with the development of imaging modalities, including ultrasonography and CT scan, imaging-based diagnosis of adrenal hemorrhage is possible. In general, non-traumatic adrenal hemorrhage revealed by CT scan characteristically presents as being round or oval, with the stranding of periadrenal fat [11]. In our case, the findings of adrenal hemorrhage were not recognized in the settings of the emergency department. In retrospect, it is apparent that the left side adrenal gland was round and accompanied by the stranding of periadrenal fat (Figure 1(b)). The final diagnosis of WFS was made possible by autopsy, with extensive bleeding necrosis of the bilateral adrenal glands. Considering this condition of WFS, acute adrenal insufficiency would be expected and, therefore, the described extensive therapeutic strategy was ineffective in this case. In general, if acute adrenal insufficiency can be diagnosed quickly in ICU settings, early administration of steroidal drugs may, in fact, be life-saving. When treating patients with severe infection diseases, it is important to unravel any existing adrenal insufficiency with the help of imaging modalities, especially CT scan.

4. Conclusion

We reported a rare case of Waterhouse-Friderichsen syndrome, presenting with purpura fulminans, resulting from an invasive pneumococcal infection. In the emergency department, it is important to be aware of adrenal insufficiency

as well as impaired splenic function whenever patients with sepsis are admitted.

Authors' Contributions

Kazumasa Emori, Nobuhiro Takeuchi and Junichi Soneda treated the patient. Kazumasa Emori and Nobuhiro Takeuchi wrote the manuscript and Nobuhiro Takeuchi revised and edited the manuscript. All authors read and approved the final manuscript.

Acknowledgment

The authors thank Himiko Kodaira, Yuichiro Koma, and Hiroshi Yokosaki of Kobe University and Kaori Mori and Kumiko Kawabuchi of Department of Laboratory Medicine, Kobe Tokusyukai Hospital. They also thank David Richard for helping them review the paper.

References

[1] R. Waterhouse, "A case of suprarenal apoplexy," The Lancet, vol. 177, no. 4566, pp. 577–578, 1911.

[2] Y. Hata, T. Chiba, M. Ohtani, S. Ishizawa, and N. Nishida, "An autopsy case of pneumococcal Waterhouse-Friderichsen syndrome with possible functional asplenia/hyposplenia," International Journal of Clinical and Experimental Pathology, vol. 8, no. 6, pp. 7518–7525, 2015.

[3] C. Vincentelli, E. G. Molina, and M. J. Robinson, "Fatal pneumococcal Waterhouse-Friderichsen syndrome in a vaccinated adult with congenital asplenia," The American Journal of Emergency Medicine, vol. 27, no. 6, pp. 751.e3–751.e5, 2009.

[4] R. Kanthan, T. Moyana, and J. Nyssen, "Asplenia as a cause of sudden unexpected death in childhood," American Journal of Forensic Medicine and Pathology, vol. 20, no. 1, pp. 57–59, 1999.

[5] M. D. Grant, H. I. Horowitz, V. Lorian, and H. R. Brodman, "Waterhouse-Friderichsen syndrome induced by pneumococcemic shock," The Journal of the American Medical Association, vol. 212, no. 8, pp. 1373–1374, 1999.

[6] P. D. Sinwar, "Overwhelming post splenectomy infection syndrome—review study," International Journal of Surgery, vol. 12, no. 12, pp. 1314–1316, 2014.

[7] K. Hansen and D. B. Singer, "Asplenic-hyposplenic overwhelming sepsis: postsplenectomy sepsis revisited," Pediatric and Developmental Pathology, vol. 4, no. 2, pp. 105–121, 2001.

[8] G. R. Corazza, L. Ginaldi, and G. Zoli, "Howell-Jolly body counting as a measure of splenic function. A reassessment," Clinical and Laboratory Haematology, vol. 12, no. 3, pp. 269–275, 1990.

[9] O. Guelloit, "Note sur trois cas de purpura infectieux foudroyant," in Union Médicale et Scientifique du Nord-Est, vol. 8, pp. 25–29, 1884.

[10] B. J. Childers and B. Cobanov, "Acute infectious purpura fulminans: a 15-year retrospective review of 28 consecutive cases," The American Surgeon, vol. 69, no. 1, pp. 86–90, 2003.

[11] A. Kawashima, C. M. Sandler, R. D. Ernst et al., "Imaging of nontraumatic hemorrhage of the adrenal gland," Radiographics, vol. 19, no. 4, pp. 949–963, 1999.

36

Increased Intracranial Pressure during Hemodialysis in a Patient with Anoxic Brain Injury

Anton Lund,[1] Mette B. Damholt,[2] Ditte G. Strange,[1] Jesper Kelsen,[3] Hasse Møller-Sørensen,[4] and Kirsten Møller[1]

[1]Department of Neuroanaesthesiology, Rigshospitalet, University of Copenhagen, Copenhagen, Denmark
[2]Department of Nephrology, Rigshospitalet, University of Copenhagen, Copenhagen, Denmark
[3]Department of Neurosurgery, Rigshospitalet, University of Copenhagen, Copenhagen, Denmark
[4]Department of Cardiothoracic Anaesthesiology, Rigshospitalet, University of Copenhagen, Copenhagen, Denmark

Correspondence should be addressed to Anton Lund; antonlund2@gmail.com

Academic Editor: Kenneth S. Waxman

Dialysis disequilibrium syndrome (DDS) is a serious neurological complication of hemodialysis, and patients with acute brain injury are at increased risk. We report a case of DDS leading to intracranial hypertension in a patient with anoxic brain injury and discuss the subsequent dialysis strategy. A 13-year-old girl was admitted after prolonged resuscitation from cardiac arrest. Computed tomography (CT) revealed an inferior vena cava aneurysm and multiple pulmonary emboli as the likely cause. An intracranial pressure (ICP) monitor was inserted, and, on day 3, continuous renal replacement therapy (CRRT) was initiated due to acute kidney injury, during which the patient developed severe intracranial hypertension. CT of the brain showed diffuse cerebral edema. CRRT was discontinued, sedation was increased, and hypertonic saline was administered, upon which ICP normalized. Due to persistent hyperkalemia and overhydration, ultrafiltration and intermittent hemodialysis were performed separately on day 4 with a small dialyzer, low blood and dialysate flow, and high dialysate sodium content. During subsequent treatments, isolated ultrafiltration was well tolerated, whereas hemodialysis was associated with increased ICP necessitating frequent pauses or early cessation of dialysis. In patients at risk of DDS, hemodialysis should be performed with utmost care and continuous monitoring of ICP should be considered.

1. Introduction

Dialysis-requiring acute kidney injury (AKI) is a common occurrence in critically ill patients and is associated with increased mortality [1]. A rare but serious complication of dialysis is the so-called dialysis disequilibrium syndrome (DDS), defined as the occurrence of acute neurological symptoms attributed to cerebral edema and increased intracranial pressure (ICP) during or following dialysis [2]. Patients with acute brain injury are at increased risk of developing DDS and present a challenge when dialysis is indicated, as the need for acute dialysis must be balanced against the risk of neurological deterioration. Here, we present a case of intracranial hypertension due to DDS in a patient with anoxic brain injury and discuss the management of hemodialysis in neurocritically ill patients.

2. Case Presentation

A 13-year-old girl with no prior medical history was admitted to the hospital after resuscitation from cardiac arrest. The patient had collapsed during physical exercise in school, and cardiopulmonary resuscitation (CPR) was initiated immediately by school personnel. Pulseless electrical activity was the first observed prehospital rhythm. The patient was intubated by the ambulance staff, and return of spontaneous circulation was achieved after 35 minutes through CPR and adrenaline administration.

Upon arrival to our emergency department, the patient was hemodynamically unstable with a mean arterial pressure (MAP) of 60–70 mmHg and heart rate of 120 bpm. Arterial blood gases showed a severe combined metabolic and respiratory acidosis with a pH of 6.7, $PaCO_2$ of 83 mmHg (11 kPa),

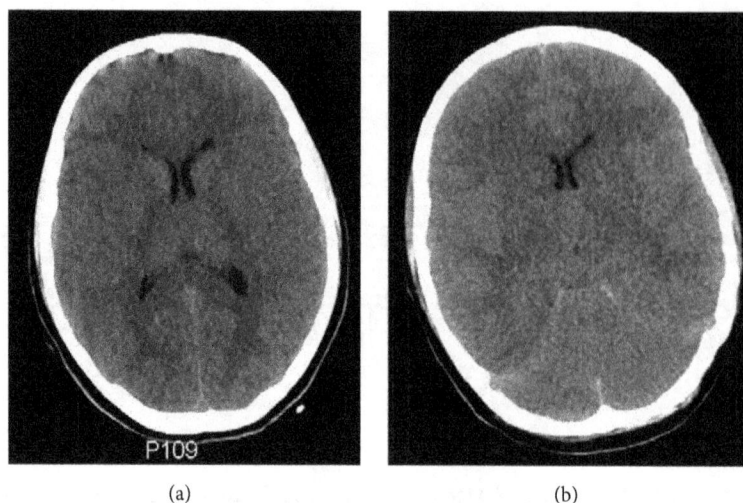

FIGURE 1: (a) Computed tomography of the brain upon arrival, showing no evidence of cerebral edema or infarction. (b) Day 3, after 7 hours of continuous renal replacement therapy: the scan now shows generalized cerebral edema with effacement of the basal cisterns and reduced grey-white matter differentiation.

and a blood lactate of 15 mmol/L on mechanical ventilation. Bedside echocardiography revealed a dilated right ventricle and a mass in the right ventricular outflow tract suggesting a venous thrombus. Computed tomography (CT) with pulmonary angiography showed multiple peripheral emboli in both lungs, and CT of the abdomen and pelvis revealed an aneurysm of the inferior vena cava as the likely source of the emboli. CT of the brain showed no evidence of cerebral edema or infarction (Figure 1(a)). However, based on the prolonged resuscitation and decreased level of consciousness, an ICP transducer was inserted to enable detection of cerebral edema during the impending deep sedation. Initial ICP readings were normal (4 mmHg).

The patient was transferred to the cardiothoracic intensive care unit (ICU) and a cerebral perfusion pressure >60 mmHg was maintained with infusion of adrenaline and noradrenaline. Targeted temperature management aiming at 36°C for 24 hours was initiated, and the patient was started on high-dose unfractionated heparin due to the pulmonary emboli. Failed attempts to cannulate both femoral arteries resulted in bilateral hematoma formation and continued bleeding from the right femoral artery despite compression necessitated surgical exploration with repair of the artery and fasciotomy.

The day after admission, the patient had been hemodynamically stabilized and weaned off vasopressors. Sedation was gradually diminished and finally turned off. The patient demonstrated eye opening upon stimulation, pupils that were equal and reactive to light, spontaneous breathing, and a normal swallowing reflex. No spontaneous movements were observed. ICP was slightly elevated at 10–17 mmHg depending on stimulation and closely related to MAP. Laboratory analyses revealed rising levels of creatinine, urea, and potassium, and diuresis was low despite stimulation with furosemide and metolazone. Myoglobin and creatine kinase were also significantly elevated, suggesting rhabdomyolysis

due to hypoxia, compartment syndrome of the right thigh, or both.

On the evening of day 3, the patient had a P-creatinine of 5.17 mg/dL (457 μmol/L), P-urea of 99 mg/dL (35.4 mmol/L), and a P-potassium of 6.0 mmol/L despite infusion of glucose and insulin. The patient was visibly hypervolemic with an estimated cumulated fluid balance of +12.5 liters. ICP was stable but slightly elevated at 16–19 mmHg, and the patient was lightly sedated with remifentanil infusion. It was decided to initiate continuous renal replacement therapy (CRRT), and a double lumen dialysis catheter was placed in the right internal jugular vein. The following dialysis settings were used: Continuous venovenous hemodiafiltration, ST100 dialyzer (Gambro; surface area 1 m², KUF 25 mL/(h·mmHg)), blood flow 120 mL/min, predilution flow 1000 mL/h (Prismocitrate, Gambro), dialysate flow 1000 mL/h (Prism0cal B22, Gambro), and postdilution flow 200 mL/h (Phoxillium, Gambro).

Approximately seven hours after start of CRRT, ICP had increased to 38 mmHg (Figure 2); the patient had developed diverging eye axes and become unresponsive to pain (Glasgow Coma Score 3). On suspicion of cerebral edema or infarction, CRRT was stopped, 50 mL of hypertonic saline (1 mmol/mL) was administered, and the patient was sedated with propofol. CT of the brain was performed and revealed diffuse cerebral edema (Figure 1(b)). ICP decreased to 20 mmHg within a few hours. Due to the neurological deterioration and unstable ICP, the patient was transferred to the neurological ICU (NICU) and sedated with thiopentone, midazolam, and fentanyl.

On day 4, an external ventricular drain (EVD) was inserted stereotaxically based on a predicted need for further hemodialysis, upon which ICP decreased from 10 to 3 mmHg. A window of cardiovascular stability and low ICP was used as an opportunity to start careful intermittent hemodialysis. Hemodialysis was chosen over peritoneal dialysis due to

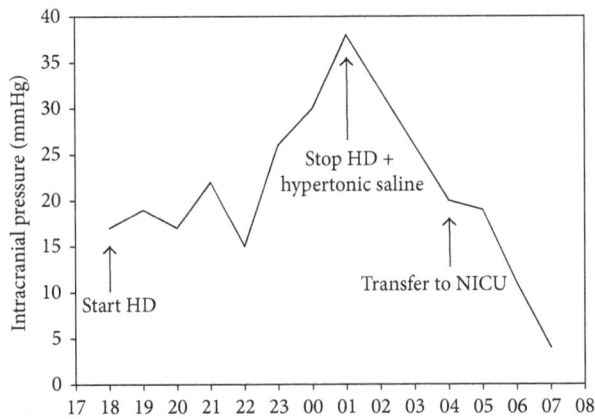

FIGURE 2: Intracranial pressure during a 13-hour period after start of continuous renal replacement therapy. x-axis denotes time of day. HD = hemodialysis; NICU = Neurointensive Care Unit.

hyperkalemia and the need for removal of large volumes of fluid, as well as the possibility of separating ultrafiltration and dialysis. P-creatinine was 5.92 mg/dL (523 μmol/L) and P-urea 95 mg/dL (34.1 mmol/L) before start of dialysis. The patient completed 3.5 hours of isolated ultrafiltration, with ultrafiltration rate gradually increasing from 250 mL/h to 1000 mL/h and a total fluid removal of 2.5 L. Subsequently, the patient underwent 1 hour of hemodialysis without complications and with no clinically significant changes in ICP. Dialysis settings were modified to reduce the dialysis dose in an attempt to prevent DDS and were as follows: H6 dialyzer (Gambro; surface area 0.6 m^2, KUF 33 mL/(h·mmHg)), dialysate sodium 148 mmol/L, potassium 2 mmol/L, bicarbonate 38 mmol/L, calcium 1.5 mmol/L, magnesium 0.5 mmol/L, and low dialysate flow at 300 mL/min and blood flow 150 mL/min with concurrent flows to reduce dialysis efficiency. On day 5, ultrafiltration and hemodialysis were repeated with similar settings. However, ICP gradually increased from 0 to 10 mmHg and the treatment was stopped prematurely. Similar problems were encountered on the following days, necessitating frequent pauses or early cessation of hemodialysis.

On day 8, an inferior vena cava filter was placed in order to prevent future episodes of pulmonary embolization. From day 10 and onwards, the patient was able to tolerate hemodialysis without increases in ICP. Hemodialysis was discontinued on day 21, as kidney function was rapidly returning. The patient was gradually weaned off sedation and mechanical ventilation; autonomic dysfunction ensued and was treated with baclofen and propranolol. On day 51 the patient was in a minimally conscious state (MCS) and was discharged from the NICU and transferred to a neurorehabilitation facility. Upon follow-up three months after discharge, she remained in MCS with signs of slow improvement.

3. Discussion

DDS occurs with a wide spectrum of clinical manifestations, ranging from mild symptoms such as headache, nausea,

vomiting, blurred vision, and muscle twitching to more severe manifestations including altered mental status, coma, seizures, and death [2]. The diagnosis is largely clinical, but the syndrome has been associated with electroencephalographic abnormalities [3], and diagnostic imaging of the brain may reveal changes consistent with cerebral edema [4]. The pathophysiology of DDS remains debated, but it likely involves an osmotic shift of water across the blood-brain barrier into the brain due to a rapid removal of urea from plasma during dialysis [5]. DDS seems to be more common in children, in patients with very high blood urea concentrations, in patients with chronic kidney disease (versus AKI), and in patients undergoing their first dialysis [2, 6]. A number of cases of DDS have been reported in patients with traumatic brain injury and intracranial hemorrhage, suggesting that patients with acute brain injury are particularly susceptible to this condition. [7–13]. Several of the mentioned risk factors were present in our patient, most notably anoxic brain injury due to prolonged cardiac arrest, which resulted in cerebral edema. In the present case, ICP monitoring aided in the detection of intracranial hypertension during CRRT and led to EVD placement and a conservative dialysis strategy.

AKI is a common complication in the course of critical illness, and dialysis is often indicated due to overhydration, hyperkalemia, or severe acidosis. To correct these disturbances in a clinically appropriate time scale, hemodialysis (as opposed to peritoneal dialysis) is often the most feasible option. In patients with acute brain injury, however, caution should be exhibited due to the risk of DDS and associated intracranial hypertension. Potential protective strategies against DDS have been proposed in the literature, including slower blood and dialysate flows, smaller surface area dialyzer membranes, and high sodium and low bicarbonate concentrations in the dialysate [14]. Furthermore, continuous therapies (i.e., CRRT) have been suggested as being safer than intermittent hemodialysis in patients at risk of DDS [15, 16]. The common rationale behind these strategies is to slow down the rate of urea clearance, to reduce the change in serum osmolality, and to maintain hemodynamic stability. In our patient, however, DDS first developed during CRRT, indicating that patients are at risk even when using continuous therapies [17]. The patient was subsequently treated with intermittent hemodialysis, in which dialysis settings were modified in an attempt to reduce the risk of DDS, including separation of ultrafiltration and dialysis and modification of dialysate electrolytes. These precautions allowed sufficient fluid removal, but hemodialysis was nonetheless complicated by recurring increases in ICP, necessitating frequent pauses or early cessation of the treatment.

Hyperosmolar therapy, a mainstay in the treatment of elevated ICP, is another potential strategy for the management of DDS. The treatment can effectively reduce cerebral edema by raising plasma osmolality, thereby removing brain extracellular fluid due to creation of an osmotic gradient across the blood-brain barrier [18]. In the present case, hypertonic saline was administered during the initial ICP crisis during CRRT and was effective in reducing ICP, although discontinuation of dialysis and increased sedation were likely important as well. As a preventive measure against

DDS, certain authors have suggested infusion of hypertonic saline during dialysis in high-risk patients [14]. A similar effect can be achieved using a high sodium dialysate, as employed in our case. There are, however, potential safety concerns with hyperosmolar therapy in the setting of renal failure, as insufficient renal excretion could put patients at risk of sodium overload and hypervolemia. Few studies have examined hyperosmolar therapy in this patient population, although a small retrospective study of hypertonic saline for treatment of elevated ICP in patients with renal failure found the treatment to be safe and effective [19].

4. Conclusion

This case highlights the inherent risks associated with hemodialysis in patients with acute brain injury. The patient in question was likely predisposed to DDS due to anoxic brain injury and cerebral edema after prolonged cardiac arrest. Increases in ICP developed both during CRRT and during careful intermittent hemodialysis, indicating that no dialysis modality confers complete protection against this complication. In high-risk patients, we suggest early start of dialysis to avoid high urea gradients during the procedure, as well as minimizing the dialysis dose. Isolated ultrafiltration seems to be well tolerated and may allow correction of fluid overload. If hemodialysis is required in the high-risk neurocritically ill patient, continuous ICP monitoring may be required to enable timely detection of and intervention against DDS.

References

[1] S. Uchino, J. A. Kellum, R. Bellomo et al., "Acute renal failure in critically ill patients: A Multinational, Multicenter Study," *Journal of the American Medical Association*, vol. 294, no. 7, pp. 813–818, 2005.

[2] N. Patel, P. Dalal, and M. Panesar, "Dialysis disequilibrium syndrome: a narrative review," *Seminars in Dialysis*, vol. 21, no. 5, pp. 493–498, 2008.

[3] H. Hampl, H. W. Klopp, N. Michels et al., "Electroencephalogram investigations of the disequilibrium syndrome during bicarbonate and acetate dialysis," *Proceedings of the European Dialysis and Transplant Association*, vol. 19, pp. 351–359, 1983.

[4] R. J. L. Walters, N. C. Fox, W. R. Crum, D. Taube, and D. J. Thomas, "Haemodialysis and cerebral oedema," *Nephron*, vol. 87, no. 2, pp. 143–147, 2001.

[5] S. M. Silver, R. H. Sterns, and M. L. Halperin, "Brain swelling after dialysis: old urea or new osmoles?" *American Journal of Kidney Diseases*, vol. 28, no. 1, pp. 1–13, 1996.

[6] A. I. Arieff, "Dialysis disequilibrium syndrome: current concepts on pathogenesis and prevention," *Kidney International*, vol. 45, no. 3, pp. 629–635, 1994.

[7] S. Yoshida, T. Tajika, N. Yamasaki et al., "Dialysis dysequilibrium syndrome in neurosurgical patients," *Neurosurgery*, vol. 20, no. 5, pp. 716–721, 1987.

[8] N. K. Krane, "Intracranial pressure measurement in a patient undergoing hemodialysis and peritoneal dialysis," *American Journal of Kidney Diseases*, vol. 13, no. 4, pp. 336–339, 1989.

[9] M. Thicoipe, H. P. Stoiber, P. Maurette, A. Leger, and J. F. Cochard, "Changes in intracranial pressure in severe head injured patients in hemodialysis," *Annales Françaises d'Anesthésie et de Réanimation*, vol. 7, pp. 336–338, 1988.

[10] C. M. Lin, J. W. Lin, J. T. Tsai et al., "Intracranial pressure fluctuation during hemodialysis in renal failure patients with intracranial hemorrhage," *Acta Neurochirurgica Supplement*, vol. 101, pp. 141–144, 2008.

[11] P. Esnault, G. Lacroix, P.-J. Cungi, E. D'Aranda, J. Cotte, and P. Goutorbe, "Dialysis disequilibrium syndrome in neurointensive care unit: the benefit of intracranial pressure monitoring," *Critical Care*, vol. 16, no. 6, article 472, 2012.

[12] Y. M. Bertrand, A. Hermant, P. Mahieu, and J. Roels, "Intracranial pressure changes in patients with head trauma during haemodialysis," *Intensive Care Medicine*, vol. 9, no. 6, pp. 321–323, 1983.

[13] M. Osgood, R. Compton, R. Carandang, W. Hall, G. Kershaw, and S. Muehlschlegel, "Rapid unexpected brain herniation in association with renal replacement therapy in acute brain injury: caution in the neurocritical care unit," *Neurocritical Care*, vol. 22, no. 2, pp. 176–183, 2015.

[14] A. Davenport, "Practical guidance for dialyzing a hemodialysis patient following acute brain injury," *Hemodialysis International*, vol. 12, no. 3, pp. 307–312, 2008.

[15] A. Davenport, "Continuous renal replacement therapies in patients with acute neurological injury," *Seminars in Dialysis*, vol. 22, no. 2, pp. 165–168, 2009.

[16] J. J. Fletcher, K. Bergman, E. C. Feucht, and P. Blostein, "Continuous renal replacement therapy for refractory intracranial hypertension," *Neurocritical Care*, vol. 11, no. 1, pp. 101–105, 2009.

[17] S. Tuchman, Z. P. Khademian, and K. Mistry, "Dialysis disequilibrium syndrome occurring during continuous renal replacement therapy," *Clinical Kidney Journal*, vol. 6, no. 5, pp. 526–529, 2013.

[18] A. Torre-Healy, N. F. Marko, and R. J. Weil, "Hyperosmolar therapy for intracranial hypertension," *Neurocritical Care*, vol. 17, no. 1, pp. 117–130, 2012.

[19] K. G. Hirsch, T. Spock, M. A. Koenig, and R. G. Geocadin, "Treatment of elevated intracranial pressure with hyperosmolar therapy in patients with renal failure," *Neurocritical Care*, vol. 17, no. 3, pp. 388–394, 2012.

37

The use of Coupled Plasma Filtration Adsorption in Traumatic Rhabdomyolysis

Mario Pezzi,[1] **Silvia Renda,**[1] **Anna Maria Giglio,**[1] **Anna Maria Scozzafava,**[1] **Simona Paola Tiburzi,**[1] **Patrizia Casella,**[1] **Fabrizio Iannelli,**[2] **and Mario Verre**[1]

[1]*Anaesthesia and Intensive Care Unit, General Hospital "Pugliese-Ciaccio", Viale Pio X, 88100 Catanzaro, Italy*
[2]*Bellco, 41037 Mirandola, Italy*

Correspondence should be addressed to Mario Pezzi; mariopezzi@yahoo.it

Academic Editor: Nicolas Nin

Severe musculoskeletal injuries induce the release of sarcoplasmic elements such as muscle enzymes, potassium, and myoglobin in the systemic circulation. The circulating myoglobin damages the glomerulus and renal tubules. Conventional haemodialysis is not able to remove myoglobin, due to its high molecular weight (17,8 kilodaltons [kDa]). We treated four traumatic rhabdomyolysis patients with Coupled Plasma Filtration Adsorption (CPFA) in order to remove myoglobin followed by 14 hours of Continuous Veno-Venous Hemofiltration (CVVH). During the treatment, all patients showed clinical improvement with a decrease in muscular (creatine kinase [CK] and myoglobin) and renal (creatinine and potassium) damage indices. One patient, in spite of full renal recovery, died of cerebral haemorrhage on the 26th day of hospital stay.

1. Introduction

Musculoskeletal damage in trauma patients includes several clinical presentations [1].

Among the various forms of rhabdomyolysis, the common pathophysiologic element is a rise in intracellular ionized calcium. The loss of transcellular calcium gradient causes a series of events which lead to cell death [2].

If rhabdomyolysis is suspected it is important to evaluate creatine kinase (CK) and myoglobin blood levels, since they represent the most sensitive markers of muscle injury. Changes in creatinine, potassium, sodium, blood urea nitrogen, total and ionized calcium, magnesium, phosphate, uric acid, albumin, and lactate blood levels may also be present. Other important investigations include acid base balance evaluation, blood cell count, and coagulation tests.

The enzyme creatine kinase is present in both skeletal and cardiac muscles in its two isoforms, MM and MB. In the skeletal muscle, MB isoenzyme accounts for 90% of total CK and its dosage is specific for muscular disorders. Normal CK blood levels are up to 170 U/L: after extended muscle injury, this value undergoes a more than fivefold increase between 2 and 12 hours after the onset of the lesion, reaches a peak (up to 100000 U/L) within 24 to 72 hours, and then decreases within 3–5 days after the resolution of the muscular lesion [3].

A fivefold elevation of serum CK in absence of cardiac or neurological disorders is diagnostic of rhabdomyolysis, and a value of more than 5000 U/L can be associated with the development of renal failure [4]. CK serum levels remain elevated longer than myoglobin, due to its relatively slow plasma clearance rate (1.5 days).

Myoglobin is a small protein with a very low hematic concentration in physiological conditions; it is composed of 153 amino acids with a single heme prosthetic group, with a molecular weight of 17,8 kDa. Myoglobin accounts for 1–3% of muscle mass dry weight and its function is to bind oxygen and facilitate its transport within muscle cells, which work under low oxygen tension conditions. Myoglobin serum levels increase within 1 hour after a musculoskeletal injury and return to baseline within 1 to 6 hours after the resolution of the lesion; its metabolism occurs by glomerular filtration, absorption in the proximal tubule by endocytosis, and proteolysis.

Coupled Plasma Filtration Adsorption

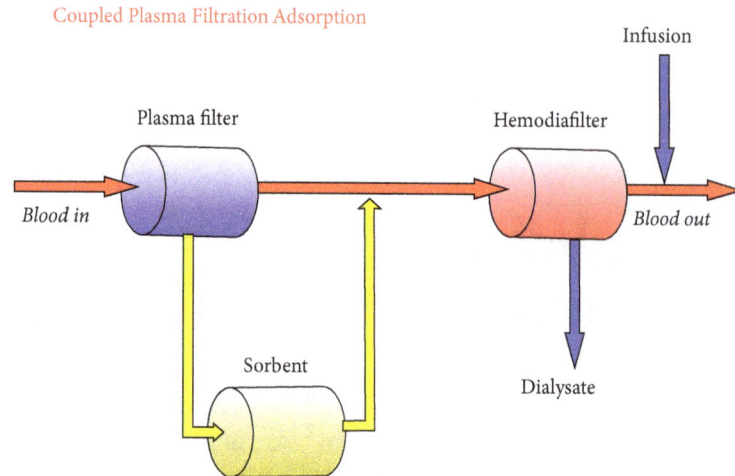

FIGURE 1

When a muscle injury takes place, free myoglobin enters the bloodstream and largely binds to haptoglobin and $\alpha2$ globulins. Myoglobin removal from the circulation is due to the reticuloendothelial system, but in rhabdomyolysis free myoglobin concentration exceeds its purifying capability [5].

The main consequence of a massive release of myoglobin in the systemic circulation is acute renal failure. The relationship between myoglobin blood levels and renal injury was demonstrated by Kasaoka et al. in a study including 30 rhabdomyolysis patients: according to these authors, the peak serum levels of CK and myoglobin were significantly higher in the group with acute renal failure than in the group with preserved renal function [6].

This phenomenon is linked to the degree of acidity of urine which is, in turn, correlated with hypovolemia. Myoglobin levels exceeding 15000 ng/mL are significantly related to the development of acute renal failure and the need for haemodialysis [7].

Correction of hypovolemia with an early and aggressive fluid resuscitation has proven to be the most important factor in preventing the development of renal failure. During the first 72 hours more than 10 litres of fluids per day may be needed, so strict monitoring of diuresis and central venous pressure is essential to avoid volume overload and pulmonary oedema. The goal should be a urine flow rate of more than 2-3 mL/kg/h; it is advisable to avoid solutions containing potassium [8]. The use of loop diuretics and mannitol may be beneficial, while the role of urine alkalinization remains controversial [9].

From November 2013 to December 2015, four patients with rhabdomyolysis came to our attention: they all presented raised serum CK and myoglobin levels and were promptly treated with fluid replacement, urine alkalinization, and forced diuresis, in order to prevent myoglobin-induced renal damage.

Since low-flow haemodialysis does not allow the elimination of substances with a molecular weight exceeding 5 kDa, the removal of high molecular weight proteins such as myoglobin requires high volume hemodiafiltration techniques [10].

To foster the removal of myoglobin, we used Coupled Plasma Filtration Adsorption (CPFA) associated with Continuous Veno-Venous Hemofiltration (CVVH). The patients were subjected to extracorporeal treatment with CPFA for 10 hours followed by CVVH for 14 hours. Two patients were subjected to three treatments in 72 hours and two patients were subjected to four treatments within 96 hours.

After control and correction of haemoglobin, platelets and antithrombin III levels, and coagulation profile, anticoagulation was obtained with a priming dose of 15000 U in 4 litres of washing liquid and a maintenance dose of 5–10 U/kg/h of unfractioned heparin, with monitoring of activated Partial Thromboplastin Time (aPTT) and Activated Clotting Time (ACT) every 4 hours. Target was aPTT (not > 60 sec) and ACT (140–200 sec). For automatic priming, the infusion liquid is used for the filling and washing. This condition predisposes the apparatus not only to the priming but also to the patient's treatment.

CPFA is an extracorporeal therapy which uses a plasma filter to separate plasma from blood, allowing the separated plasma to pass through an adsorbent cartridge for nonspecific removal of several mediators. After purification, plasma is returned to blood, which can then pass through a hemofilter for further purification by means of conventional haemodialysis, hemofiltration, or hemodiafiltration in case of acute renal failure (Figure 1). The main therapeutic goal of CPFA is to hit the excess of pro- and anti-inflammatory mediators, in order to reestablish a normal immune function [11].

In CPFA a synthetic resin made of styrene-divinylbenzene is used which interacts with the hydrophobic sites on the molecules: this type of resin is used in various processes ranging from chromatography purification to industrial food, beverage, and pharmaceutical products. This resin is suitable for extracorporeal applications for its high homogeneity, the good performance pressure-flow, and excellent mechanical and chemical stability. In addition to its mechanical properties, the choice of this particular resin was based on various other factors related to its ability to adsorb a wide variety of inflammatory mediators and its adsorption characteristics at different flow rates. The maximum of efficacy is obtained especially in case of substances with high-medium molecular weight, like myoglobin (about 18 kDa).

CPFA consists of a four-pump modular device (Lynda, Bellco®, Mirandola, Italy) with a plasma filter (0.45 m^2 polyethersulfone with an approximate cut-off of 800 kDa), a nonselective hydrophobic resin cartridge (140 mL) with a surface of approximately 700 m^2/g, and a synthetic , high-permeability hemofilter (1.4 m^2 polyethersulfone) which allows the application of convectional exchange to the whole blood once it is reconstituted in postdilution [12].

The distinctive aspect of CPFA is the application of the sorbent to the plasma rather than the whole blood. This feature brings important benefits: the lower flow of plasma allows a prolonged contact with the sorbent and reduces biocompatibility issues [12].

We used the blood flow (Qb) values that were between 200 and 250 mL/min, and the amount of reinfusion solution (Qinf) used was 35 mL/kg/h. The plasma flow value (Qs) was 15% compared to the prescribed blood flow.

In the intervals between treatments with CPFA all patients were treated with CVVH. Blood flow (Qb) between 150 and 220 mL/min has been used according to the set values of ultrafiltration, in order to obtain a fraction of filtration (FF) <20%. The amount of reinfusion solution (QR) used was 35 mL/kg/h, with a share of 30% infusion in predilution.

To make the CVVH with Lynda device Bellco is necessary to exclude the plasma filter and the sorbent cartridge and use only the hemofilter. It allows high volumes of ultrafiltrate using the filling liquid that can be administered before or after the filter. The pump ensures adequate blood flow to maintain the proportion of ultrafiltrate required.

2. Clinical Cases

2.1. Male, Aged 19. The patient presented with a gunshot wound in his left lower limb, haemorrhagic shock, muscular disintegration, left popliteal artery occlusion, and multiple venous lesions; furthermore, there was another gunshot wound in the skull with left temporal bone fracture and a retained bullet in proximity to the 5th cervical vertebral body.

The patient underwent vascular surgery after approximately 8 hours following the traumatic event. Arterial vascularization was restored, fasciotomy of the left lower limb was performed, and continuous aspiration wound dressing was placed.

During the surgery, 8 units of packed red blood cells, 4 units of fresh frozen plasma, and 4 units of platelets were administered; in the following 24 hours fluid replacement was initiated under continuous monitoring of central venous pressure: 5% glucose (3000 mL), 0,9% normal saline solution (3000 mL), and 8,4% sodium bicarbonate for urine alkalinization (500 mL) were infused. The urine output was approximately 200 mL/h.

After the surgery the patient was transferred to the Intensive Care Unit, intubated, and under mechanical ventilation and inotropic support with Dopamine.

48 hours after the traumatic event, a further increase in CK (14790 U/L) and myoglobin (7881 ng/mL) levels occurred;

the creatinine value was 1,1 mg/dL, while the potassium value was 5,2 mEq/L.

At this point Continuous Renal Replacement Therapy (CRRT) was initiated, alternating CPFA during the first 10 hours and CVVH for the remaining 14 hours.

Valid, spontaneous diuresis was present throughout the treatment, for a total of 72 hours.

Given the positive evolution of clinical course and laboratory values, CRRT was stopped. On the 9th day the patient was transferred to the Vascular Surgery Department for continuation of hospital care (Table 1, Figures 2(a) and 2(b)).

2.2. Male, Aged 55. The patient was brought to the Emergency Department after a road trauma involving a heavy vehicle, with crushing of pelvis and lower limbs. He presented haemorrhagic shock due to multiple pelvic girdle fractures, traumatic section of urethra, retroperitoneal hematoma, left femoral fracture, L2 to L5 vertebral body fractures, and crush injury of the right lower limb.

After suprapubic catheterization, the patient underwent external fixation of pelvic fractures and reduction of left femoral fracture.

Fasciotomy with confection of a continuous aspiration dressing was performed on the right lower limb. 10 units of packed red blood cells, 4 units of fresh frozen plasma, and 2 units of platelets were administered.

During the next 24 hours, under continuous monitoring of central venous pressure, 4000 mL of 5% glucose, 4000 mL of 0,9% normal saline, and 1000 mL of 8,4% sodium bicarbonate were infused; the patient also needed inotropic support with continuous infusion of Adrenaline and Dopamine.

Given the onset of acute renal failure, two sessions of haemodialysis were carried out at 48 and 72 hours after the trauma. At 96 hours, given the rising levels of serum CK and myoglobin, CRRT was commenced alternating 10 hours of CPFA with 14 hours of CVVH.

The treatment lasted 96 hours; then it was suspended due to clinical improvement and decrease of muscular and renal damage indices.

During the following days a further improvement was observed, and after one month of ICU stay the patient was transferred to a recovery department, from which he was then discharged (Table 1, Figures 2(c) and 2(d)).

2.3. Male, Aged 33. The patient presented crush injury of both lower limbs due to overturn of a quad bike, with bilateral femoral and tibial fractures, right femoral artery section, and extended muscular damage of both lower limbs.

He was initially admitted to a spoke hospital where traction was applied to lower extremities, and after approximately 12 hours he was transferred to our centre for definitive treatment of bone, muscle, and vascular injuries.

Arterial revascularization of the right lower limb, reduction of fractures and fasciotomy of both lower extremities were performed. During the surgery the patient received 10 units of packed red blood cells, 5 units of fresh frozen plasma, and 2 units of platelets.

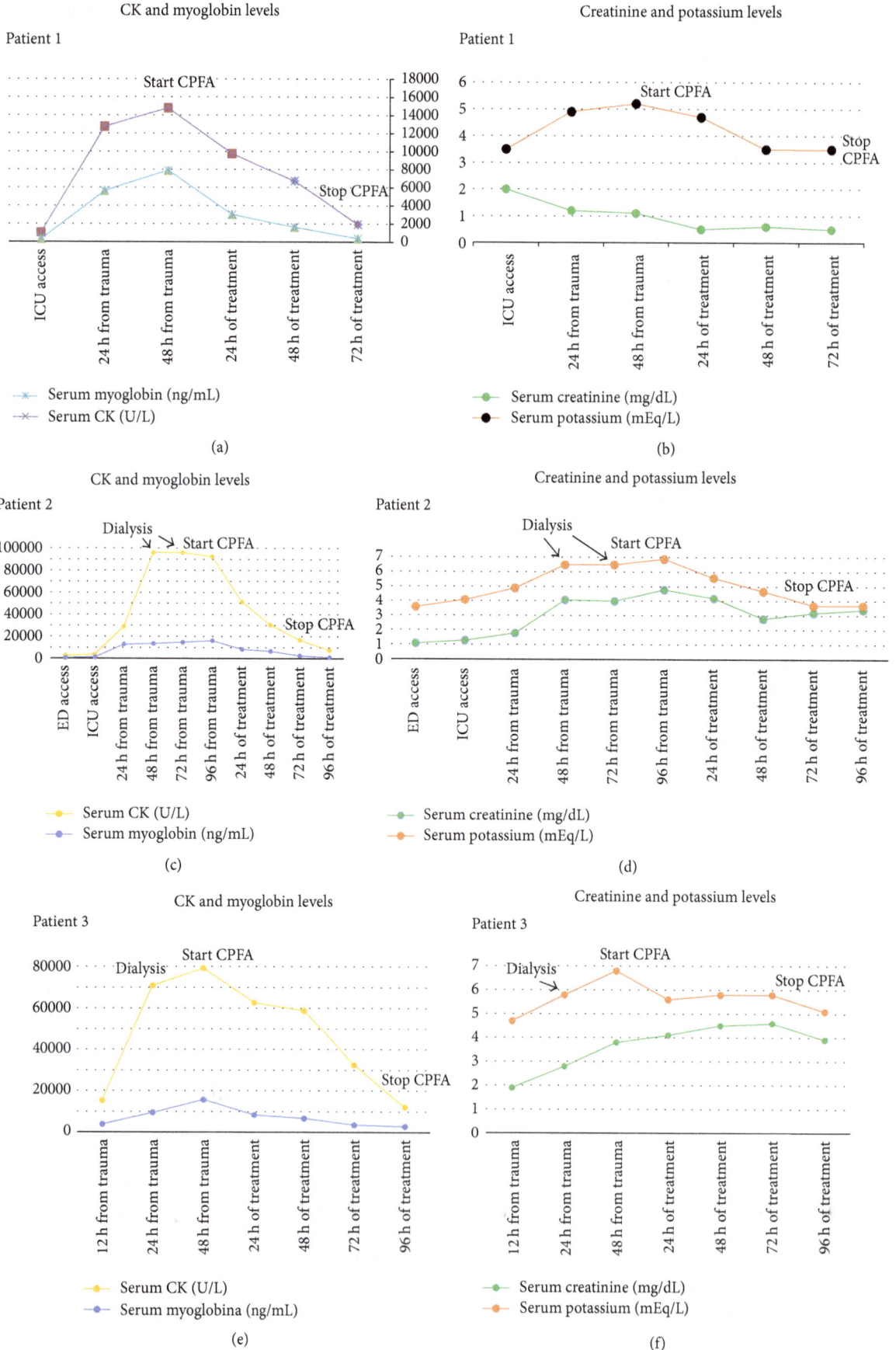

(a)

(b)

(c)

(d)

(e)

(f)

FIGURE 2: Continued.

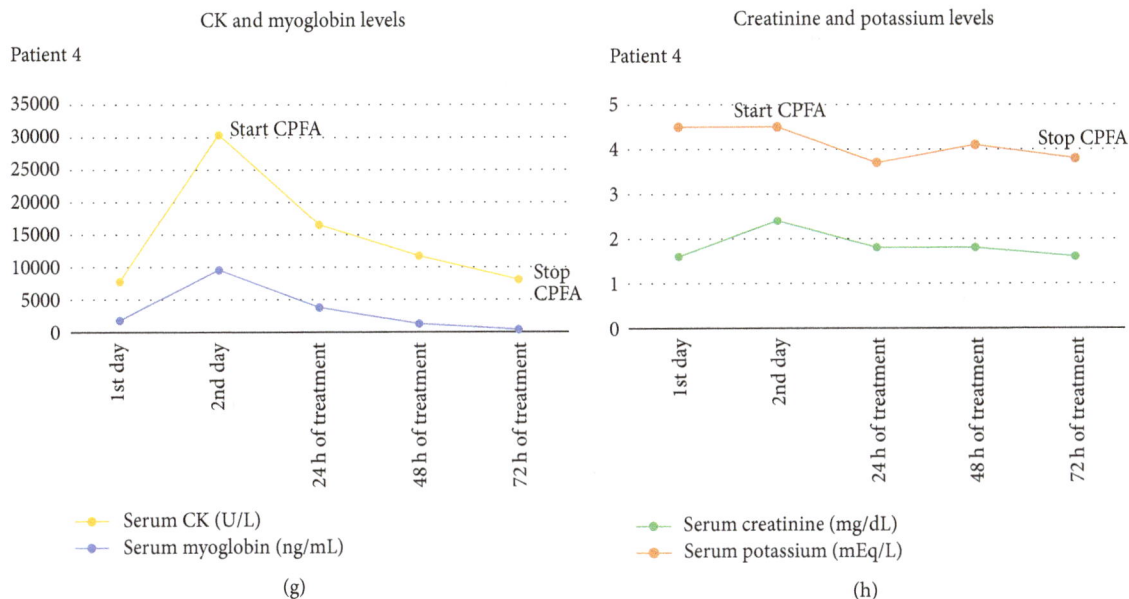

CK and myoglobin levels
Patient 4

Start CPFA

Stop CPFA

—•— Serum CK (U/L)
—•— Serum myoglobin (ng/mL)

(g)

Creatinine and potassium levels
Patient 4

Start CPFA

Stop CPFA

—•— Serum creatinine (mg/dL)
—•— Serum potassium (mEq/L)

(h)

FIGURE 2

After the surgery the patient was brought to the ICU where he remained intubated and under mechanical ventilation. During the following 24 hours, 5000 mL of 5% glucose, 5000 mL of 0,9% normal saline, and 1000 mL of 8,4% sodium bicarbonate were administered under continuous central venous pressure monitoring. The patient also required inotropic support with continuous infusion of Adrenaline and Dopamine.

Six hours after the surgical interventions the right lower limb became ischaemic again and was amputated. The left lower limb and the stump of the amputated extremity were treated with a sealed continuous aspiration dressing.

24 hours after the traumatic injury the patient became anuric, so a three-hour haemodialysis session was performed.

Since anuria persisted at 48 hours and laboratory exams showed further deterioration of renal function, CRRT therapy was started with CPFA for 10 hours and CVVH for 14 hours.

Given the improvement trend, CRRT was suspended after 96 hours of treatment and haemodialysis was restarted with a two-hour treatment on alternate days for three more days. During the following days renal function was restored completely and both respiratory and hemodynamic parameters normalized. The continuous aspiration dressing was kept in site. On the 26th day the patient suddenly died due to cerebral haemorrhage.

Enoxaparin 4000 IU was administered twice daily to the patient throughout the period of hospitalization. The autopsy showed cerebral haemorrhage with ventricular flooding and diffuse cerebral edema. It is not inconceivable that the enoxaparin had a causal role in the genesis of cerebral haemorrhage (Table 1, Figures 2(e) and 2(f)).

2.4. Male, Aged 25. The patient was transported to our Emergency Department after a 12-meter fall: he presented with multiple rib fractures, hemoperitoneum due to spleen rupture, multiple pelvic fractures, right femoral fracture, right ulnar fracture, extended muscular injury of the right upper and lower limb, and haemorrhagic shock.

He immediately underwent splenectomy and bilateral chest drain positioning. During the surgery 6 units of packed red blood cells, 4 units of fresh frozen plasma, and 2 units of platelets were given. Closed reduction of limb fractures was also performed.

During the following 24 hours the patient received 4000 mL of 5% glucose, 4000 mL of 0,9% normal saline, and 1000 mL of 8,4% sodium bicarbonate, with close monitoring of central venous pressure. Due to hemodynamic instability, inotropic support with continuous infusion of Dopamine was carried out.

In the ICU the patient underwent pharmacological sedation, several blood and hemoderivatives transfusions, mechanical ventilation, and antibiotic therapy. On the 5th day a new surgery was performed for internal fixation of femoral and elbow fractures and external fixation of pelvic fractures.

On the 1st day of stay, after splenectomy, laboratory tests showed a creatinine level of 1,6 mg/dL, a potassium level of 4,5 mEq/L, and CK and myoglobin values of 7780 U/L and 1830 ng/mL, respectively.

On the 2nd day a sharp rise in muscle damage indices was observed, with CK levels of 30389 U/L and myoglobin levels of 9562 ng/mL and concomitant increase of creatinine value (2,4 mg/dL), while potassium levels remained stable (4,5 mEq/L).

CRRT was started, alternating 10 hours of CPFA with 14 hours of CVVH. The treatment was carried out for a total of 72 hours with continuous improvement of serum CK and myoglobin levels and renal function parameters.

After 40 days of ICU stay the patient was transferred to a rehabilitation centre in good clinical conditions (Table 1, Figures 2(g) and 2(h)).

TABLE 1

	First treatment CPFA 10 h	Second treatment CPFA 10 h	Third treatment CPFA 10 h	Fourth treatment CPFA 10 h
Patient 1				
Blood flow Qb, mL/min	220	200	200	
Total plasma mL	7.500	7.000	7.250	
Plasma filtration flow rate, QS%	15	15	15	
Total dose of heparin I.U.	1.250	1.250	1.250	
Reinfusion solution Qinf, mL/min	35	35	35	
CK value U/L before CPFA	14.790	9.763	6.727	
CK value U/L after CPFA	10.725	7.659	2.512	
Myoglobin value ng/mL before CPFA	7.881	3.625	1.634	
Myoglobin value ng/mL after CPFA	4.412	1.829	823	
Patient 2				
Blood flow Qb, mL/min	250	250	220	220
Total plasma mL	9.000	8.500	8.500	8.200
Plasma filtration flow rate, QS%	15	15	15	15
Total dose of heparin I.U.	1.250	1.250	1.250	1.250
Reinfusion solution Qinf, mL/min	35	35	35	35
CK value U/L before CPFA	92.373	51.290	30.664	16.815
CK value U/L after CPFA	58.715	34.463	20.583	8.418
Myoglobin value ng/mL before CPFA	12.780	8.519	6.725	2.573
Myoglobin value ng/mL after CPFA	8.735	6.940	2.867	1.516
Patient 3				
Blood flow Qb, mL/min	250	250	250	250
Total plasma mL	9.000	9.000	8.500	8.500
Plasma filtration flow rate, QS%	15	15	15	15
Total dose of heparin I.U.	1.250	1.250	1.250	1.250
Reinfusion solution Qinf, mL/min	35	35	35	35
CK value U/L before CPFA	79.216	62.691	58.806	32.479
CK value U/L after CPFA	65.708	59.354	39.956	18.659
Myoglobin value ng/mL before CPFA	12.757	8.426	6.731	3.648
Myoglobin value ng/mL after CPFA	9.328	6.869	3.713	3.115
Patient 4				
Blood flow Qb, mL/min	220	200	220	
Total plasma mL	7.500	8.000	7.200	
Plasma filtration flow rate, QS%	15	15	15	
Total dose of heparin I.U.	1.250	1.250	1.250	
Reinfusion solution Qinf, mL/min	35	35	35	
CK value U/L before CPFA	30.389	16.495	11.699	
CK value U/L after CPFA	19.366	13.879	8.933	
Myoglobin value ng/mL before CPFA	9.562	3.815	1.318	
Myoglobin value ng/mL after CPFA	4.221	1.752	612	

3. Discussion

Acute renal failure due to myoglobinuria is the most dangerous complication of both traumatic and nontraumatic rhabdomyolysis and can be life-threatening [13].

When acute renal injury is severe enough to produce refractory hyperkalemia, metabolic acidosis, or volume overload, renal replacement therapy is indicated, mainly by intermittent haemodialysis which is able to rapidly and efficiently correct electrolyte disturbances.

Nevertheless, conventional haemodialysis is not able to remove myoglobin properly due to its high molecular weight and is generally started for renal indications: so, given its pathogenetic role in the development of acute renal injury during rhabdomyolysis, preventive extracorporeal elimination of myoglobin has been studied [9].

New "super high-flux" membranes for haemodialysis have been developed with a high cut-off pore size allowing efficient removal of middle and large size uremic toxin that cannot be removed by conventional dialysis membranes. The recent availability of a new generation of haemodialysis membranes with molecular weight cut-offs closer to that of the native kidney (65 kDa) has led to great benefits in several different clinical settings. These membranes have shown efficient removal of myoglobin in patients with rhabdomyolysis [14].

Effective removal of myoglobin by haemodialysis using a single-pass batch system and a high-flux polysulfone dialyzator (1,8 m^2 surface), able to remove substances with a molecular weight as high as 30 kDa, has been reported [15].

The use of a large pore, high cut-off membrane for haemodialysis has been described [16].

During CVVH, or hemodiafiltration, the use of high-flux, high volume (convection) filters showed good effectiveness in removing myoglobin in acute rhabdomyolysis [17].

The membrane and technique used in the process of separation of myoglobin are crucial to the success of therapy. Since standard membranes are substantially impenetrable to myoglobin, high-flux membranes should be used [18].

Experience with the use of CPFA in rhabdomyolysis, especially posttraumatic, is very limited.

Lai et al. reported the successful use of CPFA in two kidney transplant patients with post-nephrolithotomy septic shock and severe rhabdomyolysis of unknown origin [19].

Ronco suggests the use of absorption on whole blood directly or CPFA, in which the patient's plasma is reinfused once regenerated by passage through a sorbent cartridge [18].

Instead, many reports about the use of plasmapheresis exist [20].

Attempts to use plasmapheresis have resulted in higher sieving coefficients, but the final clearance is minimal because of the limitations imposed by low volume exchanges.

The affinity between plasmapheresis and CPFA is well known: these two techniques are both able to eliminate molecules with a molecular weight exceeding 15 kDa.

While plasmapheresis implies the separation of the cellular components of blood from plasma, which can be then eliminated or further filtrated (selective apheresis), CPFA consists of a combination of apheresis and haemodialysis: this technique, in fact, combines plasma separation with adsorption and postdilutional haemodialysis. The circuit includes a plasma filter (800 kDa cut-off) which initially separates plasma from the cellular components of blood and a cartridge containing a hydrophobic resin (styrene-divinylbenzene, mean diameter of single grain 75 microns, diameter of pores 30 nm, and surface area 700 m^2/g) on which plasma coming from the plasma filter is perfused at a rate of 30–40 mL/min; finally, this purified plasma passes through a hemofilter, together with the cellular components coming from the plasma filter.

The hydrophobic resin cartridge allows the removal of toxic molecules (cytokines, bilirubin, and myoglobin) without loss of nutrients such as albumin [21].

Throughout the treatment with CPFA, our patients showed a positive trend of clinical improvement with a decrease in muscular (CK and myoglobin) and renal (creatinine and potassium) damage indices.

In all patients, we began treatment with CPFA after standard therapy, intravenous fluids, urine alkalinization, surgical procedures, and diuretics. In two patients with acute kidney injury, the treatment CPFA was preceded by haemodialysis. Despite standard therapy CK and myoglobin values were increasing rapidly. In all cases already after the first treatment we observed a decrease of the values of CK and myoglobin. If CK and myoglobin values were down after the standard treatment we would not have started CPFA.

CK and myoglobin values continued to fall in the interval between treatments with CPFA. CVVH was used during the washout periods. The decrease of the blood values of CK and myoglobin was slower after the treatments with CVVH compared to the values found after treatment with CPFA (Table 1).

4. Conclusions

We treated 4 traumatic rhabdomyolysis patients with CPFA. CPFA was combined with CVVH. All patients showed a significant reduction in CK and myoglobin blood levels, along with an improvement in renal function. During the treatment, all patients maintained good respiratory and hemodynamic stability and no complications were seen.

Three patients survived and completely recovered after a rehabilitation period. One patient suddenly died on the 26th day for reasons not directly related to muscle injury or renal failure (cerebral haemorrhage).

Our experience was positive but remains limited: in order to assess the real effectiveness of CPFA in traumatic rhabdomyolysis, a multicentric study involving ICUs where major traumas are treated may be of interest. It would be useful to study with an assessment of the hourly changes in serum CK and myoglobin values during treatment in order to confirm the effectiveness of the CPFA to remove myoglobin from the blood.

References

[1] C. S. Rajagopalan, "Crush injuries and the crush syndrome," *Medical Journal Armed Forces India*, vol. 66, no. 4, pp. 317–320, 2010.

[2] S. Forcellini, F. Fabbian, Y. Battaglia, and A. Storari, "Rhabdomyolysis: role of the nephrologis," *Giornale Italiano Di Nefrologia*, vol. 31, no. 6, 2014.

[3] F. Y. Khan, "Rhabdomyolysis: a review of the literature," *Netherlands Journal of Medicine*, vol. 67, no. 9, pp. 272–283, 2009.

[4] A. L. Huerta-Alardín, J. Varon, and P. E. Marik, "Bench-to-bedside review: rhabdomyolysis—an overview for clinicians," *Critical Care*, vol. 9, no. 2, pp. 158–169, 2005.

[5] A. Jindal and S. Nayak, "Myoglobinuria and acute kidney injury," *Journal of Integrative Nephrology and Andrology*, vol. 2, no. 2, pp. 50–54, 2015.

[6] S. Kasaoka, M. Todani, T. Kaneko et al., "Peak value of blood myoglobin predicts acute renal failure induced by rhabdomyolysis," *Journal of Critical Care*, vol. 25, no. 4, pp. 601–604, 2010.

[7] V. Premru, J. Kovač, and R. Ponikvar, "Use of myoglobin as a marker and predictor in myoglobinuric acute kidney injury," *Therapeutic Apheresis and Dialysis*, vol. 17, no. 4, pp. 391–395, 2013.

[8] M. S. Sever and R. Vanholder, "Management of crush victims in mass disasters: highlights from recently published recommendations," *Clinical Journal of the American Society of Nephrology*, vol. 8, no. 2, pp. 328–335, 2013.

[9] X. Bosch, E. Poch, and J. M. Grau, "Rhabdomyolysis and acute kidney injury," *New England Journal of Medicine*, vol. 361, no. 1, pp. 10–72, 2009.

[10] F. Maduell, J. J. Sánchez-Canel, J. A. Blasco et al., "Big molecules clearance," *Nefrología*, vol. 26, pp. 469–475, 2006.

[11] A. Brendolan, C. Ronco, Z. Ricci et al., "Coupled plasma filtration adsorption: rationale, technical development and early clinical experience," *Contributions to Nephrology*, vol. 144, pp. 376–386, 2004.

[12] M. Formica, P. Inguaggiato, S. Bainotti, and M. L. Wratten, "Coupled plasma filtration adsorption," *Contributions to Nephrology*, vol. 156, pp. 405–410, 2007.

[13] N. Petejova and A. Martinek, "Acute kidney injury due to rhabdomyolysis and renal replacement therapy: a critical review," *Critical Care*, vol. 18, no. 3, article 224, 2014.

[14] V. Premru, J. Kovac, J. Buturovic-Ponikvar, and R. Ponikvar, "High cut-off membrane hemodiafiltration in myoglobinuric acute renal failure: a case series," *Therapeutic Apheresis and Dialysis*, vol. 15, no. 3, pp. 287–291, 2011.

[15] S. A. Sorrentino, J. T. Kielstein, A. Lukasz et al., "High permeability dialysis membrane allows effective removal of myoglobin in acute kidney injury resulting from rhabdomyolysis," *Critical Care Medicine*, vol. 39, no. 1, pp. 184–186, 2011.

[16] C. Albert, M. Haase, R. Bellomo, and P. R. Mertens, "High cut-off and high-flux membrane haemodialysis in a patient with rhabdomyolysis-associated acute kidney injury," *Critical Care and Resuscitation*, vol. 14, no. 2, pp. 159–162, 2012.

[17] T. Naka, D. Jones, I. Baldwin et al., "Myoglobin clearance by super high-flux hemofiltration in a case of severe rhabdomyolysis: a case report," *Critical Care*, vol. 9, no. 2, pp. 90–95, 2005.

[18] C. Ronco, "Extracorporeal therapies in acute rhabdomyolysis and myoglobin clearance," *Critical Care*, vol. 9, no. 2, pp. 141–142, 2005.

[19] Q. Lai, V. Di Pietro, S. Iesari et al., "Coupled plasma filtration adsorption in patients with a history of kidney transplantation: report of two cases," *Blood Purification*, vol. 40, no. 3, pp. 218–222, 2015.

[20] R. Bambauer, C. Bambauer, R. Latza, and R. Schiel, "Therapeutic apheresis in nephrology," *Clinical Nephrology and Urology Science*, vol. 1, article 2, 2014.

[21] E. Mancini and A. Santoro, "Plasmapheresis in intensive care," *Giornale Italiano di Nefrologia*, vol. 29, pp. S91–S102, 2012.

38

DKA-Induced Takotsubo Cardiomyopathy in Patient with Known HOCM

Ayla Gordon, Gina LaCapra, and Roberto Roberti

Overlook Medical Center, Summit, NJ, USA

Correspondence should be addressed to Ayla Gordon; ayla.gordon@atlantichealth.org

Academic Editor: Chiara Lazzeri

The first published case of Diabetic Ketoacidosis-induced Takotsubo cardiomyopathy was in 2009. Our patient is the 1st reported case of Diabetic Ketoacidosis- (DKA-) induced Takotsubo cardiomyopathy (TC) in a patient with known hypertrophic cardiomyopathy (HOCM) in the United States. In the literature, there are only two examples linking DKA to TC; however, this report focuses on the biochemical and physiological causes of TC in a patient with known HOCM and new-onset DKA. TC in previously diagnosed HOCM poses particular complications. With the above patient's baseline outflow tract obstruction due to septal hypertrophy, the acute reduction in EF due to TC resulted in transient drop in brain perfusion and, therefore, syncope.

1. Introduction

The most common documented cause of Takotsubo cardiomyopathy (TC) is a neurohormonal release of catecholamines. However, in this case report of a man presenting with syncope, we describe DKA as the physiological stressor leading to TC. Upon workup for this patient's loss of consciousness, initial labs revealed a metabolic acidotic state and a glucose level of 526 mg/dL. Troponin level was 13.8 ng/mL with EKG showing ST elevations in leads V3–V6. Emergent coronary angiography demonstrated normal coronaries with a clinical picture suggesting TC. Transthoracic echo confirmed TC. DKA was controlled by day 4 of hospital stay and repeat echo on day 5 showed documented resolution of apical ballooning. The correlation is explained physiologically; DKA increases serum catecholamines, and the metabolic acidosis that ensues prevents the healthy myocyte's stepwise chemical channel processes, most notably the sarcoplasmic reticulum's ability to release Ca++.

Typical treatment of TC is supportive in nature, and typical resolution is seen within 2 months. However, when there is a physiological underlying cause, the aim is to treat the cause first. In this case, DKA-induced physiological stress on the myocardium leads to apical stunning. When DKA was treated and glucose levels were brought within normal range, repeat echo revealed an improved EF and normal ventricular motion and, therefore, overall resolution of TC.

2. Case

The patient is a 66-year-old male with a history of hypertension, hypertrophic obstructive cardiomyopathy, Meniere's disease with intermittent lightheadedness, and gait instability that is controlled with intermittent prednisone. His usual symptoms progressively worsened with new polyuria, polydipsia, decreased oral intake, and nausea. On the day of admission, he complained of lightheadedness as he got up from the toilet and lost consciousness. He had never had a prior syncopal episode.

Initial physical exam revealed irregularly irregular heart rate at 116 bpm, respiratory rate 26, and BP 108/74 with negative orthostatics. Initial labs revealed glucose of 526 mg/dL and blood gas pH of 7.12. Troponin was 13.8 ng/mL. HgbA1c of 11.8 later revealed a new diagnosis of diabetes mellitus. EKG showed atrial fibrillation with rapid ventricular response as well as ST elevations in leads II, III, aVF, and V3–V6 (Figure 1).

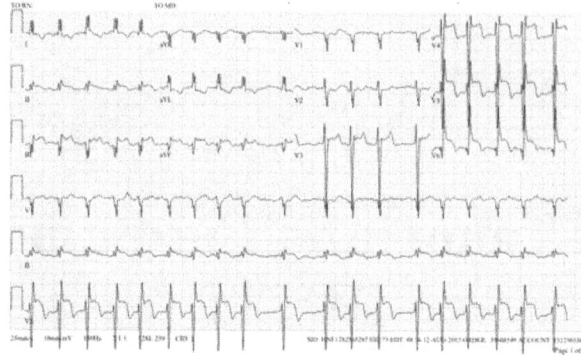

FIGURE 1: EKG showed atrial fibrillation with rapid ventricular response as well as ST elevations in leads II, III, aVF, and V3–V6.

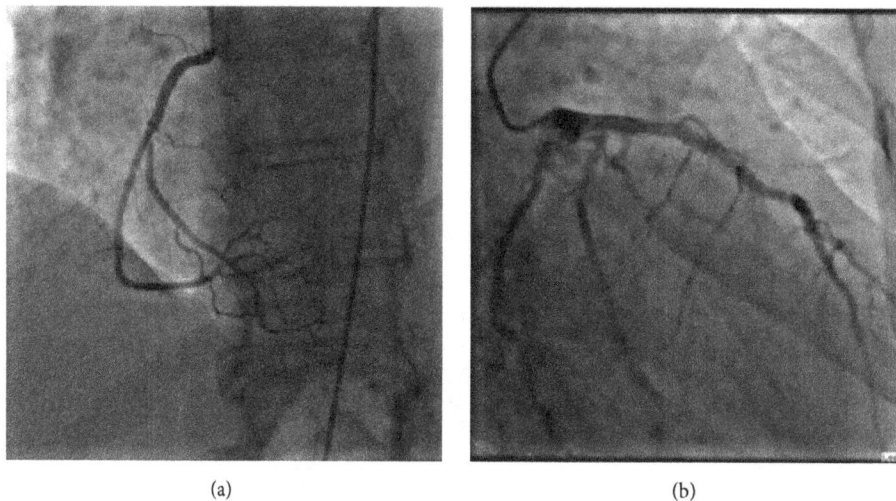

(a)

(b)

FIGURE 2: (a) and (b): cardiac catheterization on day of admission revealing no obstructive coronary artery disease in RCA and LAD, respectively.

3. Hospital Course

Patient was admitted with ST elevation MI. Emergent coronary angiography demonstrated normal coronaries (Figures 2(a) and 2(b)) with anterolateral, apical, and inferoapical dyskinesis and basal anterior and basal inferior wall hyperkinesis; ejection fraction (EF) was 20%. Clinical picture suggested TC. Transthoracic echocardiography also revealed apical hypokinesis; EF was 35–40%. Findings were consistent with TC (Figures 3(a) and 3(b)). When examining an old echocardiogram, patient had documented asymmetric septal hypertrophy, systolic anterior motion of mitral valve, and an intraventricular gradient of 32 mmhg with an EF of 75% (Figures 4(a) and 4(b)). The baseline echo showed typical characteristics of HOCM yet supported that this presentation of heart failure is a new and acute finding.

The patient was treated with an insulin drip and was started on anticoagulation. His atrial fibrillation was rate controlled with carvedilol and cardizem. Due to Diabetic Ketoacidosis (DKA) in setting of new and acute cardiomyopathy, moderate hydration was started to avoid risk of pulmonary overload. DKA was controlled by day 4 of hospital stay (Figure 5) and repeat echo on day 5 showed documented resolution of apical ballooning. EF improved to 45%. The resolution of TC with DKA treatment, seen as improvement ejection fraction and left ventricular motion improvement on echocardiogram, suggests a direct association between the two conditions.

4. Discussion

TC is a reversible heart failure with characteristic left ventricular dysfunction in the setting of ST elevations yet absence of coronary artery disease. There have been 4 classifications reported in Lithuania: Takotsubo type, reverse Takotsubo type, mid-ventricular type, and localized type [1]. In a large cohort study out of Switzerland, over 13,000 angiographies were performed with a 1.7% incidence of Takotsubo in patients presenting with acute coronary syndromes; 85% of them were women [2].

TC is believed to be caused by overactivity of the sympathetic system. The excess stress-induced catecholamines have the greatest effect on the cardiac apex due to its high

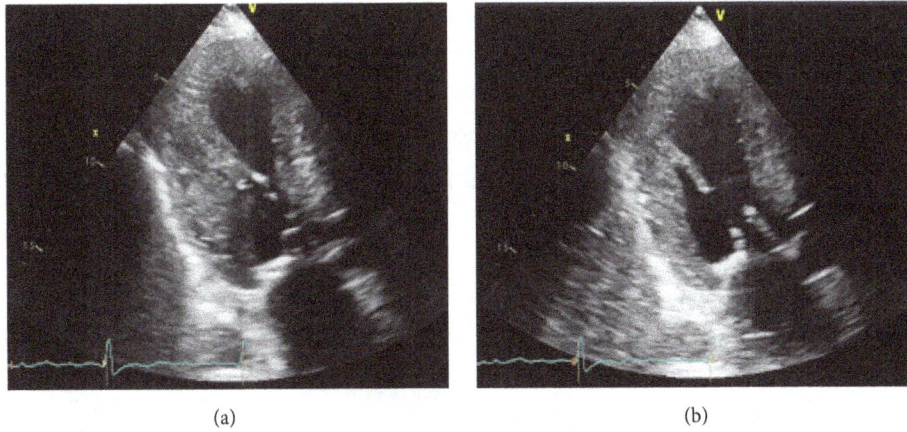
(a)   (b)

FIGURE 3: (a) and (b): echocardiogram on day of admission showing the apical ballooning typical of TC in systole and diastole, respectively.

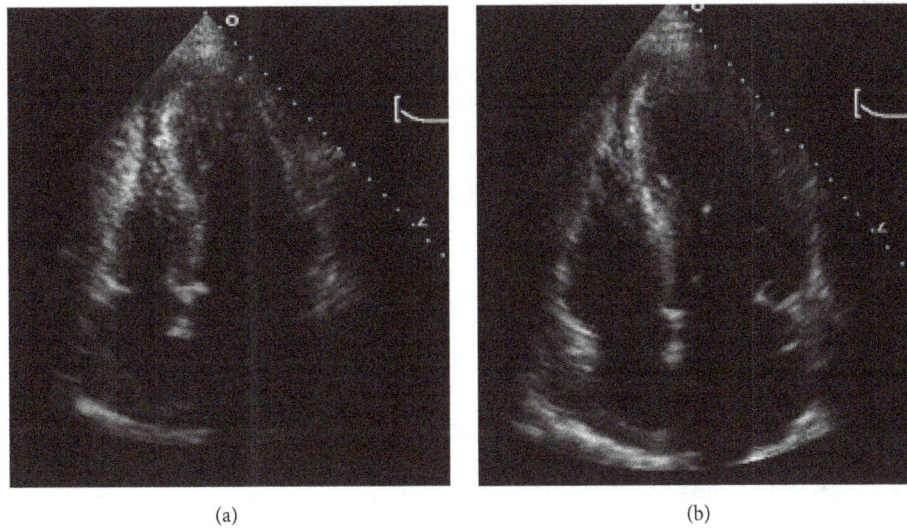
(a)   (b)

FIGURE 4: (a) and (b): patient's baseline echo showing asymmetric septal hypertrophy in systole and diastole, respectively.

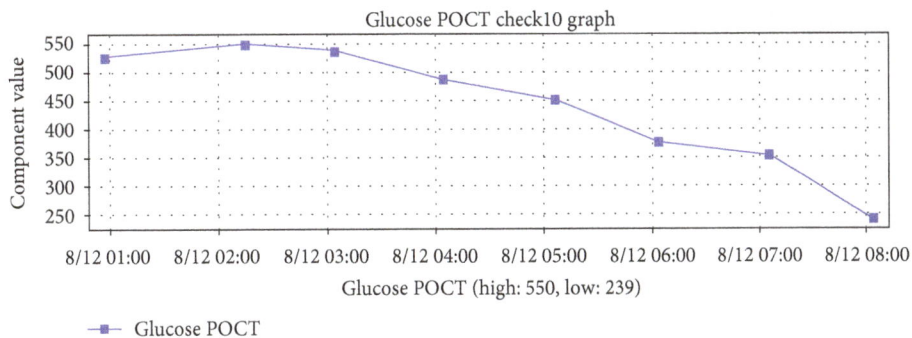

FIGURE 5: Glucose level since diagnosis of DKA.

concentration of beta-adrenoreceptors. This causes hyperstimulation of the catecholamine receptors and an inability to contract ("stunned" effect), seen as hypokinesis of the apex typically described as "apical ballooning." The most common documented cause of this type or cardiomyopathy is emotional neurohormonal stress; however, it has also been reported secondary to physiological stressors, as seen above. In this case report, we describe an association of TC with DKA being the physiological stressor.

During DKA, there is a physiological increase in other hormones such as growth hormone, cortisol, glucagon, and catecholamines which all play a part in worsening hyperglycemia [3]. In 2009, the first case of DKA-induced TC was published [4]. Our patient is the 1st reported case of DKA-induced TC in a patient with known HOCM in the United States.

In our patient, not only does DKA increase serum catecholamines, but the acidosis also contributes to the dysfunction. During DKA, hepatic oxidation of free fatty acids produces an increased amount of ketones (most commonly acetoacetate and hydroxybutyrate). Serum ketones are cardioprotective by supplying heart muscle with an energy substrate other than free fatty acids. However, when ketone concentrations become exceedingly high within the blood, the patient enters an acidotic state preventing the healthy stepwise myocyte chemical channel processes. The most affected function is the sarcoplasmic reticulum's ability to release Ca++. The ultimate effect is inhibition of normal myocyte contractility. This theory is supported by the pathological findings of sarcolipin within left ventricular myocytes during the acute phase of Takotsubo, which interrupt regulation of intracellular calcium [5].

There is a case report of a patient who had both DKA and hypothermia who developed TC [6]. In this case, hypothermia is described as the main cause of catecholamine release while coupled with an acidotic state, both causing hyperactivity of the ventricular bases and, therefore, TC. This is yet another case, where the combination of increased serum catecholamines and acidosis may result in TC.

Typical treatment of TC is supportive in nature and typical resolution is seen within 2 months [7]. However, when there is a physiological underlying cause, the aim is to treat the cause first. In this case, DKA-induced physiological stress on the myocardium leads to apical stunning. When DKA was treated and glucose levels were brought within normal range, repeat echo revealed an improved EF and normal ventricular motion and, therefore, overall resolution of TC.

TC in previously diagnosed HOCM poses particular complications. With the above patient's baseline outflow tract obstruction due to septal hypertrophy of approximately 3.2 cm, the acute presentation of dynamic LV outflow tract obstruction and reduced EF due to TC resulted in transient drop in brain perfusion and therefore syncope. Typical symptomatic presentation of TC mimics acute coronary syndromes and is usually only diagnosed after direct visualization of the apical ballooning. However, the patient's history of HOCM and new acute cardiomyopathy put him at an increased risk of cardiac shock. Due to quick reversibility of DKA-induced TC with rapid glucose control, the patient's cardiac function was able to return to baseline.

References

[1] E. Kazakauskaite, A. Jankauskas, T. Lapinskas, R. Ordiene, and E. Ereminiene, "Takotsubo cardiomyopathy: the challenging diagnosis in clinical routine," *Medicina (Lithuania)*, vol. 50, no. 1, pp. 1–7, 2014.

[2] P. Eshtehardi, S. C. Koestner, P. Adorjan et al., "Transient apical ballooning syndrome—clinical characteristics, ballooning pattern, and long-term follow-up in a Swiss population," *International Journal of Cardiology*, vol. 135, no. 3, pp. 370–375, 2009.

[3] A. E. Kitabchi, G. E. Umpierrez, J. M. Miles, and J. N. Fisher, "Hyperglycemic crises in adult patients with diabetes," *Diabetes Care*, vol. 32, no. 7, pp. 1335–1343, 2009.

[4] S. Nanda, S. Longo, S. P. Bhatt, J. Pamula, S. G. Sharma, and T. H. Dale, "Stress cardiomyopathy—a unique presentation of diabetic ketoacidosis," *Annals of Clinical Biochemistry*, vol. 46, no. 3, pp. 257–260, 2009.

[5] Y. J. Akashi, H. M. Nef, and A. R. Lyon, "Epidemiology and pathophysiology of Takotsubo syndrome," *Nature Reviews Cardiology*, vol. 12, no. 7, pp. 387–397, 2015.

[6] Y. Katayama, T. Hifumi, J. Inoue, and Y. Koido, "A case of Takotsubo cardiomyopathy induced by accidental hypothermia and diabetic ketoacidosis," *BMJ Case Reports*, Article ID 008143, 2013.

[7] Y. J. Akashi, K. Nakazawa, M. Sakakibara, F. Miyake, H. Koike, and K. Sasaka, "The clinical features of takotsubo cardiomyopathy," *Quarterly Journal of Medicine*, vol. 96, no. 8, pp. 563–573, 2003.

39

Acute Warfarin Toxicity as Initial Manifestation of Metastatic Liver Disease

Varalaxmi Bhavani Nannaka,[1] **Nihar Jani,**[2] **Masooma Niazi,**[3] **and Dmitry Lvovsky**[1]

[1]*Division of Pulmonary and Critical Care Medicine, Bronx Lebanon Hospital Center, Bronx, NY 10457, USA*
[2]*Department of Internal Medicine, Bronx Lebanon Hospital Center, Bronx, NY 10457, USA*
[3]*Department of Pathology and Histology, Bronx Lebanon Hospital Center, Bronx, NY 10457, USA*

Correspondence should be addressed to Varalaxmi Bhavani Nannaka; drnannaka@gmail.com

Academic Editor: Chiara Lazzeri

Near complete infiltration of the liver secondary to metastasis from the head and neck cancer is a rare occurrence. The prognosis of liver failure associated with malignant infiltration is extremely poor; the survival time of patients is extremely low. We present a case of acute warfarin toxicity as initial manifestation of metastatic liver disease. Our patient is a 64-year-old woman presenting with epigastric pain and discomfort, found to have unrecordable International Normalized Ratio. She rapidly deteriorated with acute respiratory failure requiring mechanical ventilation, profound shock requiring high dose vasopressor infusion, severe coagulopathy, worsening liver enzymes with worsening of lactic acidosis and severe metabolic abnormalities, and refractory to aggressive supportive care and died in less than 48 hours. Autopsy revealed that >90% of the liver was replaced by tumor masses.

1. Introduction

The coumarin derivative warfarin, which was licensed in the United States in 1954 as the first human anticoagulant [1], remains the most commonly used oral anticoagulant in North America and the United Kingdom [2, 3]. Warfarin exerts its anticoagulant effect by acting as a vitamin K antagonist and inhibiting the biosynthesis of vitamin K-dependent procoagulant factors II, VII, IX, and X [2–4].

On the basis of a study done in 5077 cases with 99,628 emergency hospitalizations, warfarin was implicated in 33.3% of such Emergency Department (ED) visits [5].

Acute liver failure (ALF) secondary to malignant infiltration of the liver is rare and is diagnosed often only after death. In the era of liver transplantation, it is important to reach a definitive diagnosis and identify the cause because liver transplantation is not indicated if malignant infiltration of the liver is present and alternative therapies may be available.

Our case presents a finding of acute warfarin toxicity as initial manifestation of metastatic liver disease in a patient with stable dose of warfarin for 1.5 years with documented stable International Normalized Ratio (INR) over the same period of time.

2. Case Presentation

A 64-year-old woman was brought to ED by a family member for generalized weakness for 10 days associated with epigastric pain and discomfort. Patient also reported having a fall one week prior to her presentation to ED. She noticed to have dark stools and red urine within few days of the fall.

Her medical history was significant for atrial fibrillation on warfarin, COPD, active smoking, and hypertension. Additional history of laryngeal cancer was present, which was treated with radiotherapy and chemotherapy four years ago. As a followup after presenting with hoarseness of voice three years ago, recurrent malignancy was ruled out with vocal cord biopsy. No personal or family history of liver disease was identified. There were no changes to her medications, which included warfarin, amlodipine, metoprolol, aspirin, and atorvastatin.

In ED, patient was tachycardic with a pulse of 160/min, afebrile, and normotensive. The patient had no evidence of acute distress or external injury. She had right subconjunctival hemorrhage, and mucous membranes were dry. Heart examination was significant for tachycardia with no murmurs, rubs, or gallops. Lungs had good bilateral air

TABLE 1: Patient's laboratory values during hospitalization until death.

Parameter	Hour (hr) 0	hr 6	hr 15	hr 18	hr 22	hr 30
PT (seconds)	>169	275.3	57.7	61.1	72	130.3
INR	Unrecordable	23.8	5.1	5.4	6.4	11.4
PTT (seconds)	92	66.8	44.3	46.7	54.1	98.9
Serum albumin (g/dL)	2.8		2.4	2.6	2.1	1.8
Alanine aminotransferase (unit/L)	420		1234	1201	1312	2179
Aspartate transaminase (unit/L)	973		2475	2344	2548	3681
Alkaline phosphatase (unit/L)	435		393	369	403	379
Total bilirubin (mg/dL)	1		1.4	1.5	1.3	1.3
Lactic acid level (mmoles/L)	13.3		6.6	17	18	15
LDH (unit/L)			8003			
Troponin (ng/mL)	0.21		0.32	0.48	0.88	1.58
CK (unit/L)	872		1059	1220	1179	1283
CK-MB (ng/mL)	40.42		44.01	53.75	66.06	72.28
CK-MB%	4.6		4.2	4.2	5.6	5.6
Haemoglobin (g/dL)	12		7.2	9.7	8.7	7.8
Bicarbonate (mEq/L)	10	13		5	6	3

entry with no wheezing, crackles, or crepitations. Abdominal examination revealed soft but mildly tender epigastrium with normal bowel sounds, whereas rectal examination showed stool mixed with dark blood. She was alert and oriented to time/place/person but appeared slightly lethargic, no focal neurological deficits on neuro examination were found.

Laboratory studies revealed anemia with hemoglobin concentration of 7.2 mg/dL with baseline values around 12 mg/dL less than 3 months ago, leukocytosis with white blood cell count of 15 k/uL, normal platelet count of 232 k/uL, prothrombin time (PT) of 169 seconds, partial thrombo-plastin time (PTT) of 92 seconds, and unrecordable INR. Chemistry showed prerenal azotemia with blood urea nitrogen levels of 54 mg/dL, creatinine of 1.3 mg/dL, bicarbonate of 10 mEq/L, and normal serum electrolytes. Liver function tests (LFTs) showed hypoalbuminemia with albumin of 2.8 g/dL, transaminitis with alanine aminotransferase (ALT) of 420 U/L, aspartate transaminase (AST) of 973 unit/L, and alkaline phosphatase (ALP) of 435 unit/L. Other significant laboratory values were elevated lactic acid to 13.3 mmoles/L, lactate dehydrogenase (LDH) level of 8003 unit/L, elevated troponin of 0.206 ng/mL, creatine kinase (CK) of 872 unit/L, and creatine kinase MB (CKMB) of 40 ng/mL with MB% of <5. Please refer to Table 1 for laboratory values during the hospitalization. Hepatitis A, B, and C serologies were negative and serum acetaminophen level was <15 ng/dL.

Her INR two weeks prior to her presentation was 2.8 with normal LFTs four weeks prior to admission. She had been on stable dose of warfarin for the past 1.5 years. Please refer to Table 2 for warfarin dosage and INR levels in the past one year.

Initial chest X-ray (Figure 1) did not show any evidence of an acute pulmonary edema or pneumonia. Computed Tomography (CT) scan of the abdomen (Figure 2) showed

TABLE 2: Warfarin dosing and INR prior to hospitalization.

Time frame	INR	Warfarin dose (mg)
2 weeks ago	2.8	4
2 months ago	2.4	4
6 months ago	2.2	4
1 year ago	2.9	4
1.5 year ago	3.7	5

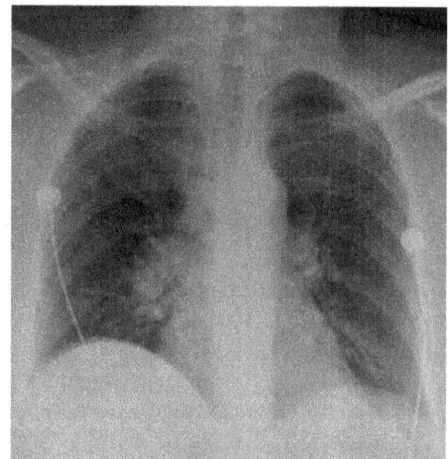

FIGURE 1: Chest X-ray.

markedly enlarged abnormal heterogeneous liver suggestive of an infiltrative process with no obvious free fluid or evidence of significant bleeding. CT scan of the head was negative for acute intracranial hemorrhage, infarction, or masses.

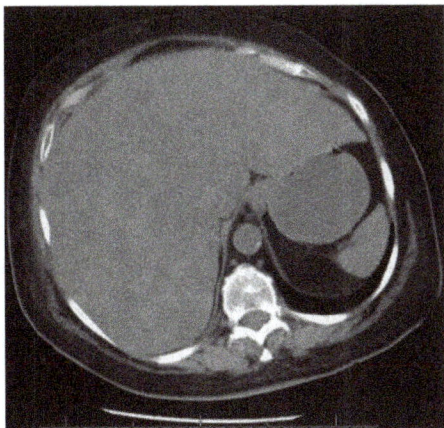

FIGURE 2: CT of the abdomen without contrast showed markedly enlarged abnormal heterogeneous liver.

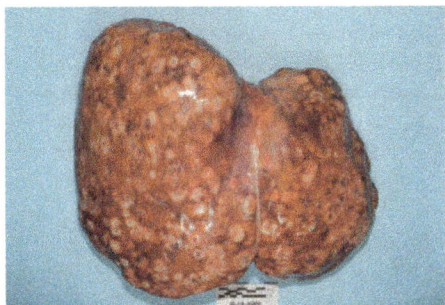

FIGURE 3: Liver weighed 4950 grams and that is enlarged with intact smooth capsule with soft tan brown parenchyma which was nearly completely replaced by multiple discrete tumor masses.

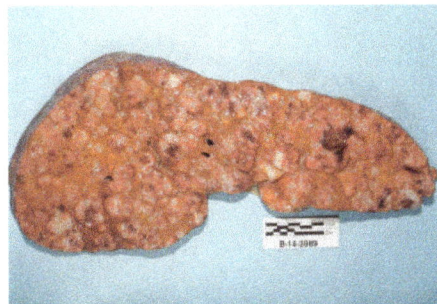

FIGURE 4: Cut section of liver with diffuse showed involvement by numerous tumor masses and nodules replacing most of the liver parenchyma.

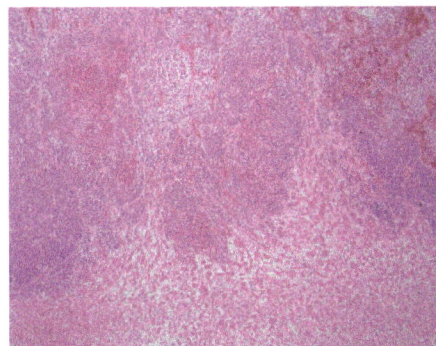

FIGURE 5: Liver diffusely involved by poorly differentiated squamous cell carcinoma (low power magnification).

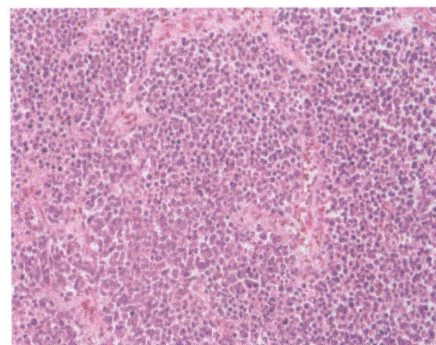

FIGURE 6: Autopsy of the liver on high magnification showing areas of poorly differentiated squamous cell carcinoma (high power magnification).

The patient had been given vitamin K and multiple transfusions of Fresh Frozen Plasma (FFP) to reverse coagulopathy.

After admission to intensive care unit (ICU), there was a rapidly progressive decline in the patient's clinical status. She developed acute respiratory failure requiring mechanical ventilation, hypotension necessitating vasoactive agents, and liver failure with worsening LFTs. In addition, she progressed to worsening of coagulopathy, elevated cardiac markers, and lactic acidosis. Her multiorgan failure did not improve with aggressive resuscitative measures, culminating in cardiac arrest and death.

Autopsy revealed that patient's liver weighed 4950 grams (Figures 3 and 4), and it was enlarged with intact smooth capsule with soft tan brown parenchyma which was nearly completely replaced by multiple discrete and near-confluent sheets of white masses, some with central punctate hemorrhage, ranging in size from approximately 0.3 to 3 cm in the greatest dimension. These tumor masses replaced nearly 90% of the total liver volume. Histopathology (Figures 5 and 6) showed poorly differentiated squamous cell carcinoma secondary to metastasis. Review of prior pathology from the time of LC surgery (Figures 7 and 8) showed moderately differentiated squamous cell carcinoma, which was histopathologically consistent with the observed metastasis in the liver.

3. Discussion

Warfarin therapy has a narrow risk-to-benefit profile. Its pharmacokinetics is complex. The effective half-life of warfarin ranges from 20 to 60 hours, with a mean of about 40 hours. The maximum dose effect occurs up to 48 hr after administration of a single dose and persists for the next 5 days. The drug is completely absorbed after oral administration, and peak concentrations occur within 4 hours. The warfarin metabolism occurs mainly in the liver. It involves the cytochrome P450, and in particular, the CYP2C9 isoenzyme. Very little is excreted unchanged in the urine and the bile [6].

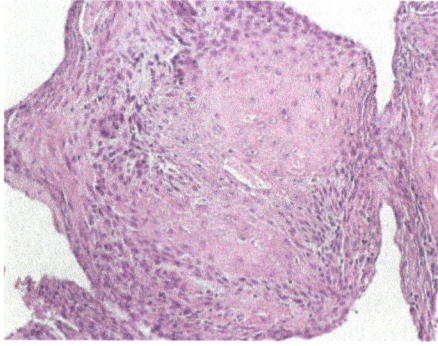

FIGURE 7: Biopsy of the vocal cord showed invasive well differentiated squamous cell carcinoma showing cohesive nests and intracytoplasmic keratinization.

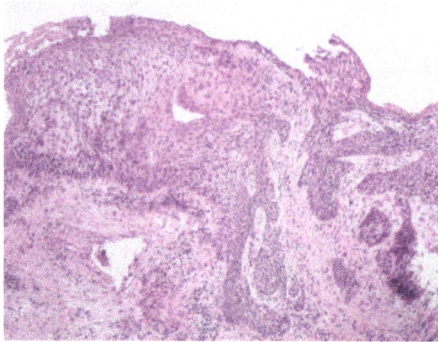

FIGURE 8: Left vocal cord mass showing deeply invasive, moderately differentiated squamous cell carcinoma.

Supratherapeutic levels of anticoagulation with warfarin result from the administration of inappropriately high doses, altered protein binding, decreased vitamin K intake, reduced synthesis, or increased clearance of vitamin K-dependent clotting factors and the simultaneous use of other compounds that interfere with warfarin metabolism. Elderly patients can also exhibit an exaggerated response to warfarin, in part because they tend to store less vitamin K than younger people [7]. Therefore, it is not surprising that the most common complication of warfarin use is adverse bleeding [8].

Before concluding that warfarin toxicity is the responsible cause for coagulopathy, many other conditions need to be considered. Differential diagnosis of prolonged PT and PTT is numerous and can be divided into inherited and acquired. Inherited causes include prothrombin, fibrinogen, factor V, X, and combined factor deficiency. Acquired causes are mostly due to impaired synthesis, loss, or increased consumption or inhibition of coagulation factors. Impaired synthesis stems from vitamin K deficiency or hepatic disease. Massive bleeding may be responsible for the loss of coagulation factors, when the intravascular volume is replaced by crystalloids, colloids, and red blood cells without replacing coagulation factors. Disseminated Intravascular Coagulation (DIC) pathophysiology is explained by increased consumption of coagulation factors. Inhibition of coagulation factors is seen with presence of inhibitor antibodies to prothrombin, fibrinogen, factor V, X, or direct thrombin inhibitor or iatrogenic with use of vitamin K antagonists (warfarin) or

with use of heparin or combined warfarin and heparin use. Warfarin is highly bound (approximately 97%) to plasma protein, mainly albumin. The high degree of protein binding is one of several mechanisms whereby other drugs interact with warfarin. Liver failure may be differentiated from vitamin K deficiency by measuring factor V, which is not vitamin K-dependent [9]. The presence of inhibiting antibodies can be confirmed by mixing studies. A diagnosis of DIC may be made using a simple scoring system based on platelet count, PT, D-dimer levels, and fibrinogen levels [10]. In the case described above, there was no evidence to suggest intentional overdose of warfarin, no use of compound that could have potentially increased the warfarin levels, and no prior history of inherited bleeding disorder. In our clinical practice, just as reported in Budnitz et al. [5], majority of coagulation abnormalities detected upon admission to our hospital are related to warfarin.

Our patient presented with severe warfarin induced coagulopathy. Results of autopsy revealed near complete infiltration of the liver with laryngeal cancer metastasis. The liver is the most common site for metastatic tumor deposits with evidence of hepatic metastasis in 36% of all patients who die from cancer [11]. Diffuse parenchymal metastasis is a rare pattern of liver metastasis. Watson reviewed the literature from the period 1868 to 1954 and reported 18 such cases [12]; Rowbotham and colleagues recognized 18 (0.44%) patients with fulminant hepatic failure (FHF) attributable to cancerous hepatic infiltration among 4020 hospital admissions [11]. The incidence of distant metastases in squamous cell carcinoma of head and neck approaches 20%–25%. The most common sites of metastases are lung (70%–75%), liver (17%–38%), and bone (23%–44%) [13]. Acute liver failure (ALF) secondary to diffuse metastatic infiltration of the liver is rare and has an extremely poor prognosis.

The mechanism of ALF in the setting of neoplastic infiltration is multifactorial. Massive cytokine release has been implicated as a cause of liver failure. Cytokine release can cause liver failure by damaging bile ducts both directly and via recruitment of effector cells, and by activation of leucocytes and hepatic sinusoidal cells, thus impeding hepatic sinusoidal microcirculation. Liver failure may also occur due to ischemia produced by tumor emboli compromising the portal venous circulation, or nonocclusive infarction of liver due to shock from other causes such as sepsis or cardiac dysfunction. The direct effect of tumor infiltration with replacement of hepatocytes is probably more important as a mechanism in nonhaematological malignancies. Indeed, FHF rarely develops in metastatic carcinomatosis in the absence of hypotension [14]. Our patient had normal LFTs four weeks prior to the development of ALF and then rapidly progressed. She has had infiltration of the liver over a period of time with no evidence of clinical or laboratory abnormalities, which then rapidly progressed to ALF as a result of further insult from hypotension and cytokine release likely secondary to sepsis or cardiac event.

Clinical presentation and laboratory findings of neoplastic infiltration of liver are vague and far from being pathognomonic. Hyperbilirubinemia may be the result of either hepatic parenchymal infiltration or extrahepatic biliary obstruction. It is well known that the increase in serum aminotransferases represents liver cell destruction and may be the only laboratory test indicating liver dysfunction prior to its clinical manifestation. But in our patient her LFTs were normal four weeks prior to admission. However, elevated serum LDH levels appear to correlate better with metastasis-related hepatic failure, since it is believed that elevated levels represent rapid tumor growth, by reflecting either the liver cell destruction process or an elevated production of LDH enzyme by neoplastic cells themselves. There are reports that correlate LDH serum levels with hepatic metastases from malignant melanoma, small cell lung cancer (SCLC) patients [15–18]. Extremely high serum LDH levels represent diffuse replacement of the liver parenchyma and are associated with a higher risk of development of FHF and a poor prognosis [19, 20]. Several authors suggest that an increase in serum LDH levels in cancer patients may prelude ALF [16, 21, 22]. These findings are well supported by the results of LFTs in our patient, who had extremely elevated serum LDH levels. Death is usually a direct consequence of the FHF, rather than the underlying malignancy. Acute warfarin toxicity on the stable dose of warfarin without any alternative cause was not a presentation in any of the reported case series. Because of the rapid progression of FHF, appropriate imaging procedures are usually difficult to perform. However, CT scan of the abdomen in our patient showed markedly enlarged liver with heterogeneity suggesting infiltrative process (Figure 2).

There have been case reports of liver metastasis-induced FHF from haematologic malignancies [23–25], breast cancer [26, 27], small cell carcinoma of lung [16, 28–30], colon cancer, urothelial cancer [31], and malignant melanoma [20, 22, 32–34]. Coagulopathy, on stable dose of warfarin, was not a presenting feature in any of these cases, but in our indexed case the main presentation was severe coagulopathy associated with ALF secondary to near complete infiltration of liver with metastatic disease. Unfortunately, the prognosis of patients with FHF resulting from malignant infiltration is dismal. The majority of patients do not survive shortly after the onset of liver failure [11, 26, 35]. According to a review by Allison et al., concerning 21 reported cases of ALF due to metastatic breast carcinoma, 18 cases died within 3 days to 7 months. Regrettably our patient died in less than 24 hours of admission to ICU.

4. Conclusion

Delayed distant metastasis is rare in head and neck cancer. ALF secondary to malignant infiltration of the liver due to delayed distant metastasis from laryngeal cancer was never reported in the literature to our best knowledge. Acute warfarin toxicity on stable dose of warfarin without any alternative cause is rare. Neoplastic infiltration of liver should be considered in the differential diagnosis when patients present with severe coagulopathy with ALF, and laboratory evidence of cellular destruction. Efforts must be made to determine the etiology of the disease, as it influences prognosis and prompt institution of specific therapies that might lead to recovery. Supportive care with close communication concerning end-of-life issues should be considered the standard of care

in patients presenting with ALF secondary to solid tumor malignancies since the prognosis is invariably poor.

References

[1] C. M. Kessler, "Urgent reversal of warfarin with prothrombin complex concentrate: where are the evidence-based data?" *Journal of Thrombosis and Haemostasis*, vol. 4, no. 5, pp. 963–966, 2006.

[2] J. P. Hanley, "Warfarin reversal," *Journal of Clinical Pathology*, vol. 57, no. 11, pp. 1132–1139, 2004.

[3] A. C. Butler and R. C. Tait, "Management of oral anticoagulant-induced intracranial haemorrhage," *Blood Reviews*, vol. 12, no. 1, pp. 35–44, 1998.

[4] G. Pindur and S. Mörsdorf, "The use of prothrombin complex concentrates in the treatment of hemorrhages induced by oral anticoagulation," *Thrombosis Research*, vol. 95, no. 4, pp. S57–S61, 1999.

[5] D. S. Budnitz, M. C. Lovegrove, N. Shehab, and C. L. Richards, "Emergency hospitalizations for adverse drug events in older Americans," *The New England Journal of Medicine*, vol. 365, no. 21, pp. 2002–2012, 2011.

[6] J. Hirsh, J. E. Dalen, D. R. Anderson et al., "Oral anticoagulants: mechanism of action, clinical effectiveness, and optimal therapeutic range," *Chest*, vol. 119, supplement 1, pp. 8S–21S, 2001.

[7] J. Hirsh, V. Fuster, J. Ansell, and J. L. Halperin, "American Heart Association/American College of Cardiology foundation guide to warfarin therapy," *Circulation*, vol. 107, no. 12, pp. 1692–1711, 2003.

[8] V. Olmos and C. M. López, "Brodifacoum poisoning with toxicokinetic data," *Clinical Toxicology*, vol. 45, no. 5, pp. 487–489, 2007.

[9] B. Bailey, D. K. Amre, and P. Gaudreault, "Fulminant hepatic failure secondary to acetaminophen poisoning: a systematic review and meta-analysis of prognostic criteria determining the need for liver transplantation," *Critical Care Medicine*, vol. 31, no. 1, pp. 299–305, 2003.

[10] K. Bakhtiari, J. C. M. Meijers, E. De Jonge, and M. Levi, "Prospective validation of the International Society of Thrombosis and Haemostasis scoring system for disseminated intravascular coagulation," *Critical Care Medicine*, vol. 32, no. 12, pp. 2416–2421, 2004.

[11] D. Rowbotham, J. Wendon, and R. Williams, "Acute liver failure secondary to hepatic infiltration: a single centre experience of 18 cases," *Gut*, vol. 42, no. 4, pp. 576–580, 1998.

[12] A. J. Watson, "Diffuse intra-sinusoidal metastatic carcinoma of the liver," *The Journal of Pathology and Bacteriology*, vol. 69, no. 1-2, pp. 207–217, 1955.

[13] J. G. Spector, D. G. Sessions, B. H. Haughey et al., "Delayed regional metastases, distant metastases, and second primary malignancies in squamous cell carcinomas of the larynx and hypopharynx," *Laryngoscope*, vol. 111, no. 6, pp. 1079–1087, 2001.

[14] P. Rajvanshi, K. V. Kowdley, W. K. Hirota, J. B. Meyers, and E. B. Keeffe, "Fulminant hepatic failure secondary to neoplastic infiltration of the liver," *Journal of Clinical Gastroenterology*, vol. 39, no. 4, pp. 339–343, 2005.

[15] H. B. Harrison, H. M. Middleton III, J. H. Crosby, and M. N. Dasher Jr., "Fulminant hepatic failure: an unusual presentation of metastatic liver disease," *Gastroenterology*, vol. 80, no. 4, pp. 820–825, 1981.

[16] B. M. McGuire, D. L. Cherwitz, K. M. Rabe, and S. B. Ho, "Small-cell carcinoma of the lung manifesting as acute hepatic failure," *Mayo Clinic Proceedings*, vol. 72, no. 2, pp. 133–139, 1997.

[17] Y. Fujiwara, K. Takenaka, K. Kajiyama et al., "The characteristics of hepatocellular carcinoma with a high level of serum lactic dehydrogenase: a case report," *Hepato-Gastroenterology*, vol. 44, no. 15, pp. 820–823, 1997.

[18] S. J. Finck, A. E. Giuliano, B. D. Mann, and D. L. Morton, "Results of ilioinguinal dissection for stage II melanoma," *Annals of Surgery*, vol. 196, no. 2, pp. 180–186, 1982.

[19] F. Tas, A. Aydiner, E. Topuz, H. Camlica, P. Saip, and Y. Eralp, "Factors influencing the distribution of metastases and survival in extensive disease small cell lung cancer," *Acta Oncologica*, vol. 38, no. 8, pp. 1011–1015, 1999.

[20] H. S. Te, T. D. Schiano, M. Kahaleh et al., "Fulminant hepatic failure secondary to malignant melanoma: case report and review of the literature," *The American Journal of Gastroenterology*, vol. 94, no. 1, pp. 262–266, 1999.

[21] R. H. Schreve, O. T. Terpstra, L. Ausema, J. S. Lameris, A. J. van Seijen, and J. Jeekel, "Detection of liver metastases. A prospective study comparing liver enzymes, scintigraphy, ultrasonography and computed tomography," *British Journal of Surgery*, vol. 71, no. 12, pp. 947–949, 1984.

[22] P. M. G. Bouloux, R. J. Scott, J. E. Goligher, and C. Kindell, "Fulminant hepatic failure secondary to diffuse liver infiltration by melanoma," *Journal of the Royal Society of Medicine*, vol. 79, no. 5, pp. 302–303, 1986.

[23] G. A. Morali, E. Rozenmann, J. Ashkenazi, G. Munter, and D. Z. Braverman, "Acute liver failure as the sole manifestation of relapsing non-Hodgkin's lymphoma," *European Journal of Gastroenterology and Hepatology*, vol. 13, no. 10, pp. 1241–1243, 2001.

[24] K. Esfahani, P. Gold, S. Wakil, R. P. Michel, and S. Solymoss, "Acute liver failure because of chronic lymphocytic leukemia: case report and review of the literature," *Current Oncology*, vol. 18, no. 1, pp. 39–42, 2011.

[25] T. M. Shehab, M. S. Kaminski, and A. S. F. Lok, "Acute liver failure due to hepatic involvement by hematologic malignancy," *Digestive Diseases and Sciences*, vol. 42, no. 7, pp. 1400–1405, 1997.

[26] H. E. Nazario, R. Lepe, and J. F. Trotter, "Metastatic breast cancer presenting as acute liver failure," *Gastroenterology and Hepatology*, vol. 7, no. 1, pp. 65–66, 2011.

[27] K. H. Allison, C. L. Fligner, and W. T. Parks, "Radiographically occult, diffuse intrasinusoidal hepatic metastases from primary breast carcinomas: a clinicopathologic study of 3 autopsy cases," *Archives of Pathology and Laboratory Medicine*, vol. 128, no. 12, pp. 1418–1423, 2004.

[28] K. Sato, Y. Takeyama, T. Tanaka, Y. Fukui, H. Gonda, and R. Suzuki, "Fulminant hepatic failure and hepatomegaly caused by diffuse liver metastases from small cell lung carcinoma: 2 autopsy cases," *Respiratory Investigation*, vol. 51, no. 2, pp. 98–102, 2013.

[29] H. Miyaaki, T. Ichikawa, N. Taura et al., "Diffuse liver metastasis of small cell lung cancer causing marked hepatomegaly and fulminant hepatic failure," *Internal Medicine*, vol. 49, no. 14, pp. 1383–1386, 2010.

[30] Y. T. Hwang, J. W. Shin, J. H. Lee et al., "A case of fulminant hepatic failure secondary to hepatic metastasis of small cell lung carcinoma," *The Korean Journal of Hepatology*, vol. 13, no. 4, pp. 565–570, 2007.

[31] M. Alcalde, M. Garcia-Diaz, J. Pecellin et al., "Acute liver failure due to diffuse intrasinusoidal metastases of urothelial carcinoma," *Acta Gastro-Enterologica Belgica*, vol. 59, no. 2, pp. 163–165, 1996.

[32] E. Bellolio, F. Schafer, R. Becker, and M. A. Villaseca, "Fulminant hepatic failure secondary to diffuse melanoma infiltration in a patient with a breast cancer history," *Journal of Postgraduate Medicine*, vol. 59, no. 2, pp. 164–166, 2013.

[33] G. G. Kaplan, S. Medlicott, B. Culleton, and K. B. Laupland, "Acute hepatic failure and multi-system organ failure secondary to replacement of the liver with metastatic melanoma," *BMC Cancer*, vol. 5, article 67, 2005.

[34] T. Fusasaki, R. Narita, M. Hiura et al., "Acute hepatic failure secondary to extensive hepatic replacement by metastatic amelanotic melanoma: an autopsy case report," *Clinical Journal of Gastroenterology*, vol. 3, no. 6, pp. 327–331, 2010.

[35] E. Athanasakis, E. Mouloudi, G. Prinianakis, M. Kostaki, M. Tzardi, and D. Georgopoulos, "Metastatic liver disease and fulminant hepatic failure: presentation of a case and review of the literature," *European Journal of Gastroenterology and Hepatology*, vol. 15, no. 11, pp. 1235–1240, 2003.

40

A Case Report of Recurrent Takotsubo Cardiomyopathy in a Patient during Myasthenia Crisis

Anusha Battineni,[1] Naresh Mullaguri,[1] Shail Thanki,[1] Anand Chockalingam,[2] and Raghav Govindarajan[1]

[1]*Department of Neurology, University of Missouri, 1 Hospital Drive, Columbia, MO 65212, USA*
[2]*Department of Cardiology, University of Missouri, 1 Hospital Drive, Columbia, MO 65212, USA*

Correspondence should be addressed to Raghav Govindarajan; govindarajanr@health.missouri.edu

Academic Editor: Michael J. Cawley

Introduction. Patients with myasthenia crisis can develop Takotsubo stress cardiomyopathy (SC) due to emotional or physical stress and high level of circulating catecholamines. We report a patient who developed recurrent Takotsubo cardiomyopathy during myasthenia crisis. Coexisting autoimmune disorders known to precipitate stress cardiomyopathy like Grave's disease need to be evaluated. *Case Report.* A 69-year-old female with seropositive myasthenia gravis (MG), Grave's disease, and coronary artery disease on monthly infusion of intravenous immunoglobulin (IVIG), prednisone, pyridostigmine, and methimazole presented with shortness of breath and chest pain. Electrocardiogram (ECG) showed ST elevation in anterolateral leads with troponemia. Coronary angiogram was unremarkable for occlusive coronary disease with left ventriculogram showing reduced wall motion with apical and mid left ventricle (LV) hypokinesis suggestive of Takotsubo stress cardiomyopathy. Her symptoms were attributed to MG crisis. Her symptoms, ECG, and echocardiographic findings resolved after five cycles of plasma exchange (PLEX). She had another similar episode one year later during myasthenia crisis with subsequent resolution in 10 days after PLEX. *Conclusion.* Takotsubo cardiomyopathy can be one of the manifestations of myasthenia crisis with or without coexisting Grave's disease. These patients might benefit from meticulous fluid status and cardiac monitoring while administering rescue treatments like IVIG and PLEX.

1. Introduction

Myasthenia gravis (MG) is a progressive autoimmune neuromuscular junction disorder that affects skeletal muscle leading to considerable morbidity and rarely mortality. Myasthenia crisis is defined as acute worsening of weakness in bulbar and respiratory muscles requiring mechanical ventilation [1]. The primary mode of treatment is immunomodulation with high-dose oral steroids, intravenous immunoglobulin (IVIG), and plasma exchange (PLEX) to clear the acetylcholine receptor autoimmune antibodies, which are responsible for neuromuscular junction dysfunction [1]. Myasthenia patients may have other coexisting autoimmune diseases like thyroiditis and polymyositis which can impact their disease course and treatment [2]. Myasthenia crisis patients may have high levels of circulating catecholamines due to physical and emotional stress, which can cause stress-induced

cardiomyopathy [3–6]. There have been several case reports of patients developing Takotsubo stress cardiomyopathy (SC) with left ventricular (LV) dysfunction during myasthenia crisis but its recurrence is rare [7]. We are reporting a patient with seropositive MG and Grave's disease who developed different variants of SC one year apart during subsequent myasthenia crisis posing a significant challenge to administering immunomodulatory treatments.

2. Case Report

A 69-year-old Caucasian female with seropositive myasthenia gravis on monthly maintenance intravenous immunoglobulin (1 gram/kg body weight) every 4 weeks and prednisone 50 mg PO daily and pyridostigmine 60 mg three times a day was transferred to the university hospital cardiology service with acute onset chest pain, palpitations, nausea,

TABLE 1: Cardiac abnormalities and thyroid function during two episodes of myasthenia gravis crisis.

MG crisis	TSH mcunit/ml	Peak troponin, ng/ml	ECG changes	Echo findings
Episode 1	7.6	0.16	ST elevation V1–V6, Q waves V1–V3	Mid ventricular variant Takotsubo stress cardiomyopathy with reduced ejection fraction (EF) of 25%
Episode 2	0.569	0.32	Deep, symmetric T inversions V1–V6	Mid and apical akinesia, EF 30% consistent with classical apical ballooning type of Takotsubo stress cardiomyopathy

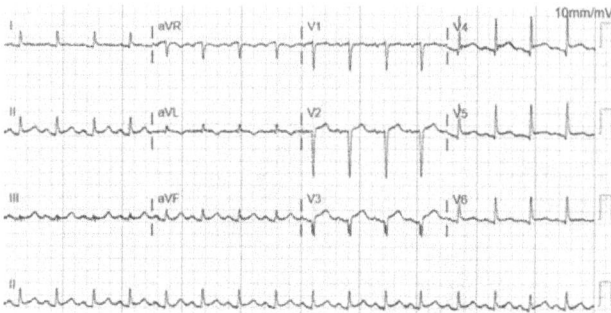

FIGURE 1: ECG during first episode of Takotsubo stress cardiomyopathy with ST elevation V1–V6, Q waves in V1–V3.

and profuse sweating on waking up in the morning at a long-term acute care (LTAC) facility. The symptoms did not relieve with multiple doses of sublingual nitrate. Her medical history is significant for hypertension, coronary artery disease status after myocardial infarction one year earlier with stent placement in left anterior descending artery (LAD), chronic obstructive pulmonary disease with a recent exacerbation with respiratory failure requiring tracheostomy, Grave's ophthalmopathy on oral methimazole 10 mg daily, and 2 packs per day smoking history. She also complained of worsening double vision, slurred speech with nasal quality, difficulty with swallowing her own saliva, and generalized weakness. Her physical examination revealed severe ophthalmoparesis in horizontal and vertical directions, worsening bilateral proptosis, facial diplegia with drooling, and nasal intonation. Wheezing was noted in the upper lobes as well as crepitations in bilateral basal regions. Cardiovascular examination revealed S3 gallop, no raised jugular venous pressure, and regular pulses. Neurological exam was consistent with generalized weakness in proximal and distal muscles with easy fatigability and absent deep tendon reflexes. Her initial ECG showed ST elevations in the anteroseptal leads (V1–V4) (Figure 1) and troponin elevation concerning for ST elevation myocardial infarction (STEMI) and she had emergent cardiac catheterization. No new coronary lesions were detected and prior stent was patent. Left ventriculogram suggested severe LV dysfunction and transthoracic echocardiogram (TTE) confirmed mid ventricular variant Takotsubo stress cardiomyopathy with reduced ejection fraction (EF) of 25% (Figure 2 and Table 1). Her TSH was elevated to 7.6 from 2.3 micro unit/ml with elevated anti-thyroglobulin and anti-thyroid peroxidase (TPO) autoantibodies suggesting worsening of Grave's disease for which endocrinology recommended

continuing high-dose oral steroids (Table 1). Neurology team was consulted for myasthenia crisis management, and they recommended PLEX and opined that the crisis was probably secondary to Grave's disease and methimazole that was started about 3 weeks earlier. She was managed conservatively with resolution of all her symptoms, ECG findings, and troponemia with 5 cycles of PLEX and was discharged back to the LTAC. The repeat TTE 4 weeks from the day of admission showed complete resolution of left ventricular dysfunction. She was continued on oral prednisone 50 mg daily and monthly IVIG (1 gram/kg body weight). One year later, she had a similar episode of ophthalmoparesis, generalized weakness with acute chest pain, troponemia with deep T wave inversions in V1–V6 leads on ECG (Figure 3) with TTE showing mid and apical akinesia, and EF 30% consistent with classical apical ballooning type of Takotsubo stress cardiomyopathy (Table 1). Her Grave's disease was well controlled with normal TPO autoantibodies and TSH (Table 1). We diagnosed her with recurrent Takotsubo stress-induced cardiomyopathy secondary to myasthenia crisis and treated her with 5 cycles of PLEX with complete resolution of the ST elevations (Figure 4) and troponemia and she was discharged to rehabilitation facility. Repeat TTE 3 weeks later showed complete normalization of LV function and wall motion (EF 60%).

3. Discussion

Myasthenia gravis is an autoimmune disorder of the neuromuscular junction predominantly in the skeletal muscles. Patients with this disease develop myasthenia crisis due to various reasons like infection, medications, and coexisting autoimmune diseases [1]. This condition and its management add significant amount of physical and psychological stress predisposing patients towards Takotsubo or stress cardiomyopathy [2–7]. Stress cardiomyopathy is a well-known complication associated with neurointensive care patients with subarachnoid hemorrhage, stroke, traumatic brain injury, and status epilepticus [8]. Rarely, certain neuromuscular junction disorders like myasthenia crisis also precipitate SC probably secondary to increased levels of circulating catecholamines [3–6, 9]. The commonest form is apical ballooning syndrome characterized by apical and mid wall akinesis and hypercontractile basal left ventricular segments [10]. Mid and basal LV segments or focal variants are also increasingly recognized now [10]. Coexistence of myasthenia gravis and Grave's disease in patients is well known and sometimes difficult to manage as treatment of one disease can worsen the

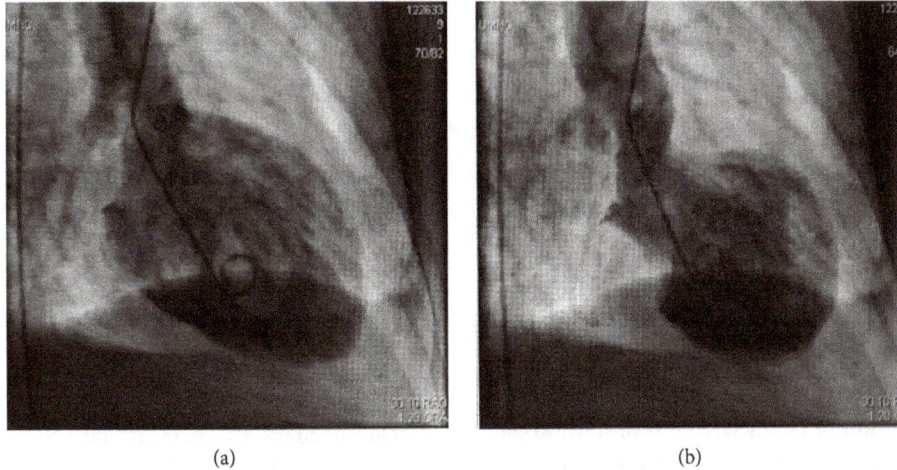

(a)   (b)

FIGURE 2: Left ventriculogram in RAO projection in diastole (a) demonstrates normal cavity contour and in systole (b) preserved basal and apical contractility with akinesia of the mid ventricle consistent with Takotsubo stress cardiomyopathy.

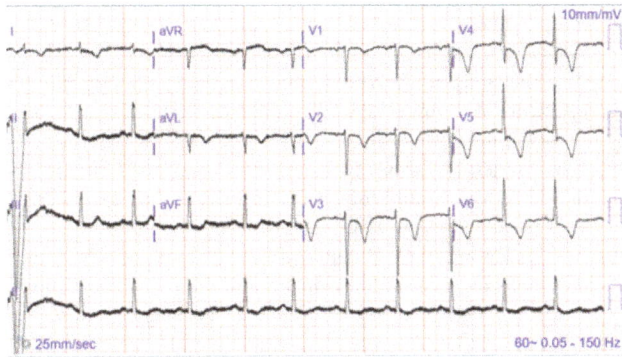

FIGURE 3: ECG during second SC episode with deep symmetrical T inversions in leads V1–V6.

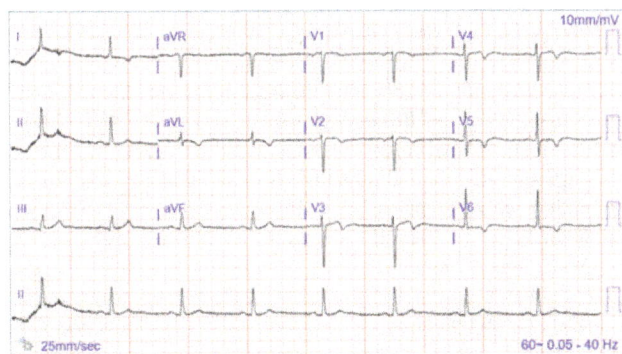

FIGURE 4: ECG 3 days later showing nonspecific ST-T wave changes only.

other like in our patient [2, 11–17]. Three weeks prior to her first episode of SC, she had worsening of her Grave's disease as manifested by proptosis and rising levels of TPO autoantibodies for which methimazole (10 mg daily) was started. Methimazole can unmask an underlying neuromuscular junction disorder in patient with Grave's disease or trigger

myasthenia crisis in patients with coexisting myasthenia gravis [18]. Both Grave's disease and myasthenia crisis were independently known to cause Takotsubo cardiomyopathy [19, 20]. In our patient, the combination of hyperthyroidism and methimazole might have triggered myasthenia crisis and subsequently SC. Over a dozen case reports describe Takotsubo cardiomyopathy complicating hyperthyroidism [19]. Coexisting coronary artery disease could cause chronic LV dysfunction with remodeling/thinning or new wall motion changes with ischemia. These factors add to the complexity, but SC can be diagnosed confidently in many instances based on carefully evaluating and recognizing SC-induced characteristic wall motion abnormalities [8, 10]. LV dysfunction improved after both diseases were managed appropriately but required prolonged hospitalization. She was continued on maintenance monthly IVIG infusions (1 gram/kg body weight) and oral prednisone (50 mg daily) and, one year later, she developed subsequent crisis and recurrence of SC. We did not find any significant trigger for her crisis after an extensive evaluation and her symptoms resolved completely with PLEX in 10 days. We think her subsequent episode of SC resolved quickly compared to the first episode as her Grave's disease was well controlled. We propose that MG patients in crisis should be screened for other autoimmune disorders like Grave's disease, which can affect neuromuscular junction and cardiac muscle. Neuromuscular specialists and intensivists managing myasthenia crisis patients should be aware of SC. If patient's cardiac symptoms like chest pain, troponemia, or ischemic ECG change during crisis, early recognition of SC and coronary artery disease can improve prognosis [20]. IVIG is contraindicated in patients with low ejection fraction as it may cause fluid overload and precipitate congestive heart failure [21]. In case reports by Gautier et al. and Anand et al., IVIG has been even shown to trigger Takotsubo cardiomyopathy [22, 23]. Cardiac complications are also known with PLEX in patients with MG with or without Takotsubo [24]. Thus, careful monitoring of fluid status and cardiac function with either IVIG or PLEX is recommended. This is especially so in older patients and in those with severe myasthenia, as they are particularly susceptible to Takotsubo cardiomyopathy and the risk of associated congestive heart failure, prolonged hospitalization, and its associated complications with either rescue treatment [20].

4. Conclusion

MG patients may have other autoimmune disorders like Grave's disease, which can worsen neuromuscular junction dysfunction and precipitate crisis. Patients who develop Takotsubo stress cardiomyopathy during myasthenia crisis require early recognition of characteristic wall motion patterns and screening for other causes like hyperthyroidism to avoid prolonged hospitalization with increased morbidity and mortality. Meticulous cardiac and fluid monitoring especially in older patients and with severe myasthenia might be beneficial in these patients as they might be at increased risk for developing recurrent stress cardiomyopathy.

Abbreviations

MG: Myasthenia gravis
ECG: Electrocardiogram
TTE: Transthoracic echocardiogram
IVIG: Intravenous immunoglobulin
PLEX: Plasma exchange
LV: Left ventricle
TPO: Thyroid peroxidase.

Disclosure

An approval from the ethics committee is not applicable to publish this case report. Data sharing is not applicable to this case report as no data sets were generated or analyzed during the current study. Anusha Battineni, Naresh Mullaguri, and Shail Thanki are co-first authors.

Authors' Contributions

Anusha Battineni (M.B.B.S.), Naresh Mullaguri (M.D.), Shail Thanki (M.D.), Anand Chockalingam (M.D.), and Raghav Govindarajan (M.D.) contributed to case report design, data collection, and manuscript writing. All authors read and approved the final manuscript. The authors contributed equally to writing this case report and formatting the images.

References

[1] L. C. Wendell and J. M. Levine, "Myasthenic crisis," *The Neurohospitalist*, vol. 1, no. 1, pp. 16–22, 2011.

[2] T. Kobayashi, H. Asakawa, Y. Komoike, Y. Nakano, Y. Tamaki, and M. Monden, "A patient with graves' disease, myasthenia gravis, and polymyositis," *Thyroid*, vol. 7, no. 4, pp. 631-632, 1997.

[3] V. Bansal, M. M. Kansal, and J. Rowin, "Broken heart syndrome in myasthenia gravis," *Muscle & Nerve*, vol. 44, no. 6, pp. 990–993, 2011.

[4] S. R. Beydoun, J. Wang, R. L. Levine, and A. Farvid, "Emotional stress as a trigger of myasthenic crisis and concomitant takotsubo cardiomyopathy: a case report," *Journal of Medical Case Reports*, article 393, 2010.

[5] S. Bijulal, S. Harikrishnan, N. Namboodiri, V. K. Ajitkumar, D. Gupta, and P. S. Mathuranath, "Tako-tsubo cardiomyopathy in a patient with myasthenia gravis crisis: a rare clinical association," *BMJ Case Reports*, 2009.

[6] J. Finsterer and C. Stöllberger, "Stress from myasthenic crisis triggers Takotsubo (broken heart) syndrome," *International Journal of Cardiology*, vol. 203, pp. 616-617, 2016.

[7] C. P. Wong and P. L. Chia, "Recurrent takotsubo cardiomyopathy precipitated by myasthenic crisis," *International Journal of Cardiology*, vol. 155, no. 1, pp. e11–e12, 2012.

[8] A. Chockalingam, "Stress cardiomyopathy of the critically ill: Spectrum of secondary, global, probable and subclinical forms," *Indian Heart Journal*, 2017.

[9] I. B. Harries, H. Levoir, C. Bucciarelli-Ducci, and S. Ramcharitar, "Takotsubo cardiomyopathy in myasthaenia gravis crisis confirmed by cardiac MRI," *BMJ Case Reports*, 2015.

[10] A. Chockalingam, G.-Y. Xie, and K. C. Dellsperger, "Echocardiography in stress cardiomyopathy and acute lvot obstruction," *The International Journal of Cardiovascular Imaging*, vol. 26, no. 5, pp. 527–535, 2010.

[11] S. Chhabra and B. Pruthvi, "Ocular myasthenia gravis in a setting of thyrotoxicosis," *Indian Journal of Endocrinology and Metabolism*, vol. 17, no. 2, pp. 341–343, 2013.

[12] D. M. Jacobson, "Acetylcholine receptor antibodies in patients with graves' ophthalmopathy," *Journal of Neuro-Ophthalmology*, vol. 15, no. 3, pp. 166–170, 1995.

[13] J. Kubiszewska, B. Szyluk, P. Szczudlik et al., "Prevalence and impact of autoimmune thyroid disease on myasthenia gravis course," *Brain and Behavior*, vol. 6, no. 10, article e00537, 2016.

[14] S. Kumar, "Management of ocular myasthenia gravis coexisting with thyroid ophthalmopathy," *Neurol India*, vol. 51, no. 2, author reply 284, pp. 283-284, 2003.

[15] K. Lakhal, Y. Blel, M. Fysekidis, K. Mohammedi, and L. Bouadma, "Concurrent Graves disease thyrotoxicosis and myasthenia gravis: The treatment of the former may dangerously reveal the latter," *Anaesthesia*, vol. 63, no. 8, pp. 876–879, 2008.

[16] D. G. Mappouras, G. Philippou, S. Haralambous et al., "Antibodies to acetylcholinesterase cross-reacting with thyroglobulin in myasthenia gravis and Graves' disease," *Clinical & Experimental Immunology*, vol. 100, no. 2, pp. 336–343, 1995.

[17] M. Marinó, R. Ricciardi, A. Pinchera et al., "Mild clinical expression of myasthenia gravis associated with autoimmune thyroid diseases," *The Journal of Clinical Endocrinology & Metabolism*, vol. 82, no. 2, pp. 438–443, 1997.

[18] M. Baretić, S. Balić, and G. Gudelj, "Myasthenic crisis as a side effect of methimazole therapy: Case report," *Acta clinica Croatica*, vol. 49, no. 1, pp. 67–71, 2010.

[19] A. E. Omar S, H. Mazek, T. Mahmoud, S. Soontrapa, and J. Suarez, "Takotsubo cardiomyopathy associated with hyperthyroidism treated with thyroidectomy," *Baylor University Medical Center Proceedings*, vol. 28, no. 2, 2015.

[20] P. Shivamurthy and M. W. Parker, "Cardiac manifestations of myasthenia gravis: a systematic review," *IJC Metabolic and Endocrine*, vol. 5, pp. 3–6, 2014.

[21] A. A. Vo, V. Cam, M. Toyoda et al., "Safety and adverse events profiles of intravenous gammaglobulin products used for immunomodulation: a single-center experience," *Clinical journal of the American Society of Nephrology*, vol. 1, no. 4, pp. 844–852, 2006.

[22] P. Gautier, R. Ravan, M. Najjar et al., "Tako-Tsubo syndrome during normal human immunoglobolin perfusion," *Annales de Cardiologie et d'Angéiologie*, vol. 60, no. 5, pp. 290–295, 2011.

[23] U. S. Anand, S. Viswanathan, and J. Arulneyam, "Pulmonary edema in myasthenic crisis," *Case Reports in Critical Care*, vol. 2013, Article ID 863620, 3 pages, 2013.

[24] M. Arai, H. Ukigai, and H. Miyata, "A case of transient left ventricular ballooning ("Takotsubo"- shaped cardiomyopathy) developed during plasmapheresis for treatment of myasthenic crisis," *Journal of Clinical Neurology*, vol. 44, no. 3, pp. 207–210, 2004.

41

Ornithine Transcarbamylase Deficiency: If at First You Do Not Diagnose, Try and Try Again

Christan D. Santos,[1] **Robert A. Ratzlaff,**[1] **Jennifer C. Meder,**[2]
Paldeep S. Atwal,[3] **and Nicole E. Joyce**[4]

[1]*Department of Critical Care Medicine, Mayo Clinic, Jacksonville, FL, USA*
[2]*Department of Nutritional Services, Mayo Clinic, Jacksonville, FL, USA*
[3]*Department of Clinical Genomics, Mayo Clinic, Jacksonville, FL, USA*
[4]*Division of Hospital Internal Medicine, Mayo Clinic, Jacksonville, FL, USA*

Correspondence should be addressed to Nicole E. Joyce; Joyce.Nicole1@mayo.edu

Academic Editor: Kurt Lenz

Ornithine transcarbamylase (OTC) deficiency is well known for its diagnosis in the neonatal period. Presentation often occurs after protein feeding and manifests as poor oral intake, vomiting, lethargy progressing to seizure, respiratory difficulty, and eventually coma. Presentation at adulthood is rare (and likely underdiagnosed); however, OTC deficiency can be life-threatening and requires prompt investigation and treatment. Reports and guidelines are scarce due to its rarity. Here, we present a 59-year-old woman with a past history of irritable bowel syndrome who underwent a reparative operation for rectal prolapse and enterocele. Her postoperative course was complicated by a bowel perforation (which was repaired), prolonged mechanical ventilation, tracheostomy, critical illness myopathy, protein-caloric malnutrition, and altered mental status. After standard therapy for delirium failed, further investigation showed hyperammonemia and increased urine orotic acid, ultimately leading to the diagnosis of OTC deficiency. This case highlights the importance of considering OTC deficiency in hospitalized adults, especially during the diagnostic evaluation for altered mental status.

1. Introduction

Ornithine transcarbamylase (OTC) deficiency (also referred to as ornithine carbamoyltransferase deficiency) is an X-linked proximal urea cycle disorder that results in a spectrum of severe neonatal-onset disease in boys, rarely in girls, and a milder adult-onset presentation. In the urea cycle, OTC combines ornithine and carbamoyl phosphate to form citrulline. Thus, an OTC enzyme deficiency leads to decreased production of citrulline, interruption of the urea cycle, increased orotic acid which is produced by excess carbamoyl phosphate, and ultimately life-threatening hyperammonemia due to the inability to excrete excess nitrogen. In females, the severity of the condition depends on the amount of X-inactivation of the pathogenic OTC allele and resultant OTC enzyme activity in the liver [1].

OTC deficiency can range from asymptomatic to severely symptomatic in heterozygous adults; those with a milder disease course often report a history of self-limiting protein intake. Acute hyperammonemic episodes can occur and are often triggered by major illness, surgery, pregnancy, corticosteroid and valproic acid administration, prolonged fasting, increased protein intake, and total parenteral nutrition (TPN) [2–6].

These hyperammonemic episodes present with neurologic abnormalities such as encephalopathy, psychosis, and delirium, which can progress to coma and death. Although limited, some reports describe the severity of this disease and emphasize the risk of death if undiagnosed. Brassier et al. [1] reviewed the long-term outcomes of 90 patients with OTC deficiency: 70% presented after the neonatal period and

9% of the late onset group (>1 month of age) died on initial presentation. Batshaw et al. [7] analyzed a larger group of patients ($n = 614$), and 66% of patients presented after the neonatal period; the overall mortality rate in the late onset age group was 11%.

2. Case Presentation

A 59-year-old woman with a history of irritable bowel syndrome and protein aversion, which led to a preferential vegetarian diet, was admitted for elective reparative surgery to treat rectal prolapse and enterocele. Her postoperative course was complicated by bowel perforation (requiring small bowel resection and end ileostomy), fecal peritonitis, intra-abdominal abscesses, septic shock, respiratory failure, tracheostomy, critical illness myopathy, protein-caloric malnutrition, and altered mental status (AMS). The patient provided written informed consent to publish these findings.

The patient's daily spontaneous awakening trials during her intensive care unit (ICU) course showed a positive evaluation on the Confusion Assessment Method for the ICU, score of +3 on the Richmond Agitation and Sedation Scale, and inability to follow 2-step commands, which led to an initial diagnosis of delirium. After standard delirium treatment was unsuccessful, further ICU investigation yielded normal renal, thyroid, and liver function. However, she had a markedly elevated ammonia level (100 mcmol/L, normal 0–30). Noncontrast head computed tomography and magnetic resonance imaging of the brain were negative for acute intracranial process.

Electroencephalography showed no evidence of nonconvulsive status epilepticus. Urine orotic acid and plasma amino acid panel were ordered to investigate her unexplained hyperammonemia. Her urine orotic acid level was elevated (3.2 mmol/mol creatinine, normal 0.4–1.2) but the plasma glutamine (normal 371–957 nmol/ml), ornithine (normal 38–130 nmol/ml), citrulline (normal 17–46 nmol/ml), arginine (normal 30–120 nmol/ml), and argininosuccinic acid (normal <2 nmol/ml) were within normal ranges. Nitrogen scavengers were not initiated at this time since there were no abnormalities in the rest of the urea cycle panel, ammonia began to trend down, and her mental status subsequently improved.

Because of prolonged mechanical ventilation and weaning failure, the patient received a standard polymeric enteral formula with a modular protein supplement. This was transitioned to an isotonic enteral formula after her ileostomy output increased. Her enteral nutrition was inconsistent during her ICU stay because of intestinal perforation, multiple planned procedures, intermittent high doses of vasopressors, and fluctuating doses of propofol.

On day 25 in the hospital, she was transferred to the step-down unit at her baseline mental state. Her appetite remained poor as she continued to experience bloating, nausea, and high gastric residual volume resulting in intermittent enteral and oral feeding. Trials of antiemetics, appetite stimulants, nutrition supplements, and diet adjustments were unsuccessful.

In the days approaching discharge, she had acute neurologic changes overnight, including visual hallucinations, hyperreflexia, clonus, generalized high-frequency low-amplitude tremors, nystagmus, and delirium. During the same night, she received the longest period of continuous enteral feeding since admission.

After this sudden neurologic decline on the step-down unit, OTC deficiency as a diagnosis was investigated further and empiric treatment was immediately initiated. Urine organic acid and acylglycines, quantitative plasma amino acid, and quantitative plasma acylcarnitine panels were ordered to screen for inborn errors of metabolism. This additional testing confirmed increased orotic acid, low citrulline, and elevated ammonia levels. The constellation of elevated urine orotic acid, low citrulline, persistent hyperammonemia with normal liver function, ketonuria, feeding difficulty, and neurologic changes were so highly suspicious of OTC deficiency; a confirmation of diagnosis by means of liver biopsy was not performed.

3. Treatment

This patient's management was based on consultation with a biochemical geneticist and focused on 4 main areas: restriction of protein, promotion of anabolism, administration of nitrogen-scavenging medications, and monitoring. Protein intake was withheld for 24 hours at treatment onset and then limited to 0.5 g/kg per day with a calorie goal of 30 kcal/kg. In this case, protein restriction could not be achieved through the available enteral formulas in the inpatient setting. TPN was initiated with dextrose (100 g), a lipid emulsion (28 g), and standard essential amino acids (25 g). Rohr recommends 30% to 50% of total protein be given as essential amino acids, a provision that is important for preventing chronic protein insufficiency [8].

To stimulate the urea cycle, intravenous arginine was initiated at a continuous rate of 600 mg/kg per day, along with 10% dextrose in normal saline at 125 cc/hr [6]. A glucose goal of 100 to 150 mg/dL was maintained with an insulin drip.

Ammonia scavenger therapy with intravenous sodium benzoate and sodium phenylacetate was initiated. Hemodialysis can be used for refractory hyperammonemia, but this intervention was not needed by our patient [6]. While receiving these interventions, her serum sodium and ammonia levels were monitored every 4 hours and her serum amino acid levels were monitored every 48 hours.

This course was continued until she became neurologically stable, at which time her oral discharge regimen was initiated. This regimen included a specially ordered, protein-free infant formula mixed with almond milk. She was instructed to consume 3 portions of this supplement daily, with a protein intake goal of less than 25 g per day. She received nutritional education regarding the effects of protein in patients with OTC deficiency and the importance of protein restriction. She was discharged with oral arginine (500 mg, 3 times per day). On follow-up, she was transitioned to oral citrulline (1.3 g, 3 times per day) (3 g/m^2) and sodium phenylbutyrate (4.5 g, 3 times per day) (10 g/m^2).

TABLE 1: Differential diagnosis of altered mental status.

Origin of AMS	Differential diagnosis
Infection	Urinary tract infection, pneumonia, bacteremia, meningitis, encephalitis, brain abscess, neurosyphilis, fever
Withdrawal	Alcohol, sedative-hypnotic drugs, barbiturates, benzodiazepines
Acute metabolic condition	Acid-base disturbance, electrolyte imbalance, liver or renal failure
Trauma	Head injury, surgery, burns, heat stroke, hypothermia
Central nervous system pathology	Subdural hematoma, epidural hematoma, subarachnoid hemorrhage, hydrocephalus, seizure, stroke, tumor, demyelinating lesion, transient ischemic attack
Hypoxia or cardiopulmonary condition	Hypoxemia, hypotension or shock, arrhythmia, anemia, carbon monoxide poisoning, methemoglobinemia
Vitamin deficiency	Thiamine (Wernicke encephalopathy), niacin, vitamin B12
Endocrinopathy	Hyperadrenocorticism, hypoadrenocorticism, hyperglycemia, hypoglycemia, hyperthyroidism, hypothyroidism, hypercalcemia
Acute vascular condition	Hypertensive encephalopathy, stroke, arrhythmia, shock, thrombotic thrombocytopenic purpura, mesenteric ischemia
Toxin or drug toxicity	Sedatives, narcotics, anticholinergics, antipsychotics, neuroleptic malignant syndrome, serotonin syndrome, illicit drugs
Heavy metal poisoning	Lead, arsenic, manganese, mercury, thallium

4. Outcome and Follow-Up

After prompt initiation of OTC specific treatment including nitrogen scavengers and restricted protein, her neurologic symptoms improved over 48 hours, and by 72 hours, she had returned to her baseline mental and neurologic state. Her inpatient oral intake adequately met goals, and TPN was discontinued. She was transitioned to a short-term rehabilitation facility, and on discharge to home, she was eating a regular-texture oral diet and supplementing with low-protein formula. Unfortunately, this diet was not sustained over several weeks, and she had failure to thrive. She was readmitted to the hospital for reinitiation of TPN in addition to oral diet. Upon final discharge, outpatient follow-up included consultations with a geneticist and genetic dietician.

5. Discussion

This case depicts a unique diagnosis (OTC) to a common clinical dilemma (AMS). The most common causes of AMS are cerebrovascular, traumatic, metabolic, infectious, psychiatric, and endocrine in origin [9]. Table 1 includes the broad range of disorders that can result in AMS.

OTC deficiency is not routinely considered during an investigation of AMS; however, early diagnosis and treatment are imperative to prevent severe neurologic injury and death [6]. For our patient, OTC deficiency was considered in the differential diagnosis because of her persistent hyperammonemia and nutritional history (preferential vegetarian diet) and the consistent failure of traditional delirium therapies. This case exemplifies the important role of multidisciplinary collaboration and communication in managing this uncommon deficiency in a urea cycle enzyme. During this patient's course, consultants from the departments of intensive care, neurology, internal medicine, nutrition, and genetics all had pivotal roles in diagnosing and treating this patient's disease.

Abbreviations

AMS: Altered mental status

ICU: Intensive care unit

OTC: Ornithine transcarbamylase

TPN: Total parenteral nutrition.

References

[1] A. Brassier, S. Gobin, J. B. Arnoux et al., "Long-term outcomes in Ornithine Transcarbamylase deficiency: A series of 90 patients," *Orphanet Journal of Rare Diseases*, vol. 10, no. 1, article no. 58, 2015.

[2] M. A. Chiong, B. H. Bennetts, S. I. Strasser, and B. Wilcken, "Fatal late-onset ornithine transcarbamylase deficiency after coronary artery bypass surgery," *Medical Journal of Australia*, vol. 186, no. 8, pp. 418-419, 2007.

[3] W. T. Hu, O. H. Kantarci, J. L. Merritt II et al., "Ornithine transcarbamylase deficiency presenting as encephalopathy during adulthood following bariatric surgery," *JAMA Neurology*, vol. 64, no. 1, pp. 126–128, 2007.

[4] S. Lipskind, S. Loanzon, E. Simi, and D. W. Ouyang, "Hyperammonemic coma in an ornithine transcarbamylase mutation carrier following antepartum corticosteroids," *Journal of Perinatology*, vol. 31, no. 10, pp. 682–684, 2011.

[5] N. Marcus, O. Scheuerman, V. Hoffer, E. Zilbershot-Fink, J. Reiter, and B. Z. Garty, "Stupor in an adolescent following Yom Kippur fast, due to late-onset ornithine transcarbamylase deficiency," *Israel Medical Association Journal*, vol. 10, no. 5, pp. 395-396, 2008.

[6] J. Häberle, N. Boddaert, A. Burlina et al., "Suggested guidelines for the diagnosis and management of urea cycle disorders," *Orphanet Journal of Rare Diseases*, vol. 7, no. 1, article 32, 2012.

[7] M. L. Batshaw, M. Tuchman, M. Summar, and J. Seminara, "A longitudinal study of urea cycle disorders," *Molecular Genetics and Metabolism*, vol. 113, no. 1-2, pp. 127–130, 2014.

[8] L. E. Bernstein, F. Rohr, and J. R. Helm, *Nutrition Management of Inherited Metabolic Diseases*, Springer International Publishing, Cham, 2015.

[9] S. T. Wilber, "Altered mental status in older emergency department patients," *Emergency Medicine Clinics of North America*, vol. 24, no. 2, pp. 299–316, 2006.

A Rare Clinical Course of Seronegative Pulmonary-Renal Syndrome

M. Fröhlich-Gildhoff,[1] W. J. Jabs,[2] C. Berhold,[1] M. K. Kuhlmann,[2] U. Ketterer,[1] S. Kische,[1] and H. Ince[1]

[1]Department of Cardiology and Intensive Care Medicine, Vivantes Klinikum im Friedrichshain, Landsberger Allee 49, 10249 Berlin, Germany
[2]Department of Nephrology, Vivantes Klinikum im Friedrichshain, Landsberger Allee 49, 10249 Berlin, Germany

Correspondence should be addressed to M. Fröhlich-Gildhoff; moritzfg@aol.com

Academic Editor: Zsolt Molnar

Purpose. Pulmonary-renal syndrome (PRS) is characterized by diffuse alveolar hemorrhage and rapidly progressive glomerulonephritis mainly due to autoimmune etiologies. Seronegative PRS is a challenging entity to the clinician, since early diagnosis may be missed leading to delayed appropriate treatment. *Materials and Methods.* We present the clinical course of a 77-year-old patient who was admitted under the suspected diagnosis of pneumogenic sepsis and septic renal failure with fever, dyspnea, and elevated CRP levels. The diagnosis of pulmonary-renal syndrome was initially missed because of the absence of autoantibodies in all serological findings. *Results.* Despite delayed initiation of immunosuppressive therapy and a prolonged period of dialysis and extracorporeal membrane oxygenation the patient recovered well and was released to a rehabilitation center with nearly normalized creatinine levels. The diagnosis of PRS was established by renal biopsy. *Conclusion.* This case illustrates the important differential diagnosis of seronegative pulmonary-renal syndrome in patients with pulmonary and renal impairment.

1. Introduction

Pulmonary-renal syndrome (PRS) is a rare clinical condition defined by rapidly progressive glomerulonephritis (RPGN) and diffuse alveolar hemorrhage (DAH). Its etiology is mainly autoimmune and can be categorized by serological findings (ANCA; anti-GBM antibodies) and renal or pulmonary biopsy. In over 90% of the cases autoantibodies (ANCA, anti-GBM) can be detected, making unclassified PRS a diagnostically challenging entity to the clinician.

We hereby present a case in which the diagnosis of seronegative PRS was established by a pauci-immune RPGN in renal biopsy, in a patient that had undergone immunosuppressive treatment eight months before admission to our hospital due to PRS, positive for both ANCA- and anti-GBM antibodies.

2. Case Report

We report the case of a 77-year-old German woman, who presented to our emergency department due to dyspnea, cough, hemoptysis, and fever.

Initial vital signs were as follows: RR 165/60, heart rate 89 bpm, SpO$_2$ 96%, respiratory rate 28/min, and temperature 38.8°C.

Her past medical history included Goodpasture's syndrome, chronic obstructive pulmonary disease, smoking, high blood pressure, diabetes mellitus type II, and hyperlipidemia.

Eight months before admission the patient had suffered a dialysis-dependent acute kidney failure and an acute respiratory distress syndrome with long-term ventilation, caused by diffuse alveolar hemorrhage. Diagnosis of Goodpasture's syndrome was established by positive serological tests for anti-GBM antibodies and responded well to immunosuppressive therapy with corticoids and cyclophosphamide. Renal biopsy had not been performed, although ANCA also had been tested positive and therefore polyangiitis would have been a likely differential diagnosis. Due to persistent leucopenia and reoccurring infections cyclophosphamide therapy was stopped four months before admission to our hospital and had been replaced by 10 mg prednisolone per day.

On admission to our hospital laboratory results showed an elevation of C-reactive protein level (CRP 94 mg/L) and moderate renal impairment (creatinine 1,3 mg/dL, GFR 38 mL/min) without alterations in white or red blood cell count. Pulmonary radiography showed opacities in the left lower and middle lung zone and antibiotic treatment (Piperacillin/Tazobactam, Ciprofloxacin) was initiated under the suspected diagnosis of pneumonia under immunosuppression.

After progressive worsening of the patient's status with continuous dyspnea even under noninvasive ventilation (FiO$_2$ 1.0), a further increase in CRP (264 mg/L) under escalated antibiotic treatment (vancomycin, Clarithromycin, and Voriconazole), and deteriorated renal function (creatinine 2.7 mg/dL), she was admitted to our intensive care unit on day 6 after hospitalization.

A chest-CT scan showed progressive, diffuse bilateral infiltrates, corresponding to a further decline of the respiratory situation and leading to intubation on day 12 (see Figure 1). Bronchoscopy, performed on day 13, showed signs of pulmonary hemorrhage with microbiological findings of C. albicans and no abnormal results in cytological testing.

Laboratory testing for Goodpasture's syndrome (anti-GBM ELISA, Alegria®, Orgentec) on days 5, 26, and 49 as well as vasculitis (MPO-ANCA, PR3-ANCA; ELISA Orgentec and ANAM; immunofluorescence) on days 13, 26, and 49 repeatedly showed negative results. The negative test results hereby differed from the serological testing in the patient's fulminant Goodpasture's syndrome which had occurred eight months earlier.

A further deterioration in pulmonary function with failing oxygenation under highly invasive ventilation protocols resulted in the application of a system of extracorporeal membrane oxygenation (ECMO, CARDIOHELP®, Maquet) on day 16; tracheotomy had been performed on day 26.

Failing kidney function required the initiation of continuous venovenous hemodialysis (CVVHD) from day 25. Urinary testing showed unselective proteinuria of 2300 mg/g creatinine (of which albumin 1462 mg/L) consistent with glomerular damage and mild hematuria (erythrocytes 97/μL) as well as leukocyturia (50/μL). Microscopic exploration showed hyaline cylinders.

In spite of high CRP levels (290 mg/L) we suspected a relapse of a pulmonary-renal syndrome with pulmonary hemorrhage rather than an infection because of low PCT levels and a drop of hemoglobin from 12.6 to 8.1 g/dL within 8 days due to alveolar bleeding. Moreover, the patient showed no clinical improvement under long-lasting broad antibiotic treatment.

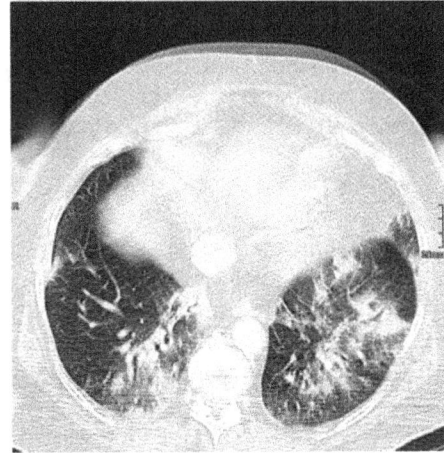

FIGURE 1: Illustrating diffuse bilateral infiltrates of the lung.

Despite repeatedly negative results in laboratory testing for anti-GBM and ANCA a therapy with methylprednisolone (1 g/d) was started on day 26, continued for three days, and followed by a therapy with prednisolone 80 mg per day. It was accompanied by the start of plasma exchange for the duration of 6 days as well as the application of 750 mg of cyclophosphamide on day 31. Under this regime of immunosuppressive therapy the pulmonary and renal function rapidly improved leading to the termination of ECMO therapy and the alternation from CVVHD to intermittent hemodialysis on day 33, which had to be continued until day 50. CRP levels also dropped significantly from 290 to 36 mg/L.

The course of the patient was then complicated by a pneumogenic septic shock with the detection of MRSA in a bronchoalveolar lavage and blood cultures. The situation was stabilized under an escalation of the antibiotic regime to vancomycin and imipenem.

After septic thrombopenia and the impaired hemostatic situation had been improved, renal biopsy was performed on day 44 and revealed scarred intra- and extracapillary glomerulonephritis (crescents) of the pauci-immune type, coherent with rapidly progressive glomerulonephritis and polyangiitis. It also showed diffuse potentially reversible tubular damage and mild benign nephrosclerosis. Despite repetitive dilutions no linear deposition of IgG was observed on the basement membrane by immunofluorescence microscopy.

After the diagnosis of RPGN had histologically been established immunosuppressive therapy was continued with MabThera (Rituximab 1000 mg on days 65 and 79).

Under antibiotic and immunosuppressive therapy the patient's status continually improved. The mobilization of the patient, which initially was complicated by a proximal tetraparesis due to critical illness myopathy (MRI-scan on day 53 showed no signs of myelopathy), eventually showed progress and she could be released to a rehabilitation center on day 104 after admission with a maintenance dosage of prednisolone of 15 mg/d.

Pulmonary function had normalized entirely by the date of discharge. The kidneys showed only moderate impairment (creatinine 1.27 mg/dL; GFR 41 mL/min). The urinalysis showed persistent proteinuria of 888 mg/g creatinine with no further hematuria, probably due to scarred glomeruli.

3. Discussion

Pulmonary-renal syndrome (PRS) is rare and describes the clinical cooccurrence of renal impairment due to glomerulonephritis and a decrease in pulmonary function due to diffuse alveolar hemorrhage. The underlying causes of PRS are heterogeneous and contain a group of autoimmune disorders, which are mainly classified by the detection of antibodies, renal or lung biopsy, or cytological findings in bronchoalveolar lavage. They mainly include ANCA-associated small vessel vasculitis (such as Wegener's granulomatosis, microscopic polyangiitis, and Churg-Strauss vasculitis), Goodpasture's syndrome, systemic lupus erythematosus, Henoch-Schönlein purpura, or cryoglobulinemia. Other rare causes of PRS include drug-induced vasculitis (e.g., propylthiouracil) and subacute endocarditis.

As a particularly deleterious cause for PRS Goodpasture's syndrome is defined by the occurrence of antibodies against the alpha3-NC1-domain of collagen IV in the glomerular or alveolar basement membrane and typical linear deposition of IgG (rarely IgA) observed in part of the basement membrane by immunofluorescence microscopy.

Studies suggest that over 90% of patients with PRS present with one or more antibodies (ANCA, anti-GBM) in the serum, making PRS with no detection of antibodies as in the above-mentioned case very rare [1–3], albeit there have been reports of seronegative relapses in anti-GBM disease after immunosuppressive therapy [4].

In this case two differential diagnoses for the underlying clinical condition seemed possible: a seronegative relapse of anti-GBM disease—which initially had only been diagnosed by circulating antibodies but without renal biopsy—as well as a seronegative ANCA-vasculitis with RPGN and diffuse alveolar hemorrhage.

In the renal biopsy, scarred crescents without linear deposition of IgG along the basement membrane emphasize the possibility of a seronegative ANCA-vasculitis with RPGN. A significant improvement of renal function as in our patient seems to make the diagnosis of an ANCA-associated vasculitis more probable, as anti-GBM diseases like Goodpasture's syndrome usually lead to severe renal impairment and long-term dialysis [5, 6], particularly when treatment is delayed. On the other hand, there have been suggestions that a seronegative anti-GBM disease with predominant pulmonary involvement, as in our case, might be more common than generally suspected and case reports of seroconversion to seronegativity in anti-GBM diseases treated with immunosuppression exist [4]. Additionally, a correlation between cigarette smoking and pulmonary hemorrhage in patients with anti-GBM disease has been demonstrated by Donaghy and Rees [7].

Even though testing by commercially available ELISA-kits, as in our case, is generally considered to be a highly sensitive method for the detection of anti-GBM, the possibility of existing anti-GBM in very low concentrations remains. Furthermore, no tests other than ELISA (e.g., immunoblot, indirect immunofluorescence) have been performed. Importantly, an incidence of 2-3% of seronegative anti-GBM has been estimated by the British reference laboratory for anti-GBM antibodies [8].

The prognosis of PRS derives from simple center experience with low patient numbers. Gallagher et al. observed a 36% early mortality in their single-center study ($n = 14$) with a mean follow-up of four years [9]. Predictors of poor prognosis are crescents in >50% of glomeruli in renal biopsy, serum creatinine levels >5-6 mg/dL, oliguria, or the need for acute dialysis on admission. The early establishment of the correct diagnosis followed by prompt immunosuppressive therapy and plasma exchange are pivotal points in the treatment of PRS.

Diagnosis was missed early in our case due to the complete absence of antibodies, delaying renal biopsy which was performed after immunosuppressive therapy had been started on day 26. The observation of almost complete convalescence of renal and pulmonary function despite delayed disease-specific treatment makes this case very interesting.

Clinical data concerning the course of patients with seronegative PRS is scarce and in most cases the disease leads to end-stage renal failure [1, 10, 11]. As in PRS with a detection of specific antibodies or typical findings in renal or pulmonary biopsy, treatment with corticoids and cyclophosphamide is the basis of any therapy for patients with a suspected seronegative PRS. In some cases plasma exchange has been described to have beneficial effects on patients with seronegative and therefore uncategorizable PRS [12].

4. Conclusion

Seronegative pulmonary-renal syndrome is a rare but potentially life-threatening clinical condition. As the diagnostic process is complicated by the absence of antibodies, end-stage renal disease and even death have been reported as a common consequence of seronegative PRS. This case illustrates the rare instance of renal and pulmonary recovery after therapy with corticosteroids, cyclophosphamide, plasma exchange, and Rituximab, notwithstanding the temporary necessity for renal and pulmonary supportive therapy by dialysis and ECMO.

Competing Interests

The authors declare that there are no competing interests regarding the publication of this paper.

Authors' Contributions

M. Fröhlich-Gildhoff and W. J. Jabs contributed equally.

References

[1] H. Yamaguchi, A. Shirakami, T. Haku et al., "Pulmonary-renal syndrome with negative ANCAs and anti-GBM antibody," *Case Reports in Nephrology*, vol. 2013, Article ID 434531, 6 pages, 2013.

[2] R. Sexena, P. Bygren, B. Arvastson, and J. Wieslander, "Circulating autoantibodies as serological markers in the differential diagnosis of pulmonary renal syndrome," *Journal of Internal Medicine*, vol. 238, no. 2, pp. 143–152, 1995.

[3] J. L. Niles, E. P. Böttinger, G. R. Saurina et al., "The syndrome of lung hemorrhage and nephritis is usually an ANCA-associated condition," *Archives of Internal Medicine*, vol. 156, no. 4, pp. 440–445, 1996.

[4] D. J. Serisier, R. C. W. Wong, and J. G. Armstrong, "Alveolar haemorrhage in anti-glomerular basement membrane disease without detectable antibodies by conventional assays," *Thorax*, vol. 61, no. 7, pp. 636–639, 2006.

[5] F. Madore, J. M. Lazarus, and H. R. Brady, "Therapeutic plasma exchange in renal diseases," *Journal of the American Society of Nephrology*, vol. 7, no. 3, pp. 367–386, 1996.

[6] P. Biesenbach, R. Kain, K. Derfler et al., "Long-term outcome of anti-glomerular basement membrane antibody disease treated with immunoadsorption," *PLoS ONE*, vol. 9, no. 7, article e103568, 2014.

[7] M. Donaghy and A. J. Rees, "Cigarette smoking and lung haemorrhage in glomerulonephritis caused by autoantibodies to glomerular basement membrane," *The Lancet*, vol. 322, no. 8364, pp. 1390–1393, 1983.

[8] A. D. Salama, T. Dougan, J. B. Levy et al., "Goodpasture's disease in the absence of circulating anti-glomerular basement membrane antibodies as detected by standard techniques," *American Journal of Kidney Diseases*, vol. 39, no. 6, pp. 1162–1167, 2002.

[9] H. Gallagher, J. T. C. Kwan, and D. R. W. Jayne, "Pulmonary renal syndrome: a 4-year, single-center experience," *American Journal of Kidney Diseases*, vol. 39, no. 1, pp. 42–47, 2002.

[10] S. C. West, N. Arulkumaran, P. W. Ind, and C. D. Pusey, "Pulmonary-renal syndrome: a life threatening but treatable condition," *Postgraduate Medical Journal*, vol. 89, no. 1051, pp. 274–283, 2013.

[11] Y. Uji, T. Shimizu, T. Yoshioka, H. Yamamoto, Y. Endo, and T. Tani, "A case report of pulmonary-renal syndrome treated with continuous hemodiafiltration and hemodialysis," *Therapeutic Apheresis and Dialysis*, vol. 10, no. 5, pp. 467–471, 2006.

[12] C.-C. Wang, J.-C. Shiang, M.-K. Tsai et al., "Prompt plasmapheresis successfully rescue pulmonary-renal syndrome caused by ANCA-negative microscopic polyangiitis," *Clinical Rheumatology*, vol. 28, no. 12, pp. 1457–1460, 2009.

43

Anasarca, Fever, Thrombocytopenia, Organomegaly, and Multiorgan Failure in a 24-Year-Old Pregnant Woman

Guillaume Morel,[1] Joy Mootien,[2] Philippe Guiot,[2] and Khaldoun Kuteifan[2]

[1]Service d'Hématologie, CHU de Strasbourg, 67000 Strasbourg, France
[2]Service de Réanimation Médicale, GHRSMA, 68100 Mulhouse, France

Correspondence should be addressed to Khaldoun Kuteifan; kuteifank@ghrmsa.fr

Academic Editor: Petros Kopterides

TAFRO syndrome is a distinct idiopathic multicentric Castleman disease characterized by the association of thrombocytopenia, anasarca, fever, reticulin fibrosis, and organomegaly. We report the first case occurring in a Caucasian pregnant woman. At 34 weeks of gestation, our patient presented with all clinical and biological symptoms compatible with a TAFRO syndrome. Tough quick cesarean section was performed as symptoms got worse with onset of multiorgan failure requiring mechanical ventilation for acute respiratory distress, continuous renal replacement, and vasopressors. Nine days after ICU admission, steroid boluses were started and allowed spectacular clinical and biological improvement. As systemic inflammatory manifestations are important, TAFRO syndrome can be mistaken with severe autoimmune diseases, systemic infections, hematological malignancies, or hemophagocytic lymphohistiocytosis.

1. Background

Castleman disease is a nontumoral lymphoproliferative disorder initially described by Castleman and Towne in 1954 [1] usually characterized as either unicentric (UCD) or multicentric Castleman disease (MCD). UCD is an isolated lymph adenopathy without symptoms except those due to the tumoral mass while MCD is defined by the presence of diffuse lymph adenopathy and hepatosplenomegaly associated with systemic inflammatory manifestations: fever, asthenia, and weight loss. Laboratory abnormalities commonly include elevated inflammatory markers, microcytic anemia, hypergammaglobulinemia, and hypoalbuminemia [2]. Coombs test can also be positive. MCD is highly associated with HIV infection and these patients are also coinfected by HHV8 [3]. There is also a cohort of MCD patients without HIV and HHV8 coinfection defined as idiopathic multicentric Castleman disease (iMCD) [4]. TAFRO syndrome is a distinct subtype of iMCD characterized by the association of thrombocytopenia, anasarca, fever, reticulin fibrosis, and organomegaly [5]. The first description of TAFRO syndrome was published in 2010 by Takai et al. [6] who reported the case

of three patients presenting these symptoms with histological findings compatible with iMCD. Some case reports or case series followed this first description. We report hereby the first case of TAFRO syndrome occurring in a Caucasian pregnant woman.

2. Case Report

A Caucasian 24-year-old woman, gravida 1, para 1 at 34 weeks of gestation, presented to our obstetric emergency department. The patient had no medical history and the pregnancy period was going well. One week before admission to our hospital, she noticed progressive weight gain associated with bilateral lower leg oedema. She also reported dyspnea, chest tightness, anorexia, and asthenia. The blood pressure was normal. Clinical exam also revealed hyperreflexia, hepatosplenomegaly, and diffuse supracentimetric lymph adenopathy. Laboratory tests were remarkable for moderate thrombocytopenia (138×10^9/L) and hyponatremia (125 mmol/L) as well as an increase of C-reactive protein (194 mg/L) and uric acid (607 μmol/L). Renal impairment

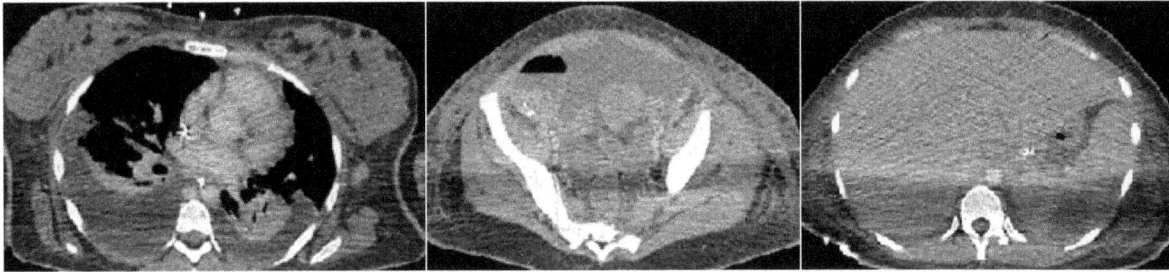

FIGURE 1: Computerized tomography scan showing bilateral pleural effusion and ascites. Presence of a right axillary adenopathy and hepatosplenomegaly.

was not observed though the patient was oliguric. Dipstick urine test did not reveal proteinuria.

Finally, three days after her admission a cesarean section was performed due to the bad tolerance. She gave birth to a girl weighting 2,650 grams with Apgar scores of 3 and 9. The surgery was smooth but the presence of ascites was noticed. The next days, chest pain and hyperreflexia disappeared but edema got worse with a total weight gain of 10 kg. Respiratory distress came out and the patient was oliguric despite diuretics as well as fever and thrombocytopenia got deeper to 50×10^9/L associated with epistaxis. Computerized tomography scan showed diffuse superficial and deep lymphadenopathy, pleural effusions, ascites, and massive hepatosplenomegaly (Figure 1).

Two days later the patient was transferred to our intensive care unit, requiring mechanical ventilation for acute respiratory distress and continuous renal replacement for acute renal failure. She also became hypotensive and needed pressor support. Hemodynamic monitoring revealed hyperdynamic and vasoplegic profile. Myocardial function was preserved at transthoracic echocardiography. Table 1 shows the evolution of biological parameters during ICU hospitalization.

First-line large spectrum antibiotics (Piperacillin-Tazobactam and Ciprofloxacin) were started but fever and inflammatory syndrome kept going. A second line antibiotic was then introduced (Meropenem, Vancomycin, and Amikacin) together with Caspofungin two days later. All blood, protected samples of lower respiratory tract secretions and urinary cultures were sterile. Serological tests for HIV, Hepatitis B and C virus, CMV (for both IgM and IgG), EBV (for both IgM and IgG), HTLV1, and Parvovirus were negative. PCR blood test did not reveal viral replication for CMV and HHV8. Exhaustive immune tests were also not contributive, and the serum complement was normal. Neither monoclonal nor polyclonal elevation of gamma globulin was found. Only serum level of IL-6 was increased (842 pg/mL). Bone marrow biopsy revealed a hypercellular marrow with megakaryocytic hyperplasia associated with the presence of reticulin fibrosis. Tumoral burden was assessed by positron emission tomography using [18F] fluorodeoxyglucose and showed diffuse supra- and infradiaphragmatic adenopathy. All tumoral lymph nodes were smaller than two centimeters and the metabolic activity was low (Figure 2).

The diagnosis of TAFRO-like syndrome was proposed. Nine days after ICU admission, steroid boluses of 1 g of methylprednisolone per day during three days were started followed by 1,5 mg/kg/day.

Spectacular clinical and biological improvement followed steroid introduction. Fever disappeared and blood pressure became normal allowing the weaning of pressor support. We also noticed a decline of pleural effusions and ascites which conduced to respiratory improvement and we preceded extubation eleven days later. Dialysis was stopped at day 30 as the renal function improved. Tumoral infiltration also declined. ICU acquired neuromyopathy was observed but got better with intensive kinesitherapy. Finally thirty-eight days after ICU admission the patient was transferred to internal medicine unit and rehabilitation started.

3. Discussion

Diagnostic criteria of TAFRO syndrome [7] include presence of histological criteria (compatible with pathological findings of lymph node as TAFRO-iMCD and negative LANA-1 for HHV8), three of five major criteria (thrombocytopenia, anasarca, fever, reticulin fibrosis, and organomegaly), and one of two minor criteria (hyper/normoplasia of megakaryocytes in bone marrow or high levels of serum ALP without markedly elevated serum transaminase) which are needed to meet the diagnosis of TAFRO syndrome. Our patient met all the major and minor criteria but unfortunately we could not have a histological analysis of a lymph adenopathy. However we had considered this diagnostic and started treatment by steroids. Moreover we quickly observed a significant improvement of hemodynamic, respiratory, and hematological and renal parameters which strengthened our diagnosis.

As systemic inflammatory manifestations are important, TAFRO syndrome can be mistaken with severe autoimmune diseases [8], systemic infections, hematological malignancies, or hemophagocytic lymphohistiocytosis. These syndromes were proposed but none of them were absolutely compatible with the diagnostic. There was no evidence for underlying autoimmune disease which could explain systemic inflammation or renal failure. C-reactive protein was high but all microbiological cultures serology and PCR were negative and ruled out a possible systemic infection. On the other hand, a tumoral syndrome was present but bone marrow biopsy did

TABLE 1: Evolution of biological tests in ICU.

	Day 0 Admission in ICU	Day 4 Pressor support	Day 7 Dialysis	Day 9 Steroids	Day 12	Day 16 Stop pressor support	Day 20 Stop ventilation	Day 30 Stop dialysis
Leucocyte count (G/L)	17,3	27,9	24,1	36,4	38,1	23,5	27,9	19,8
Hemoglobin (g/dL)	9,2	6,9	8,6	8,1	7,6	7,9	8,2	7,8
Platelets (G/L)	54	30	26	22	30	59	183	116
Serum creatinine (μmol/L)	75	137	151	153	99	86	73	60
Fibrinogen (mg/dL)	930	780	790	530	520	640	610	410
C-reactive protein (mg/dL)	34,3	28,9	31,4	29,5	21,4			2,9
Serum ferritin (ng/mL)	526	939		1053				261
Triglycerides (mg/dL)	240							430
Albumin (g/dL)	1,6	1,8	2	2,4	2,5			2,9
Aspartate amino-transferase (IU/L)		7	6	9	43	134	46	35
Alanine amino-transferase (IU/L)		21	32	52	131	155	81	18
Alkaline phosphatase (IU/L)		479	355	176	204	655	949	261
Lactate dehydrogenase (IU/L)		240	443	497	505			161
Blood lactate (mmol/L)	1,25	0,6	2,7	2,7	2,2	2,1	1,4	3

Reference Ranges. Leucocyte count (4,0–10 G/L), hemoglobin (11–16 g/dL), platelets (150–450 G/L), serum creatinine (45–90 μmol/L), fibrinogen (200–400 mg/dL), C-reactive protein (0–0,4 mg/dL), serum ferritin (12–180 ng/mL), triglycerides (43–148 mg/dL), albumin (3,2–5,5 g/dL), aspartate amino-transferase (0–40 (IU/L)), alanine amino-transferase (0–40 IU/L), alkaline phosphatase (115–359 IU/L), lactate dehydrogenase (85–250 IU/L), and blood lactate (0,6–2,1 mmol/L).

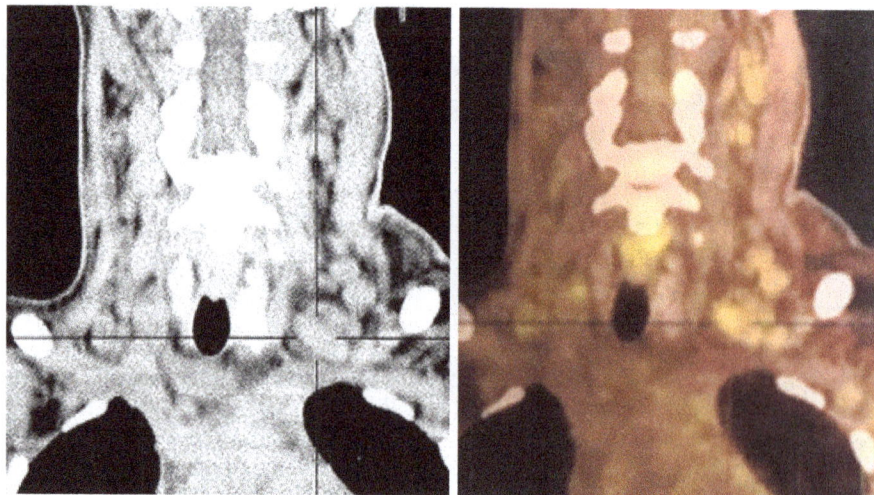

FIGURE 2: Positron emission tomography using [18F] fluorodeoxyglucose showing diffuse infracentimetric supra and infradiaphragmatic adenopathy with low metabolic activity.

not find tumoral infiltration and PET scanner revealed small lymph nodes with low metabolic activity and consequently not compatible with an aggressive lymphoproliferative disorder. Furthermore H-score [9] was not increased, particularly due to the low ferritin level, and excluded the probability of hemophagocytic lymphohistiocytosis. Finally only TAFRO-like syndrome was the compatible diagnostic.

First-line steroid is the usual treatment for TAFRO syndrome [10] and can bring about sustained remissions. In case of relapse or refractory disease, several immuno-suppressive drugs have been proposed and also associated with successful disease control. For example Cyclosporine A [11] may be an alternative therapy for refractory TAFRO syndrome. Anti-IL-6 receptor monoclonal antibodies such as Tocilizumab have demonstrated effectiveness [12] leading to durable remission. Cytotoxic chemotherapies based on lymphoma protocols showed responses in TAFRO syndrome [13] or iMCD patients but is associated with chemotherapy-linked side effects and relapse is common. Rituximab, which is also used in iMCD, may be effective for disease control in TAFRO syndrome [14].

References

[1] B. Castleman and V. W. Towne, "Case records of the Massachusetts general hospital; weekly clinicopathological exercises; founded by Richard C. Cabot," *The New England Journal of Medicine*, vol. 251, no. 10, pp. 396–400, 1954.

[2] J. D. Soumerai, A. R. Sohani, and J. S. Abramson, "Diagnosis and management of Castleman disease," *Cancer Control*, vol. 21, no. 4, pp. 266–278, 2014.

[3] E. E. Mylona et al., "Multicentric Castleman's disease in HIV infection: a systematic review of the literature," *AIDS Reviews*, vol. 10, pp. 25–35, 2008.

[4] D. C. Fajgenbaum, F. van Rhee, and C. S. Nabel, "HHV-8-negative, idiopathic multicentric Castleman disease: novel insights into biology, pathogenesis, and therapy," *Blood*, vol. 123, no. 19, pp. 2924–2933, 2014.

[5] H. Kawabata, K. Takai, M. Kojima et al., "Castleman-Kojima disease (TAFRO syndrome) : a novel systemic inflammatory disease characterized by a constellation of symptoms, namely, thrombocytopenia, ascites (anasarca), microcytic anemia, myelofibrosis, renal dysfunction, and organomegaly : a status report and summary of Fukushima (6 June, 2012) and Nagoya meetings (22 September, 2012)," *Journal of Clinical and Experimental Hematopathology*, vol. 53, no. 1, pp. 57–61, 2013.

[6] K. Takai, K. Nikkuni, H. Shibuya, and H. Hashidate, "Thrombocytopenia with mild bone marrow fibrosis accompanied by fever, pleural effusion, ascites and hepatosplenomegaly," *[Rinshō ketsueki] The Japanese journal of clinical hematology*, vol. 51, no. 5, pp. 320–325, 2010.

[7] Y. Masaki, H. Kawabata, K. Takai et al., "Proposed diagnostic criteria, disease severity classification and treatment strategy for TAFRO syndrome, 2015 version," *International Journal of Hematology*, 2016.

[8] N. Iwaki, D. C. Fajgenbaum, C. S. Nabel et al., "Clinicopathologic analysis of TAFRO syndrome demonstrates a distinct subtype of HHV-8-negative multicentric Castleman disease," *American Journal of Hematology*, vol. 91, no. 2, pp. 220–226, 2016.

[9] L. Fardet, L. Galicier, O. Lambotte et al., "Development and validation of the hscore, a score for the diagnosis of reactive hemophagocytic syndrome," *Arthritis and Rheumatology*, vol. 66, no. 9, pp. 2613–2620, 2014.

[10] M. Inoue, M. Ankou, J. Hua, Y. Iwaki, and M. Hagihara, "Complete resolution of TAFRO syndrome (thrombocytopenia, anasarca, fever, reticulin fibrosis and organomegaly) after immunosuppressive therapies using corticosteroids and cyclosporin A: a case report," *Journal of Clinical and Experimental Hematopathology*, vol. 53, no. 1, pp. 95–99, 2013.

[11] Y. Konishi, S. Takahashi, K. Nishi et al., "Successful treatment of TAFRO syndrome, a variant of multicentric Castleman's disease, with cyclosporine a: Possible pathogenetic contribution of interleukin-2," *Tohoku Journal of Experimental Medicine*, vol. 236, no. 4, pp. 289–295, 2015.

[12] H. Kawabata, S.-I. Kotani, Y. Matsumura et al., "Successful treatment of a patient with multicentric castleman's disease who presented with thrombocytopenia, ascites, renal failure and myelofibrosis using tocilizumab, an anti-interleukin-6 receptor antibody," *Internal Medicine*, vol. 52, no. 13, pp. 1503–1507, 2013.

[13] S. Tedesco, L. Postacchini, L. Manfredi et al., "Successful treatment of a Caucasian case of multifocal Castleman's disease with TAFRO syndrome with a pathophysiology targeted therapy - a case report," *Experimental Hematology and Oncology*, vol. 4, no. 1, article 3, 2015.

[14] S. Hiramatsu, K. Ohmura, H. Tsuji et al., "Successful treatment by rituximab in a patient with TAFRO syndrome with cardiomyopathy," *Japanese Journal of Clinical Immunology*, vol. 39, no. 1, pp. 64–71, 2016.

44

Severe Undifferentiated Vasoplegic Shock Refractory to Vasoactive Agents Treated with Methylene Blue

Farheen Manji,[1,2] **Benjamin Wierstra,**[1,3] **and Juan Posadas**[1,3]

[1]*University of Calgary and Alberta Health Services, Calgary, AB, Canada*
[2]*Department of Medicine, University of Calgary, Calgary, AB, Canada*
[3]*Department of Critical Care, University of Calgary, Calgary, AB, Canada*

Correspondence should be addressed to Farheen Manji; farheen.manji@ahs.ca

Academic Editor: Moritoki Egi

Methylene blue is a phenothiazine-related heterocyclic aromatic molecule presently used in the treatment of methemoglobinemia. Recently, it has been implicated in the treatment of severe refractory vasoplegic shock caused by anaphylaxis, sepsis, or postcardiopulmonary bypass. We present a case of a 27-year-old male with profound vasoplegic shock of unknown etiology which was refractory to vasopressors who responded within hours to a single dose of methylene blue. Additionally, we review the evidence of methylene blue's role in the treatment of shock. This case illustrates a diagnostic approach and treatment options in the setting of undifferentiated vasodilatory shock and outlines a new and emerging role for methylene blue in this clinical setting.

1. Introduction

Vasodilatory shock is a state of hypoperfusion characterized by a significant decrease of vasomotor tone and consequently a decrease of systemic vascular resistance [1]. There are many prevailing theories regarding the pathophysiology of vasodilation that center around the inappropriate activation of vasodilator mechanisms and the dysregulation of vasoconstriction. One such mechanism involves excessive production of nitric oxide (NO) and upregulation of cyclic guanosine $3',5'$-monophosphate (cGMP) which results in dephosphorylation of myosin and subsequent vasodilation [1]. Vasodilatory shock has multiple etiologies including sepsis, anaphylaxis, adrenal insufficiency, drug-induced shock, and postcardiopulmonary bypass vasoplegia [1]. Treatment usually includes addressing the underlying cause and the provision of supportive care including intravenous fluids and vasoactive agents [2]. In addition to conventional therapies, there has been research into inhibiting the cellular pathways at the level of NO and cGMP to prevent vasodilation and tissue hypoperfusion [2]. One such therapy for refractory vasodilatory shock is methylene blue which is a guanylyl cyclase inhibitor and inhibits production of cGMP and therefore inhibits dephosphorylation of myosin, decreasing vasodilation [1].

We present the case of a 27-year-old male with profound vasoplegic shock refractory to vasoactive agents in the setting of intravenous methamphetamine use who responded within hours to methylene blue therapy. Additionally, we review the current literature on the use of methylene blue in the setting of distributive shock of various etiologies including anaphylaxis, sepsis, and postcardiac bypass.

2. Case Presentation

A 27-year-old with past medical history of polysubstance abuse, including methamphetamines, cocaine, opioids, and alcohol, presented to the emergency department after two days of intravenous methamphetamine use with generalized malaise, nausea, dizziness, and blurry vision. He denied fever, chills, chest pain, or shortness of breath. He had no recent sick contacts. He purchased his methamphetamines from his regular dealer but did admit to feeling unwell a few hours after injecting it.

His vitals on arrival to the emergency department were a temperature of 36.1 Celsius, heart rate of 122 bpm, blood

TABLE 1: Bloodwork on initial presentation to the emergency department.

	At admission	Normal range
Hemoglobin	128	137–180 g/L
White blood cell	8.6	4.0–11.0 × 10^9/L
Platelets	66	150–400 × 10^9/L
Sodium	129	133–145 mmol/L
Potassium	3.7	3.3–5.1 mmol/L
Chloride	94	98–111 mmol/L
Bicarbonate	15	21–31 mmol/L
Creatinine	418	50–120 μmol/L
Total bilirubin	47	0–24 μmol/L
INR	2.2	0.9–1.1
PTT	39.2	27–37 s
Lactate dehydrogenase (LDH)	377	100–235 U/L
Ferritin	754	30–400 μg/L
D-Dimer	>10	<0.46 mg/L
Fibrinogen	1.1	1.6–4.1 g/L
Creatinine kinase	929	0–195 U/L
Lactate	8.0	<2 mmol/L
Random cortisol	626	nmol/L
Arterial pH	7.20	7.35–7.45
Arterial pCO2	21	35–45 mmHg
Arterial pO2	61	80–100 mmHg
Arterial bicarbonate	9	24–26 mmgHg

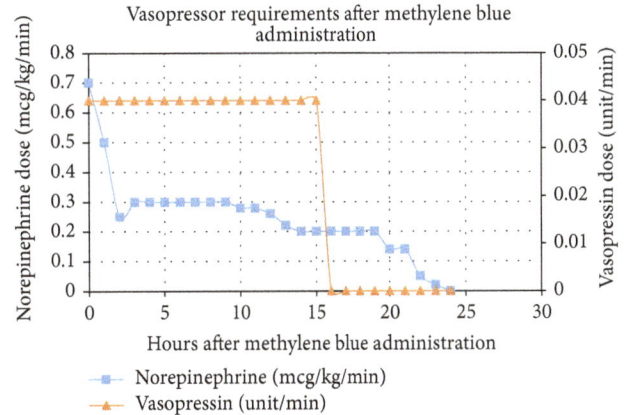

FIGURE 1: Vasopressor requirements hours after methylene blue administration.

pressure of 80/60 mmHg with O2 saturation of 92% on room air. On examination, his extremities were warm. He was alert and oriented to person, place, and time. His neurological exam revealed no motor or sensory deficits. His neck was supple. His cardiovascular exam revealed a regular tachycardia but no murmur. His respiratory exam was unremarkable. His abdomen was mildly tender in the right upper quadrant.

His initial laboratory work is shown in Table 1. In summary, he presented with a mild normocytic anemia, new thrombocytopenia, and new renal failure with a urinalysis showing no casts with trace blood and protein. He had coagulation abnormalities consistent with disseminated intravascular coagulation (DIC). His initial arterial blood gas showed a primary metabolic acidosis secondary to lactic acidosis with a partially compensated by a respiratory alkalosis. Computed Tomography (CT) scan of his head, chest, abdomen, and pelvis was only significant for mild atelectasis in the posterior aspect of both lower lobes and splenomegaly (measured at 15.8 cm, normal < 12 cm). An echocardiogram revealed normal right and left ventricular function with no hemodynamically significant valvular disease. One out of three sets of blood cultures was positive for coryneform bacilli at 65 hours which was thought to be a contaminant. HIV and hepatitis serologies were negative.

In the emergency department, his blood pressure declined to 62/34 mmHg. He was given three liters of normal saline initially with no response in blood pressure. He was then started on escalating doses of norepinephrine

up to 0.9 mcg/kg/min after which his blood pressure increased to 70/40 mmHg. Epinephrine was then added at 0.2 mcg/kg/min, resulting in his blood pressure increasing to 100/50 mmHg. He was empirically started on piperacillin-tazobactam and vancomycin. Given that he had no biochemical evidence of adrenal insufficiency, steroids were not given. Upon transfer to the ICU, the patient was intubated and his hemodynamic profile remained tenuous with his blood pressure dropping to 74/26 mmHg. His norepinephrine was increased to 1 mcg/kg/min, epinephrine was increased to 0.35 mcg/kg/min, and vasopressin was added at 0.04 unit/min. Forty-eight hours into his admission, his lactate normalized but he was still requiring 0.9 mcg/kg/min of norepinephrine and 0.04 unit/min of vasopressin to maintain a mean arterial pressure greater than 60 mmHg. He was given methylene blue dosed at 2 mg/kg for a total dose of 190 mg once. His blood pressure and vasoactive agent requirements are illustrated in Figure 1 in relation to the number of hours after methylene blue administration. Within two hours of administration, the norepinephrine dosage was halved, within 15 hours, he was weaned off vasopressin and within 24 hours, he was off vasoactive support completely and successfully extubated.

No septic or anaphylactic etiology was identified as a cause of the patient's distributive shock. There was no clinical or biochemical evidence of adrenal insufficiency. He denied any overdoses of medications known to commonly cause vasoplegic shock such as calcium channel blockers. As such, the etiology of his shock remained undifferentiated.

3. Discussion

Methylene blue is a phenothiazine-related heterocyclic aromatic molecule that has a long history of use, dating back to the 1800s for treatment of malaria and more commonly, methemoglobinemia [3]. Recently, there has been emerging use of methylene blue in the treatment of refractory distributive shock via inhibition of the nitric-oxide cyclic guanosine monophosphate pathway (Figure 2) [1]. An initial insult results in an increase in nitric oxide synthase and nitric

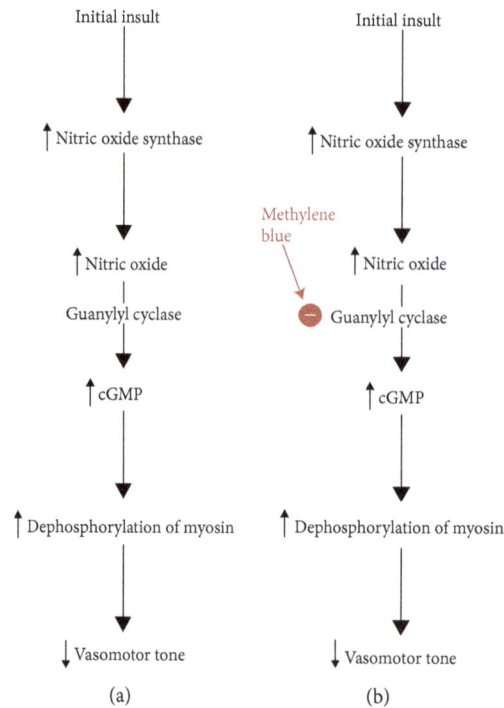

FIGURE 2: (a) The biochemical pathway of vasodilatory shock as a result of upregulation of the nitric oxide-cGMP pathway. (b) Methylene blue's site of action, as a guanylyl cyclase inhibitor, resulting in increased vasomotor tone.

oxide which, via guanylyl cyclase, increases cGMP, and downstream signaling, ultimately resulting in dephosphorylation of myosin and vasodilation [1].

Various in vitro and in vivo animal studies have shown methylene blue as a selective inhibitor of cGMP, counteracting its downstream vasodilatory effects in shock [3]. Clinically, the most well-established use of methylene blue in shock is with patients after cardiac bypass surgery with a range of observational data as well as randomized controlled trials [4]. While not proven as a first line agent, it has been shown to improve systemic vascular resistance if therapy with norepinephrine fails [4]. There have been case reports and series demonstrating the efficacy of methylene blue in cases of anaphylactic shock with resolution of hypotension within one hour of administration [3]. In septic shock, several small randomized control trials support the use of methylene blue, suggesting improved hemodynamics through increase in mean arterial pressure and systemic vascular resistance but no mortality benefit, likely a factor of the small sample sizes [5]. The use of methylene blue in drug-induced vasoplegic shock has very little data to corroborate its regular use; some observational studies have shown a benefit in hemodynamics while others have showed no change. A recent systematic analysis reviewed 17 cases of drug-induced shock described in the literature, most commonly as a result of calcium channel blocker overdose, which showed that there was varying evidence for the use, efficacy, and dosing of methylene blue [6].

There are various dosing regimens for treating shock with methylene blue. Overall experimental and clinical data suggest that 1-2 mg/kg as a single one-time dose is effective [3]. There are other regimens which include continuous infusions

and repeat boluses but there is no evidence suggesting that those are more efficacious. Consideration must also be taken of the side effect profile for methylene blue. It can commonly cause dizziness, tremors, nausea, vomiting, and discoloration of bodily fluids [3]. Less commonly, it can cause an acute hemolytic anemia or precipitation of serotonin syndrome [3]. Higher doses of methylene blue are associated with more serious adverse effects [3].

Our patient presented with severe undifferentiated vasoplegic shock that was not of septic or anaphylactic etiology and was refractory to vasoactive agents. Based on a literature search, there is minimal evidence for use of methylene blue in patients who present with a vasoplegic syndrome that is not postcardiac bypass or due to sepsis or anaphylaxis. There are no case reports or observational studies describing the use of methylene blue in undifferentiated vasoplegic shock. The patient's hemodynamics improved within hours of administration of methylene blue and he was completely off vasoactive support within twenty-four hours (Figure 1). This case report further adds to the growing body of literature that methylene blue has a significant role in the treatment of vasoplegic shock but additionally highlights its effects on shock that is of an unclear etiology, having ruled out sepsis, anaphylaxis, and adrenal insufficiency.

4. Conclusion

Methylene blue has growing evidence of its use as an adjunctive therapy in refractory vasoplegic shock caused after cardiac bypass or by sepsis or anaphylactic shock. This case report suggests that, in patients with severe undifferentiated vasoplegic shock that is unresponsive to vasoactive agents, there is potentially a role for use of a single dose of methylene blue as a rescue therapy.

References

[1] F. H. Epstein, D. W. Landry, and J. A. Oliver, "The pathogenesis of vasodilatory shock," *New England Journal of Medicine*, vol. 345, no. 8, pp. 588–595, 2001.

[2] L. Hosseinian, M. Weiner, M. A. Levin, and G. W. Fischer, "Methylene blue," *Anesthesia & Analgesia*, vol. 122, no. 1, pp. 194–201, 2016.

[3] D. H. Jang, L. S. Nelson, and R. S. Hoffman, "Methylene blue for distributive shock: a potential new use of an old antidote," *Journal of Medical Toxicology*, vol. 9, no. 3, pp. 242–249, 2013.

[4] R. L. Levin, M. A. Degrange, G. F. Bruno et al., "Methylene blue reduces mortality and morbidity in vasoplegic patients after cardiac surgery," *The Annals of Thoracic Surgery*, vol. 77, no. 2, pp. 496–499, 2004.

[5] C. A. Paciullo, D. McMahon Horner, K. W. Hatton, and J. D. Flynn, "Methylene blue for the treatment of septic shock," *Pharmacotherapy*, vol. 30, no. 7, pp. 702–715, 2010.

[6] B. J. Warrick, A. P. Tataru, and S. Smolinske, "A systematic analysis of methylene blue for drug-induced shock," *Clinical Toxicology*, vol. 54, no. 7, pp. 547–555, 2016.

45

Acute Liver and Renal Failure: A Rare Adverse Effect Exclusive to Intravenous form of Amiodarone

Robin Paudel,[1] **Prerna Dogra,**[1] **Saurav Suman,**[1] **Saurav Acharya,**[2] **and Jyoti Matta**[2]

[1]*Department of Internal Medicine, University of Kentucky, Lexington, KY, USA*
[2]*Department of Internal Medicine, Jersey City Medical Center, Jersey City, NJ, USA*

Correspondence should be addressed to Robin Paudel; robinpaudel@uky.edu

Academic Editor: Tuuli Metsvaht

Amiodarone is an antiarrhythmic drug which is highly effective against a wide spectrum of ventricular tachyarrhythmias making it irreplaceable in certain group of patients. We report an unusual case of acute liver and renal failure within 24 hours of initiation of intravenous (IV) amiodarone which resolved after stopping the medication. The mechanism of acute liver and renal toxicity is not clearly known but is believed to be secondary to amiodarone induced (relative) hypotension, idiosyncratic reaction to the drug, and toxicity of the vector that carries the medication, polysorbate-80. In this case review, we discuss the hyperacute drug toxicity caused by IV amiodarone being a distinctly different entity compared to the adverse effects shown by oral amiodarone and support the suggestion that oral amiodarone can be safely administered even in patients who manifest acute hepatitis with the IV form.

1. Introduction

Amiodarone is a class III antiarrhythmic drug highly effective against a wide spectrum of ventricular tachyarrhythmias. We report an unusual case of acute liver and renal failure within 24 hours of initiation of intravenous (IV) amiodarone. Despite wide popularity and efficacy of amiodarone in the treatment of various kinds of cardiac arrhythmias, little is understood about the mechanisms by which IV amiodarone can lead to acute liver and renal failure. As a result, most of the physicians end up withholding this medication altogether. In this case review, we discuss the hyperacute drug toxicity caused by IV amiodarone being a distinctly different entity-compared to the adverse effects shown by oral amiodarone and support the suggestion that oral amiodarone can be safely administered even in patients who manifest acute hepatitis with the IV form.

2. Case Summary

65-year-old Caucasian male with past medical history of Coronary Artery Disease (CAD) status post Coronary Artery Bypass Graft Surgery (CABG), Ischemic Cardiomyopathy status post Automatic Implantable Cardioverter Defibrillator (AICD), hypertension, and dyslipidemia presented to the emergency room (ER) with complaints of multiple AICD shocks. In the ER, he was hemodynamically stable and in no acute distress. His physical examination was unremarkable and had no signs of decompensated heart failure. His initial set of labs at presentation that included Complete Blood Count (CBC), Basic Metabolic Panel (BMP), and Liver Function Test (LFT) were within normal limits. Echocardiogram showed severely dilated left ventricle with ejection fraction of 23%. Patient was loaded with amiodarone 150 mg IV followed by amiodarone drip (1 mg/min for first 6 hours and then 0.5 mg/min for next 18 hours). Patient received total of 1050 mg. Patient was continued on his home medications (Docusate 100 mg three times a day as needed, aspirin 81 mg daily, clopidogrel 75 mg daily, famotidine 20 mg two times a day, escitalopram 10 mg daily, valsartan 80 mg daily, metoprolol succinate 100 mg daily, ezetimibe 10 mg daily, and simvastatin 80 mg daily). In addition, he also received enoxaparin 40 mg daily and zolpidem 5 mg daily.

His BP at presentation was 140/88(MAP 105) which dropped to the lowest, 90/60(MAP 70), over the initial 5 to 6 hours of starting amiodarone and remained in that range

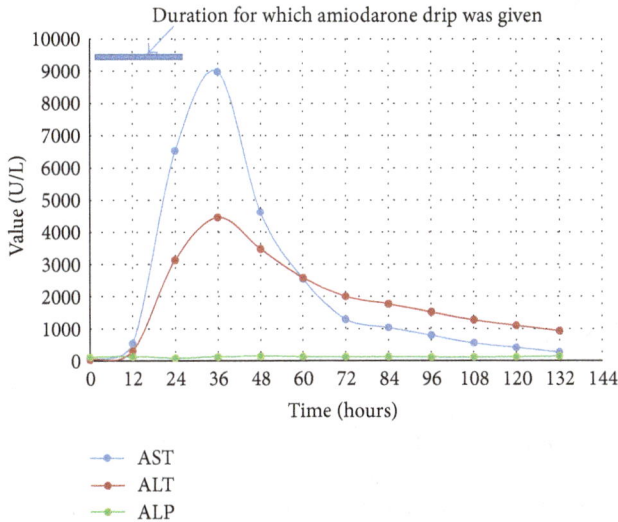

FIGURE 1: Elevation of liver enzymes after IV amiodarone.

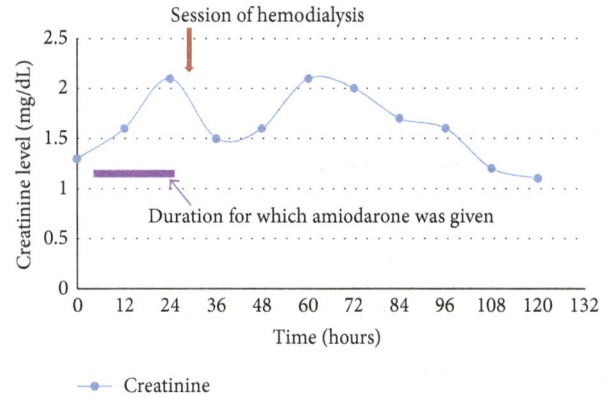

FIGURE 2: Worsening renal function after IV amiodarone.

for 2 to 3 hours. It then improved to MAP of 70–75 but remained lower than his baseline MAP around 100. During the last one-third duration of the amiodarone drip, patient had another period of hypotension with the lowest systolic BP of 86 and diastolic BP of 49 with MAP ranging from 61 to 75 lasting for a period of 3 hours. All other causes of hypotension including sepsis, hypovolemia, and cardiac arrhythmia were ruled out. His blood pressure began to improve 2 hours after stopping amiodarone. However, labs showed dramatic changes. Lab works done one day after starting amiodarone showed marked increase in WBC, potassium, LFTs (Figure 1), and creatinine (Figure 2). Patient became oliguric and hyperkalemic requiring emergent hemodialysis. Ultrasound of the right upper quadrant of the abdomen showed normal liver architecture, workup for viral hepatitis was negative, and sepsis was ruled out.

Patient was monitored in the hospital over 5 days for downward trend of LFTs and creatinine and was discharged home with arrangements for further follow-up plans. After one month, oral amiodarone was started which was well tolerated by the patient with follow-up lab works done at 6 months showing normal values.

3. Discussion

Amiodarone is an iodinated-benzofuran class III antiarrhythmic drug which is highly effective against a wide spectrum of ventricular tachyarrhythmias. Amiodarone is notoriously known to cause various adverse effects including but not limited to liver toxicity, hypo- or hyperthyroidism, QT prolongation, Atrioventricular (AV) block, severe hypotension, Acute Respiratory Distress Syndrome (ARDS), cardiogenic shock, pulmonary fibrosis, and visual disturbance. Amiodarone, being extremely lipophilic, enters the tissues easily and accumulates in the cells including hepatocytes. With a half-life of around 6 months, most of the common serious adverse effects are mainly seen on long term use, oral route being the mode of administration. Amiodarone is initially given at a higher dosage orally or IV termed as the loading dose followed by a daily maintenance dose orally. While most of the known toxic effects of amiodarone is seen on prolonged oral use, most acute adverse effects are observed with the intravenous use of the medication. For unknown reasons, few of the rare side effects that include acute liver failure, cardiac arrest, ARDS, renal injury, and hypotension are almost exclusively seen with the intravenous administration of amiodarone and not with oral loading or maintenance dosing of amiodarone [1–4]. We have presented one such rare case of acute liver and renal failure secondary to intravenous amiodarone administration. The diagnosis of amiodarone toxicity was made based on a thorough drug history excluding any other hepatotoxic agents and other causes of hepatitis, complete physical examination, laboratory investigation, and the temporal relationship with amiodarone administration and rapid improvement in liver/renal function after stopping amiodarone.

Hepatotoxicity caused by *oral* amiodarone is well documented with around 15–20% patients on amiodarone shown to have elevation in levels of transaminases [2, 5–7]. It can lead to 1.5- to 4-fold increase in the level of amino transferases (AST/ALT) while there will be minimal increase in Gamma Glutamyl Transferase (GGT) and generally no change in the level of bilirubin and alkaline phosphatase [5]. Despite elevation of the liver enzymes, clinically significant liver injury warranting discontinuation of amiodarone remains low at around 1%.

On the other hand, *intravenous (IV)* amiodarone toxicity can raise AST/ALT up to 100–200-fold (*AST of 8981 and ALT of 4450 in our case*) within a day of infusion which then reverses quickly after discontinuation of amiodarone except for a few reported cases of fatal hepatotoxicity [8, 9]. There have been case reports where patients who manifested acute hepatotoxicity when started on IV amiodarone tolerated the oral amiodarone quite well and manifested acute toxicity when IV form was reintroduced [10, 11]. While the toxicity from chronic oral amiodarone is believed to be due to direct damage to the lipid bilayers and the disturbance of lysosomal and mitochondrial function, the acute toxicity due to IV amiodarone is believed to be due to different mechanisms like hypersensitivity reaction, relative hypotension causing ischemic liver injury [10, 12, 13], toxicity of the vehicle (polysorbate-80) [11, 14, 15], and idiosyncratic toxicity. Centrilobular necrosis and collapse with minimal inflammation and no appreciable fat as seen in these patients with acute liver toxicity with intravenous amiodarone toxicity suggest ischemic cause of liver injury. Ischemic liver injury is understood to be caused by relative hypotension in the setting of congestive hepatopathy secondary to underlying congestive heart failure which most of the patients needing amiodarone would probably have. Our patient did not have increase in eosinophils count in the blood which points against hypersensitivity reaction. The fact that the mean arterial pressure (MAP) dropped on average by 30–40 mm Hg compared to his baseline favors the etiology being ischemic. His BP remained low throughout the course of amiodarone administration only to improve after stopping amiodarone.

There is also some literature suggestive of the vehicle polysorbate-80 as the cause behind the acute toxicity seen in intravenous amiodarone administration [11, 14, 15]. Polysorbate-80 or polyoxyethylene-sorbitan-20 monooleate ($C_{64}H_{124}O_{26}$) is a vehicle used to make the stable solution form of amiodarone for intravenous use. Polysorbate-80 has been shown to have similar hepatotoxic and nephrotoxic effect, popularly known as *E-ferol syndrome* [14–19] seen in the infants who get intravenous form of vitamin E which contains polysorbate-80 and polysorbate-20.

Not much has been studied about the kidney injury seen in amiodarone. Fogoros et al. [5] reported that about 8.8% of patients on oral amiodarone had an elevation of creatinine with a mean increase of 0.81 mg/dL with one among them requiring discontinuation of the medication. The mechanism behind renal injury due to amiodarone is not clearly understood with renal failure secondary to rhabdomyolysis and cardiorenal syndrome due to drop in blood pressure being the proposed mechanisms. In our patient, cardiorenal syndrome is the most likely mechanism.

Although acute toxic effect due to intravenous amiodarone is rare, but occurred once, it creates a true dilemma in the physician's mind regarding its future use in the patient. While failure to recognize acute toxicity of IV amiodarone can be detrimental, unnecessary avoidance of amiodarone can preclude a patient from getting a potentially lifesaving medication. Our case, for instance, presented with 16 episodes of sustained ventricular tachycardia, 10 of them being terminated by AICD firing and the need for effective antiarrhythmic cannot be overemphasized.

Etiology behind acute toxicity associated with IV amiodarone is still not completely understood. However, irrespective of the etiology, taking into consideration that the acute toxicity of IV amiodarone is a distinctly different entity from the chronic toxicities of oral amiodarone, we support the recommendation not to withhold the potentially lifesaving oral amiodarone after the patient has an acute toxicity due to IV amiodarone. Oral amiodarone can be safely started once the liver enzymes normalize [10, 11, 15], as done in our patient, although further monitoring of the liver enzymes is recommended once the patient is started on oral amiodarone.

Additional Points

Objective. We report a case of acute liver and renal failure induced by intravenous amiodarone and review of similar cases.

Competing Interests

The authors declare that they have no competing interests.

References

[1] L. Donaldson, I. S. Grant, M. R. Naysmith, and J. S. J. Thomas, "Acute amiodarone-induced lung toxicity," *Intensive Care Medicine*, vol. 24, no. 6, pp. 626–630, 1998.

[2] B. McGovern, H. Garan, E. Kelly, and J. N. Ruskin, "Adverse reactions during treatment with amiodarone hydrochloride," *The British Medical Journal*, vol. 287, no. 6386, pp. 175–180, 1983.

[3] S. Kumar, S. Bangalore, R. Kumari, H. Grosu, and R. Jean, "Amiodarone-induced acute respiratory distress syndrome masquerading as acute heart failure," *Journal of Emergency Medicine*, vol. 43, no. 5, pp. e311–e314, 2012.

[4] E. Liverani, A. Armuzzi, F. Mormile, M. Anti, G. Gasbarrini, and N. Gentiloni, "Amiodarone-induced adult respiratory distress syndrome after nonthoracotomy subcutaneous defibrillator implantation," *Journal of Internal Medicine*, vol. 249, no. 6, pp. 565–566, 2001.

[5] R. N. Fogoros, K. P. Anderson, R. A. Winkle, C. D. Swerdlow, and J. W. Mason, "Amiodarone: clinical efficacy and toxicity in 96 patients with recurrent, drug-refractory arrhythmias," *Circulation*, vol. 68, no. 1, pp. 88–94, 1983.

[6] L. Harris, W. J. McKenna, E. Rowland, D. W. Holt, G. C. Storey, and D. M. Krikler, "Side effects of long-term amiodarone therapy," *Circulation*, vol. 67, no. 1, pp. 45–51, 1983.

[7] J. H. Lewis, R. C. Ranard, A. Caruso et al., "Amiodarone hepatotoxicity: prevalence and clinicopathologic correlations among 104 patients," *Hepatology*, vol. 9, no. 5, pp. 679–685, 1989.

[8] A. L. F. Chan, H. J. Hsieh, Y.-A. Hsieh, and S.-J. Lin, "Fatal amiodarone-induced hepatotoxicity: a case report and literature review," *International Journal of Clinical Pharmacology and Therapeutics*, vol. 46, no. 2, pp. 96–101, 2008.

[9] J.-G. Li, T.-C. Yang, D.-M. Yu, and T.-H. Ren, "Fatal acute liver failure after intravenous amiodarone administration," *Journal of the Formosan Medical Association*, vol. 114, no. 3, pp. 294–296, 2015.

[10] Amiodarone, http://livertox.nlm.nih.gov/Amiodarone.htm#casereport.

[11] A. E. Rätz Bravo, J. Drewe, R. G. Schlienger, S. Krähenbühl, H. Pargger, and W. Ummenhofer, "Hepatotoxicity during rapid intravenous loading with amiodarone: description of three cases and review of the literature," *Critical Care Medicine*, vol. 33, no. 1, pp. 128–246, 2005.

[12] N. Gluck, M. Fried, and R. Porat, "Acute amiodarone liver toxicity likely due to Ischemic hepatitis," *Israel Medical Association Journal*, vol. 13, no. 12, pp. 748–752, 2011.

[13] M. Nasser, T. R. Larsen, B. Waanbah, I. Sidiqi, and P. A. McCullough, "Hyperacute drug-induced hepatitis with intravenous amiodarone: case report and review of the literature," *Drug, Healthcare and Patient Safety*, vol. 5, no. 1, pp. 191–198, 2013.

[14] A. Rhodes, J. B. Eastwood, and S. A. Smith, "Early acute hepatitis with parenteral amiodarone: a toxic effect of the vehicle?" *Gut*, vol. 34, no. 4, pp. 565–566, 1993.

[15] P. R. James and S. M. C. Hardman, "Acute hepatitis complicating parenteral amiodarone does not preclude subsequent oral therapy," *Heart*, vol. 77, no. 6, pp. 583–584, 1997.

[16] K. E. Bove, N. Kosmetatos, K. E. Wedig et al., "Vasculopathic hepatotoxicity associated with E-Ferol syndrome in low-birth-weight infants," *The Journal of the American Medical Association*, vol. 254, no. 17, pp. 2422–2430, 1985.

[17] J. B. Arrowsmith, G. A. Faich, D. K. Tomita, J. N. Kuritsky, and F. W. Rosa, "Morbidity and mortality among low birth weight infants exposed to an intravenous vitamin E product, E-Ferol," *Pediatrics*, vol. 83, no. 2, pp. 244–249, 1989.

[18] V. Lorch, M. D. Murphy, L. R. Hoersten, E. Harris, J. Fitzgerald, and S. N. Sinha, "Unusual syndrome among premature infants: association with a new intravenous vitamin E product," *Pediatrics*, vol. 75, no. 3, pp. 598–602, 1985.

[19] W. J. Martone, W. W. Williams, M. L. Mortensen et al., "Illness with fatalities in premature infants: association with an intravenous vitamin E preparation, E-Ferol," *Pediatrics*, vol. 78, no. 4, pp. 591–600, 1986.

46

Acute Hypoxic and Refractory Respiratory Failure Induced by an Underlying PFO: An Unusual Case of Platypnea Orthodeoxia and Transient Complication after Transcatheter Closure

Carlos Salazar[1] and Romeo A. Majano[2]

[1]Department of Internal Medicine, Weiss Memorial Hospital, 4646 N. Marine Drive, Chicago, IL 60640, USA
[2]Miami Cardiac and Vascular Institute, South Miami Hospital, Baptist Health, 6200 SW 73 Street, South Miami, FL 33143, USA

Correspondence should be addressed to Carlos Salazar; salazarcarcamo77@gmail.com

Academic Editor: Gerhard Pichler

Platypnea orthodeoxia (PO) is an infrequent condition of dyspnea with hypoxemia, increased by adopting an upright position and is relieved in decubitus. This condition may occur in patients with hidden intracardiac shunts, usually across a persistent foramen ovale (PFO). The incidence of PFO in general population is quite common, around 27%; however, the concurrent presentation with PO, especially in acute refractory respiratory failure, is extremely rare. PFO closure in this setting is still the treatment of choice with significant improvement or complete resolution of symptoms after closure with an overall periprocedural complication in the first 24 hours of approximately less than 5%. A transient ST-segment elevation in the inferior leads is present in extremely rare occasions and most likely is induced by either an air embolism or a mechanically provoked spasm of coronary arteries. We report a case of an 83-year-old woman in acute hypoxic and refractory respiratory failure in whom PO was identified, most likely induced by a hidden PFO. The patient underwent percutaneous transcatheter closure and developed immediate chest pain, transient hemodynamic instability, and ST-segment elevation in the inferior leads; nevertheless, our patient recovered completely with rapid resolution of respiratory failure with no adverse clinical sequelae.

1. Introduction

Platypnea orthodeoxia (PO) is an uncommon presentation of an underlying disorder consisting of hypoxemia and dyspnea upon assuming an upright position and is relieved by decubitus [1]. This condition can be secondary to an intracardiac shunt, a pulmonary vascular shunt, or a ventilation–perfusion mismatch. A right-to-left shunt through a persistent foramen ovale (PFO) may produce a significant desaturation of arterial blood when the patient changes from decubitus to a sitting or standing position [2]. Most PFOs are not expected to cause sufficient right-to-left shunting to elicit hypoxemia due to higher left atrial pressure and greater compliance of the right atrium and ventricle. A spontaneous or induced increase in pulmonary artery pressure (PAP) may produce a sufficient increase in the

right atrial pressure to promote a right-to-left shunt ensuing hypoxemia [3]. The incidence of PFO is quite common in general population with an overall incidence of 27% and with a mean diameter of 4.9 mm; however, the concurrent presentation with PO in the context of acute refractory respiratory failure is extremely rare [4, 5]. Transient periprocedural complications in the first 24 hours following PFO closure are uncommon and the pathophysiological mechanisms have not been yet described. We present a case of a patient in acute hypoxic and refractory respiratory failure exhibiting PO due to a right-to-left shunt through a previously undiagnosed PFO. The patient was treated with percutaneous transcatheter PFO closure and presented chest pain, transient hemodynamic instability, and ST-segment elevation after this procedure. The patient recovered completely and there were no adverse clinical sequelae.

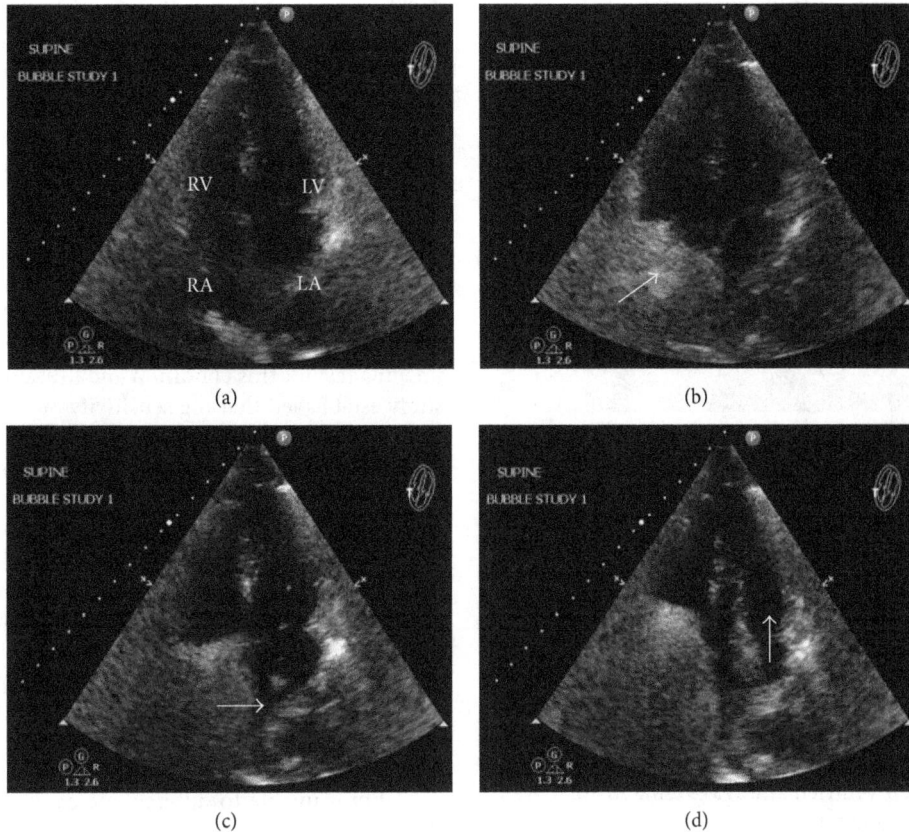

FIGURE 1: Agitated saline contrast study showing (a) 4 chambers prior contrast infusion. (b) Agitated saline entering the RA. (c) and (d) *Arrows* demonstrating right-to-left shunt into the LA and LV. *RV*: right ventricle; *LV*: left ventricle; *RA*: right atria; *LA*: left atria. Arrows throughout indicate direction of the agitated saline flow.

2. Case Report

An 83-year-old woman with diabetes mellitus type 2, essential hypertension, and hyperlipidemia came to the emergency department with history of 3 days of progressive cough and shortness of breath and 1 day of pressure-like chest pain and anxiety. She did not have a history of smoking. Initial physical examination revealed a patient in severe respiratory distress. Oxygen saturation (O_2 Sat) was 94% with a nonrebreather mask at 80% FIO_2 and cardiovascular examination revealed a soft 2/6 holosystolic murmur located in the left sternal border, without gallops. Diffused rales were auscultated in both lung fields. The rest of examination and vital signs were unremarkable.

ABG analysis showed acute respiratory alkalosis with moderate hypoxemia and laboratory panels including complete blood count, electrolytes, and troponins were within normal limits. Electrocardiogram (ECG) was normal; chest X-ray and chest computed tomography angiography exhibited diffuse interstitial ground-glass opacities bilaterally suggestive of pulmonary edema and no filling defects ruling out pulmonary embolism. The patient was transferred to the Intensive Care Unit for close monitoring and treated with bilevel positive airway pressure and intravenous diuretics demonstrating a slight clinical improvement; however, hypoxemia persisted and orthodeoxia was identified. O_2 Sat

decreased significantly from 91% in decubitus to 86% when adopting a sitting position.

Echocardiography (TTE) showed ejection fraction 50–55% with RVSP 63 and a slightly positive agitated saline contrast test (ASCT) consistent with an interatrial shunting. Transesophageal echocardiography (TEE) was performed showing a positive interatrial communication; nevertheless, images were inconclusive to further evaluate and to determine the precise location of this interatrial defect due to suboptimal echocardiographic images. Cardiac magnetic resonance was not definitive for the presence of an atrial septal defect. Coronary computed tomography angiography was recommended and exhibited mild nonobstructive coronary atherosclerosis and nonspecific pulmonary vascular congestion with no evidence of atrial septal defect or an unroofed coronary sinus.

Decision was made to clarify the diagnosis with a right heart catheterization and intracardiac echocardiography, which revealed an intact interatrial septum with an evident PFO. An absent "step up" in saturation ruled out a left-to-right shunt. A TTE with ASCT was repeated and performed in reversed Trendelenburg position demonstrating a strongly and obvious right-to-left shunt through a PFO (Figure 1). The defect was emergently closed using an 18 mm Amplatzer Cribriform Septal Occluder (Figure 2). The patient expressed sudden severe chest pain after the procedure. ECG exhibited

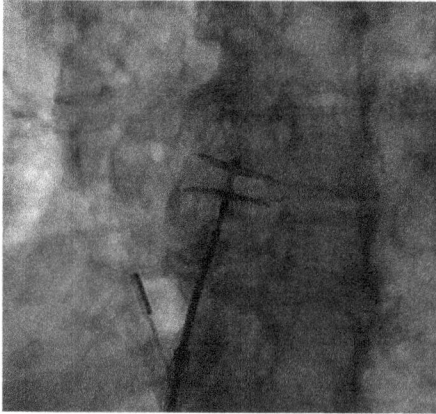

FIGURE 2: Fluoroscopic positioning and deployment of 18 mm Amplatzer Cribriform Septal Occluder.

ST-segment elevation in leads II, III, and aVF, followed by a significant decrease in the mean arterial pressure. Bedsides ultrasonography showed proper device position and no cardiac tamponade was noted. Intra-aortic balloon pump was inserted for hemodynamic support and vasopressors were started. A right coronary artery air embolism was suspected; therefore a coronary angiogram was performed and showed no abnormalities. Left ventricular angiogram and aortogram were within normal parameters.

The patient stabilized with resolution of chest pain and normalization of the ECG changes and became normotensive. A TTE was repeated showing normal left ventricle function, no evidence of pericardial effusion, and no wall motion abnormalities. The patient remained hemodynamically stable, vasopressors were weaned off, and the intra-aortic balloon pump was removed. The patient experienced a positive outcome with complete resolution of respiratory failure with low requirements of oxygen therapy. The patient was discharged to home saturating 98% on room air.

3. Discussion

The exact pathophysiological mechanism of PO is not well understood; however, it could be explained by several hypotheses on the basis of positional modifications that favor a shunting phenomenon through an atrial communication. These modifications might increase a right-to-left shunt through a PFO with significant desaturation of arterial blood when the patient stands up or bends over [6]. PFO size tends to be enhanced with increasing age, from a mean of 3.4 mm in the first decade to 5.8 mm in the 10th decade of life [4]. Standing upright might stretch the interatrial communication of the PFO thus allowing more streaming of venous blood from the inferior vena cava through the defect [7]. Another explanation could be a preferential vena caval blood flow directed towards the atrial septum during an upright position, such as in patients with prominent Eustachian valve. In patients with chronic hypoxemia, low mixed venous oxygen tension of blood returning to the pulmonary arteries induces a pulmonary vasoconstriction that increases right

atrial pressure and it is believed that it could create a greater gradient of pressures between both atria, supporting a right-to-left shunt through an interatrial communication [8].

PO in the setting of a PFO can be presented with a concomitant increase in PAP; nevertheless, in some cases in which a preferential flow phenomenon has been detected, patients present with normal atrial pressure and PAP but with severe right-to-left shunt [9]. These anatomic abnormalities together with a pulmonary hypertension could deteriorate in an acute, refractory, and dangerous manner a patient's oxygenation status if the diagnosis of a PFO and immediate treatment is not considered. It is imperative to select an initial imaging test for this condition and Muratori et al. in a recent study established that the sensitivity of TTE with ASCT can be improved using provocative measures like valsalva maneuvers [10]. TEE is the gold standard technique for the visualization of atrial septal anatomy, but there might be some technical challenges in eliciting an adequate increase in right atrial pressure during imaging due to varying degree of patient sedation and participation [11]. In our patient, no positional changes were assessed during imaging testing, the strength of the right-to-left shunt through the PFO could have been physiologically reduced during decubitus position and consequently extremely difficult to detect. Transcranial Doppler is another imaging tool with high sensitivity that can be used to screen and quantitate shunt severity; unfortunately, this modality is unable to differentiate cardiac from pulmonary shunts [12].

Percutaneous transcatheter closure is still the treatment of choice for PFO presenting with PO. Guérin et al. demonstrated in 78 patients an immediate increase in saturation and significant decrease in dyspnea following percutaneous occlusion of PFO [13]. A recent study confirmed that 64.8% of patients presenting with PFO and PO had improvement or complete resolution of their dyspnea after transcatheter closure [14]. There have been some studies that have identified that the overall periprocedural complications in the first 24 hours in 276 patients following PFO closure were of 4%. A transient (<3 min) ST-segment elevation, in the inferior leads was present in 1.4%, most likely induced by either an air embolism or a mechanically induced spasm of the coronary arteries [15]. Some authors have reported similar transient events during transseptal catheter procedures such as atrial fibrillation ablation and have hypothesized that following manipulation of the interatrial septum could stimulate left atrial ganglion plexuses causing an imbalance in autonomic innervation, which leads to coronary artery spasm and ST-segment elevation [16]. A recent multicenter, randomized, superiority trial evaluated the procedural complications from PFO closure and demonstrated that atrial fibrillation was only present in 5.9% in comparison to the nonintervention group [17]. Other potential complications of percutaneous device placement can include access difficulties, device embolisation or malposition, pericardial effusion secondary to perforation of the atrium or pulmonary veins, or device thrombus formation [18]. There is no supporting data in literature about sudden chest pain immediately after transcutaneous closing of PFO. A small number of patients have had device removal due to chest pain, presenting late after implantation, of which 18% were associated with nickel allergy present in Amplatzer devices [19]. This would not explain the immediate hemodynamic collapse seen in our patient.

We suspect that the transient hemodynamic instability and ST-segment elevation were probably due to catheter manipulation of the atrial septum or a small air embolism to the right coronary artery, sufficient enough to induce an autonomic imbalance and a possible coronary artery vasospasm. Despite this brief episode of instability, the patient's respiratory failure and chest pain resolved completely and there were no adverse clinical sequelae.

4. Conclusion

A PFO as the main cause of acute hypoxic respiratory failure is rare and usually it is not sufficient to cause right-to-left shunting to elicit desaturation. Refractory hypoxemia associated with positional anatomic modifications might favor a shunting phenomenon through an atrial communication. If orthostatic desaturation is detected, it should warrant further investigation. Patients with refractory hypoxemia and suspicious echocardiographic findings should prompt an evaluation with positional changes to facilitate identification of a PFO as a potentially treatable cause of respiratory failure. A noninvasive, safe, and initial diagnosis can be performed by TTE using ASCT moving the patient from a supine to an upright position or by using a tilt-table. Therefore, the shunt can be localized at the atrial level and directly visualized. The transient hemodynamic compromise seen in our patient appeared to be a complication of PFO closure and more studies should be performed to elucidate the exact pathophysiologic mechanism. Physicians should be aware of this transient immediate complication after PFO closure.

References

[1] J. Tobis and M. Shenoda, "Percutaneous treatment of patent foramen ovale and atrial septal defects," *Journal of the American College of Cardiology*, vol. 60, no. 18, pp. 1722–1732, 2012.

[2] C. Blanche, S. Noble, M. Roffi et al., "Platypnea-orthodeoxia syndrome in the elderly treated by percutaneous patent foramen ovale closure: A case series and literature review," *European Journal of Internal Medicine*, vol. 24, no. 8, pp. 813–817, 2013.

[3] J. B. Seward, D. L. Hayes, H. C. Smith et al., "Platypnea-orthodeoxia: Clinical profile, diagnostic workup, management, and report of seven cases," *Mayo Clinic Proceedings*, vol. 59, no. 4, pp. 221–231, 1984.

[4] P. T. Hagen, D. G. Scholz, and W. D. Edwards, "Incidence and size of patent foramen ovale during the first 10 decades of life: an autopsy study of 965 normal hearts," *Mayo Clinic Proceedings*, vol. 59, no. 1, pp. 17–20, 1984.

[5] J. T. Knapper, J. Schultz, G. Das, and L. S. Sperling, "Cardiac platypnea-orthodeoxia syndrome: an often unrecognized malady," *Clinical Cardiology*, vol. 37, no. 10, pp. 645–649, 2014.

[6] T. O. Cheng, "Mechanisms of platypnea-orthodeoxia: what causes water to flow uphill?" *Circulation*, vol. 105, no. 6, p. e47, 2002.

[7] G. P.-W. Chen, S. L. Goldberg, and E. A. Gill Jr., "Patent foramen ovale and the platypnea-orthodeoxia syndrome," *Cardiology Clinics*, vol. 23, no. 1, pp. 85–89, 2005.

[8] C. Marshall and B. Marshall, "Site and sensitivity for stimulation of hypoxic pulmonary vasoconstriction," *Journal of Applied Physiology*, vol. 55, pp. 711–716, 1983.

[9] P. Kubler, H. Gibbs, and P. Garrahy, "Platypnoea-orthodeoxia syndrome," *Heart*, vol. 83, no. 2, pp. 221–223, 2000.

[10] M. Muratori, G. Italiano, E. Innocenti et al., "P594Contrast transthoracic echocardiography as a gatekeeper for patent foramen ovale closure," *European Heart Journal - Cardiovascular Imaging*, vol. 17, pp. ii109–ii113, 2016.

[11] K. Marriott, V. Manins, A. Forshaw, J. Wright, and R. Pascoe, "Detection of right-to-left atrial communication using agitated saline contrast imaging: Experience with 1162 patients and recommendations for echocardiography," *Journal of the American Society of Echocardiography*, vol. 26, no. 1, pp. 96–102, 2013.

[12] A. N. Mahmoud, I. Y. Elgendy, N. Agarwal, J. M. Tobis, and M. K. Mojadidi, "Identification and Quantification of Patent Foramen Ovale–Mediated Shunts," *Interventional Cardiology Clinics*, vol. 6, no. 4, pp. 495–504, 2017.

[13] P. Guérin, V. Lambert, F. Godart et al., "Transcatheter closure of patent foramen ovale in patients with platypnea-orthodeoxia: Results of a multicentric French registry," *CardioVascular and Interventional Radiology*, vol. 28, no. 2, pp. 164–168, 2005.

[14] M. K. Mojadidi, R. Gevorgyan, N. Noureddin, and J. M. Tobis, "The effect of patent foramen ovale closure in patients with platypnea-orthodeoxia syndrome," *Catheterization and Cardiovascular Interventions*, vol. 86, no. 4, pp. 701–707, 2015.

[15] M. U. Braun, D. Fassbender, S. P. Schoen et al., "Transcatheter closure of patent foramen ovale in patients with cerebral ischemia," *Journal of the American College of Cardiology*, vol. 39, no. 12, pp. 2019–2025, 2002.

[16] B. H. Le, J. N. Black, and S. K. Huang, "Transient ST-Segment Elevation during Transseptal Catheterization for Atrial Fibrillation Ablation," *Texas Heart Institute Journal*, vol. 37, no. 6, pp. 717–721, 2010.

[17] J. Mas, G. Derumeaux, B. Guillon et al., "Patent Foramen Ovale Closure or Anticoagulation vs. Antiplatelets after Stroke," *The New England Journal of Medicine*, vol. 377, no. 11, pp. 1011–1021, 2017.

[18] J. N. Johnson, M. L. Marquardt, M. J. Ackerman et al., "Electrocardiographic changes and arrhythmias following percutaneous atrial septal defect and patent foramen ovale device closure," *Catheterization and Cardiovascular Interventions*, vol. 78, no. 2, pp. 254–261, 2011.

[19] S. K. Verma and J. M. Tobis, "Explantation of patent foramen ovale closure devices: A multicenter survey," *JACC: Cardiovascular Interventions*, vol. 4, no. 5, pp. 579–585, 2011.

47

Veno-Arterial Extracorporeal Membrane Oxygenation for Septic Cardiomyopathy due to *Legionella* Pneumonia after Influenza Virus Infection

Motohiro Asaki ⓘ, Takamitsu Masuda, and Yasuo Miki

Department of Emergency Medicine, Emergency and Critical Care Center, Fujieda Municipal General Hospital, Shizuoka, Japan

Correspondence should be addressed to Motohiro Asaki; motohiro.asaki@gmail.com

Academic Editor: Anita J. Reddy

A 57-year-old man presented to the emergency department with fever and progressive altered level of consciousness of 5 days' duration. Three days before admission, influenza A was diagnosed at a clinic. On admission, his vital signs were unstable. Pneumonia was diagnosed through chest computed tomography, and urinary *Legionella* antigen test was positive. A diagnosis of septic shock due to *Legionella* and influenza pneumonia was made, and critical care management was initiated, including mechanical ventilation and vasopressors. However, tachycardia did not improve, left ventricular ejection fraction was 20%, and circulatory insufficiency progressed. Therefore, considering the involvement of septic cardiomyopathy and cardiogenic shock, veno-arterial extracorporeal membrane oxygenation (VA-ECMO) was initiated for circulation assistance on day 3 since admission. Tachycardia and myocardial dysfunction improved by day 8, and VA-ECMO was withdrawn. Subsequently, nutrition management and rehabilitation were performed, and the patient was transferred to a recovery hospital on day 108. VA-ECMO may be beneficial when concomitant with circulatory assistance in uncontrollable cases of septic cardiomyopathy using catecholamines and β-blockers. It may be necessary to adopt VA-ECMO at an appropriate time before the patient progresses to cardiopulmonary arrest.

1. Introduction

Legionella pneumonia occasionally leads to severe septic shock and multiple organ dysfunction and is known to follow a lethal course. In 2008, Von Baum et al. reported that the mortality rate of *Legionella* pneumonia was 14% [1]. Furthermore, reversible myocardial depression in patients with septic shock was first described in 1984 by Parker et al., as septic cardiomyopathy [2]. Veno-arterial extracorporeal membrane oxygenation (VA-ECMO) is an extracorporeal circulation device used for severe cardiogenic shock, and Brechot et al. reported the effectiveness of VA-ECMO on septic shock with cardiovascular dysfunction [3]. This case report describes the successful treatment of severe *Legionella* pneumonia that led to septic shock and severe septic cardiomyopathy by timely and proper introduction of VA-ECMO.

2. Case Presentation

A previously healthy 57-year-old man presented to the emergency department with fever and progressive altered mental status for 5 days. Three days before admission, he was diagnosed with influenza A at a clinic, for which oseltamivir was prescribed. Upon arrival at the emergency department, his vital signs were unstable: respiratory rate, 40 breaths/min; heart rate, 153 beats/min (irregular); blood pressure, 96/70 mmHg; body temperature, 39.9°C; and Glasgow Coma Scale (GCS), 11/15 (E3V3M5). On physical examination, an oral mucosa was dry and coarse crackles in the left lung were documented, but there were no heart murmur and no lower edema. Blood examination results were as follows: white blood cell count (10100/μL); hemoglobin (15.7 d/L); platelet count (12.8 × 10^3 /μL); C-reactive protein (36.82 mg/dL); creatine kinase (3181 IU/L);

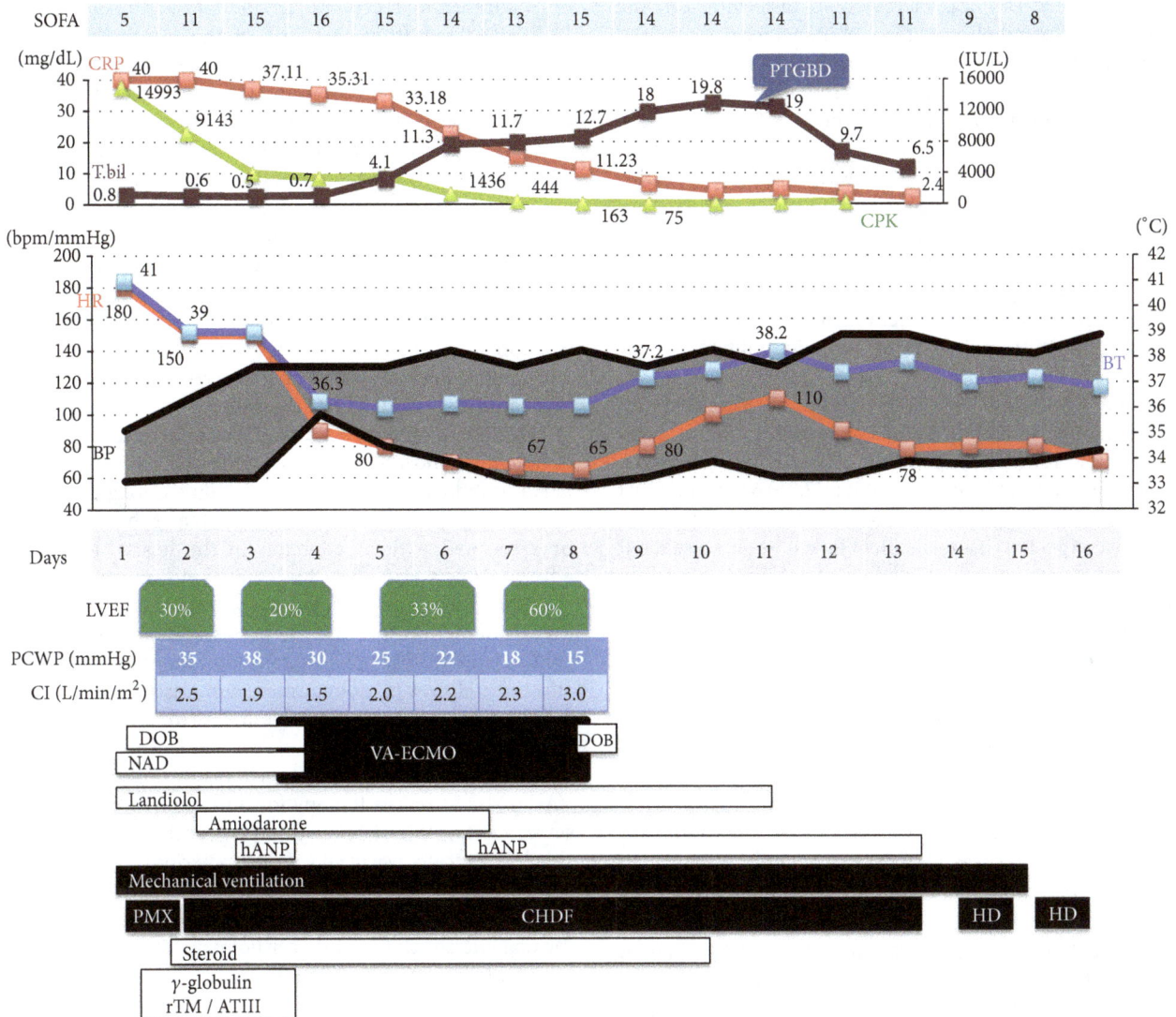

FIGURE 1: Patient's clinical course in the intensive care unit.

procalcitonin (19.58 ng/mL); and brain natriuretic peptide (123 pg/mL). Urinary *Legionella* antigen test was positive, while rapid influenza A and B antigen tests were both negative. Arterial blood gas analysis yielded the following findings: pH 7.54, pCO$_2$ 25.8 mmHg, pO$_2$ 81.2 mmHg (O$_2$ 10 L/min reserver mask), HCO$_3$$_-$ 21.1 mmol/L, and lactate 2.0 mmol/L. A consolidation was observed in the left lung field by chest X-ray and chest computed tomography (CT). Electrocardiogram initially documented atrial fibrillation (AF), while echocardiogram revealed left ventricular ejection fraction (LVEF) of approximately 30%. Due to the presence of *Legionella*, pneumonia, and qSOFA of 3 points, it was diagnosed with *Legionella* pneumonia and septic shock. He was transferred to the intensive care unit (ICU), intubated, and started with mechanical ventilation management and intensive care. His progress in the ICU is shown in Figure 1.

Tazobactam/piperacillin and levofloxacin for *Legionella* pneumonia and peramivir for suspected influenza pneumonia were initiated intravenously. For septic shock, noradrenaline at 0.06 µg/kg/min, hydrocortisone at 200 mg/day, and intravenous immunoglobulin were started. In view of AF, landiolol was started at 1 µg/kg/min and then increased to 10 µg/kg/min. Moreover, due to the low ventricular contractility, additional dobutamine at 3 µg/kg/min was initiated. The patient was then given polymyxin B-immobilized fiber and continuous hemodiafiltration (CHDF) for acute kidney injury (AKI) and suspected endotoxin shock (endotoxin level was later observed to be high, at 139.7 pg/mL). On day 3 of hospitalization, we performed cardioversion several times for AF and there was a temporary return to normal sinus rhythm (SR); however, it immediately returned to AF. Transthoracic echocardiography showed that LVEF worsened to 15%, and the left ventricular end-diastolic/systolic diameter (LVDd/Ds) was increased to 61/55 mm. On the night of day 3, metabolic and respiratory acidosis progressed due to circulatory failure (pH 7.138, pO$_2$ 70.4 mmHg, pCO$_2$ 68.4 mmHg, BE -8.7 mmol/L, lactate 2.4 mmol/L) (ventilator mode: pressure control ventilation: FiO2 70%, RR 20/min, PEEP 9 cmH$_2$O, PC 15 cmH$_2$O). Thus, the patient was diagnosed with cardiogenic shock due to septic cardiomyopathy. This required introduction of VA-ECMO and catecholamines were discontinued. Subsequently, the acidemia ameliorated and hemodynamic circulation stabilized. AF reverted to normal SR on day 5. And on day 7, LVEF recovered to 60%. Therefore, it stabilized hemodynamics by infusion, a little catecholamine, and VA-ECMO was discontinued on day 8.

While VA-ECMO was in progress, the patient developed progressive jaundice; this appeared to be a complication of VA-ECMO because of mechanical hemolysis (on day 7, total/direct bilirubin: 13.3/9.6 mg/dL, LDH 3077 IU/L, Hb: 8.1 g/dL). Therefore, after VA-ECMO withdrawal, we expected that total bilirubin will be decreased, but no improvement was observed (max total/direct bilirubin: 19.8/15.8 mg/dL). Cholecystitis was detected via an abdominal echography. Following percutaneous transhepatic gallbladder drainage performed on day 11, the bilirubin level declined. Subsequently, on day 15, the patient's general condition stabilized, and he was extubated. However, CHDF was switched to hemodialysis (HD) as the patient's anuric state due to AKI persisted. After 16 days, the patient was discharged from the ICU.

An arteriovenous fistula was created as a continuation of maintenance HD was necessary. Although, in the ICU, the patient had been on initiated enteral nutrition (EN), he was unable to tolerate EN due to intestinal dysfunction advancement. Therefore, he was initiated on total parenteral nutrition. Long-term rehabilitation intervention was also required due to ICU-acquired weakness (ICU-AW), because of long-term sedation and muscle relaxation during extracorporeal support. After 70 days, dialysis was discontinued; the patient was able to eat independently at approximately 90 days. He was transferred to a recovery hospital on day 108 and underwent complete social reintroduction at 5 months after discharge from our hospital.

3. Discussion

In the present case report, we treated a 57-year-old man with severe *Legionella* pneumonia using VA-ECMO. Interestingly, through this case we could properly judge VA-ECMO adaptation by evaluating appropriate shock.

Septic cardiomyopathy (or sepsis-induced cardiomyopathy) has been recognized in sepsis treatment since first reported by Parker in 1984 [1]. In a study by Sato et al. [4], the following characteristics were stated as clinical features: left ventricular dilatation, depressed left ventricular ejection fraction, and recovery within 7-10 days. The causes of septic cardiomyopathy are chemical mediators, specifically endotoxin, cytokines, and nitric oxides, as well as induced mitochondrial dysfunction and downregulation

of β-adrenergic receptors. In the present case, although LVEF declined from the time of the hospitalization, left ventricular expansion was not initially considered; treatment was initiated based on the opinion that vasoplegic shock and intravascular depletion were the main cause. However, on day 4, LVDd/Ds showed clear left ventricular expansion at 61/55 mm, and the patient was diagnosed with severe septic cardiomyopathy.

We needed to determine the possibility of acute myocarditis. There was no elevation in myocardial enzyme levels (troponin I 0.228 ng/ml on day 3 and CK-MB 12 IU/L on day 4), and myocardial edema and pericardial effusion were not observed on echocardiogram even when left ventricular dysfunction occurred. Therefore, acute myocarditis was judged to be negative.

During treatment, Gattinoni et al. reported that using dobutamine and dopamine as support for the cardiac index failed to reduce morbidity and mortality among critically ill patients [5]. Morelli et al. suggested that β-blockade could be associated with a reduction in the heart rate without adverse effects and that this could help improve survival [6]. The effectiveness of β-blokers for sepsis is still under discussion, but in this case the use of landiolol for heart rate control from the time of hospitalization may have been a little effective. However, dobutamine administered for cardiac dysfunction with uncontrollable tachycardia may have been an exacerbating factor.

There are several case reports on the successful use of VA-ECMO as rescue therapy for unresponsive patients with severe cardiogenic shock with septic cardiomyopathy. Septic shock is typically warm shock due to peripheral vasodilation and peripheral vascular hyperpermeability. However, among shocks associated with sepsis, diagnosis of the involvement of cardiogenic shock (= septic cardiomyopathy) in addition to septic shock is key to judging the introduction of VA-ECMO. Sato et al. reported that mechanical support with ECMO might be a therapeutic option; however, further studies are required to confirm whether it is truly effective in septic cardiomyopathy [4].

The timing of VA-ECMO introduction is also controversial. ECMO is considered an invasive and excessive introduction that may worsen prognosis due to complications. In this case, we decided to introduce VA-ECMO because it was judged that there was a high possibility of falling into CPA by prolongation of shock, based on the progression of both respiratory and metabolic acidosis. Securing an artery/vein for VA-ECMO is necessary; however, doing this following cardiopulmonary arrest (CPA) will lead to a puncture without pulsation, thus increasing the frequency of punctures and complications associated with it. Therefore, it is important to secure an artery/vein sheath prior to the introduction of VA-ECMO and introduce it in the state of shock before CPA.

In conclusion, we treated a patient with severe *Legionella* pneumonia using VA-ECMO. We wish to highlight the importance of timely and appropriate introduction of VA-ECMO, with the recognition of the involvement of septic cardiomyopathy by evaluating cardiac function in septic shock.

Abbreviations

AT III:	Antithrombin III
BP:	Blood pressure
BT:	Body temperature
CHDF:	Continuous hemodiafiltration
CPK:	Creatine kinase
CRP:	C-reactive protein
DOB:	Dobutamine
hANP:	Human atrial natriuretic peptide
HD:	Hemodialysis
HR:	Heart rate
LVEF:	Left ventricular ejection fraction
NAD:	Noradrenalin
PMX:	Polymyxin-B-immobilized fiber
PTGBD:	Percutaneous transhepatic gallbladder drainage
rTM:	Recombinant human soluble thrombomodulin
SOFA:	Sepsis-related organ failure assessment
T. bil:	Total bilirubin
VA-ECMO:	Veno-arterial extracorporeal membrane oxygenation
PCWP:	Pulmonary capillary wedge pressure
CI:	Cardiac index.

Acknowledgments

We would like to thank Editage (https://www.editage.jp) for English language editing. No funds were received in support of this work.

References

[1] H. Von Baum, S. Ewig, R. Marre et al., "Community-acquired Legionella pneumonia: new insights from the German competence network for community acquired pneumonia," *Clinical Infectious Diseases*, vol. 46, no. 9, pp. 1356–1364, 2008.

[2] M. M. Parker, J. H. Shelhamer, S. L. Bacharach et al., "Profound but reversible myocardial depression in patients with septic shock," *Annals of Internal Medicine*, vol. 100, no. 4, pp. 483–490, 1984.

[3] N. Bréchot, C.-E. Luyt, M. Schmidt et al., "Venoarterial extracorporeal membrane oxygenation support for refractory cardiovascular dysfunction during severe bacterial septic shoc," *Critical Care Medicine*, vol. 41, no. 7, pp. 1616–1626, 2013.

[4] R. Sato and M. Nasu, "A review of sepsis-induced cardiomyopathy," *Journal of Intensive Care*, vol. 3, article 48, 2015.

[5] L. Gattinoni, L. Brazzi, P. Pelosi et al., "A trial of goal-oriented hemodynamic therapy in critically ill patients. SvO2 Collaborative Group," *The New England Journal of Medicine*, vol. 333, no. 16, pp. 1025–1032, 1995.

[6] A. Morelli, C. Ertmer, M. Westphal et al., "Effect of heart rate control with esmolol on hemodynamic and clinical outcomes in patients with septic shock: a randomized clinical trial," *The Journal of the American Medical Association*, vol. 310, no. 16, pp. 1683–1691, 2013.

48

Significant Bradycardia in Critically Ill Patients Receiving Dexmedetomidine and Fentanyl

Channing Hui,[1] Maria Cardinale,[2] and Balaji Yegneswaran[3]

[1]*Rutgers-Robert Wood Johnson Medical School, Department of Emergency Medicine, One Robert Wood Johnson Place, MEB 389, New Brunswick, NJ 08901, USA*
[2]*Ernest Mario School of Pharmacy, Rutgers University, 160 Frelinghuysen Rd., Piscataway Township, NJ 08854, USA*
[3]*Saint Peter's University Hospital, 254 Easton Ave., New Brunswick, NJ 08901, USA*

Correspondence should be addressed to Channing Hui; huich@rwjms.rutgers.edu

Academic Editor: Ricardo Oliveira

Purpose. To report a case series of three patients who developed significant bradycardia while receiving the combination of dexmedetomidine and fentanyl for sedation and analgesia. *Materials and Methods.* This is a case series of patients obtained from a mixed medical, surgical, and cardiac ICU in a community teaching hospital. Three intubated patients receiving fentanyl and dexmedetomidine infusion developed sudden bradycardia requiring intervention. In all three cases, adjustments to therapy were required. *Results.* All three patients experienced significant bradycardia, with a heart rate less than 50 bpm, and one patient briefly developed asystole. In Case 1, the fentanyl infusion rate was reduced by 67% and the dexmedetomidine infusion rate was reduced by 25%. In Case 2, the sedation was changed to midazolam, and in Case 3, both fentanyl and dexmedetomidine were discontinued. In all three cases, there were no further incidences of significant bradycardia following intervention. *Conclusions.* Fentanyl used in combination with dexmedetomidine can result in clinically significant bradycardia. Further study is warranted to identify risk factors and elucidate the mechanisms that result in life-threatening bradycardia.

1. Introduction

The current pain, agitation, and delirium guidelines encourage the use of fentanyl with sedation strategies using nonbenzodiazepine sedatives [1]. Dexmedetomidine is an effective sedative that is often used in conjunction with opioids such as fentanyl in the critical care and anesthesia setting. Bradycardia and hypotension are well-known associations with dexmedetomidine, yet no human studies have examined the occurrence of drug-induced bradycardia secondary to the combination of dexmedetomidine and fentanyl. One study demonstrated attenuation of the tachycardia response to flexible bronchoscopy with the combination of dexmedetomidine-fentanyl compared to propofol-fentanyl [2]. Here we report three cases in which a synergistic interaction between fentanyl and dexmedetomidine may have contributed to clinically relevant bradycardia.

2. Case Series

2.1. Case 1. Patient was a 59-year-old male with a past medical history of cirrhosis, ulcerative colitis, esophageal varices with previous banding, hypertension, and hyperlipidemia. He had advanced alcoholic cirrhosis, with a Model for End-Stage Liver Disease (MELD) score of 17, and was admitted with a large right pleural effusion secondary to ascites. His initial pharmacologic management included furosemide, spironolactone, albumin, midodrine, pantoprazole, lactulose, rifaximin, and antibiotics for a possible pneumonia. During his admission, he received nadolol for portal hypertension, with his heart rate averaging between 55 and 85 bpm, but this was discontinued on hospital day four.

Despite multiple thoracenteses, he ultimately required intubation on hospital day six secondary to worsening respiratory failure. His weight and select values at this time are

TABLE 1: Select demographic data and labs at time of bradycardia.

	Case 1	Case 2	Case 3
Weight (kg)	77	86.8	93.4
Body mass index (BMI)	29.3	25.1	29.9
Serum creatinine (mg/dL)	1.10	1.78	0.61
Serum CO_2 (mEq/L)	28	20	27
Blood urea nitrogen (mg/dL)	28	41	24
Albumin (g/dL)	1.9	2.6	4.1
Protein (g/dL)	5.4	5.3	4.6
ALT (units/L)	7	4	48
AST (units/L)	29	37	46
Alkaline phosphatase (units/L)	60	164	74
INR	2.12	1.14	1.03
aPTT (seconds)	37.3	24.1	30.6

ALT: alanine aminotransferase; AST: aspartate aminotransferase; INR: international normalized ratio; aPTT: activated partial thromboplastin time.

provided in Table 1. He was initially sedated with propofol alone, which was changed to dexmedetomidine after a few hours due to persistent agitation. Dexmedetomidine was titrated to a Richmond Agitation Sedation Scale (RASS) score of −2. During this time, his heart rate remained between 50 and 65 bpm. Approximately 30 hours later, while receiving dexmedetomidine 0.4 mcg/kg/hour, fentanyl was added at 25 mcg/hour for an elevated pain assessment score. As fentanyl was titrated up to 150 mcg/hour, his heart rate decreased into the range of 40 to 47 bpm. Once the fentanyl rate was decreased to 75 mcg/hour, the heart rate began to increase to 50 bpm. As both infusion rates were decreased, the heart rate steadily improved further. Ultimately, the patient was maintained on dexmedetomidine 0.3–0.6 mcg/kg/hour and fentanyl 50–100 mcg/hour, and his heart rate remained between 55 and 70 bpm. His blood pressure remained stable throughout the entire duration of mechanical ventilation. The patient remained intubated until hospital day 11, when he again became agitated, requiring dexmedetomidine to be increased from 0.5 mcg/kg/hour to 0.6 mcg/kg/hour and fentanyl to be increased to 100 mcg/hour to 200 mcg/hour. Within two hours, his heart rate decreased from 60 bpm to 48 bpm. His heart rate remained between 45 and 48 bpm until he was transferred later that afternoon to a liver transplant center. The patient had no other medications or precipitating factors that would be expected to contribute to bradycardia.

2.2. Case 2. Patient was a 75-year-old male with a history of metastatic breast cancer, cholangiocarcinoma, atrial fibrillation, and hyperthyroidism who was initially admitted to the hospital with abdominal pain and found to have a yeast infection in his peritoneal fluid. After seven days in the hospital, he was transferred to the ICU for septic shock due to *E. coli* bacteremia. Despite vasopressor therapy, the patient remained in a persistent shock state and subsequently developed multiorgan failure. Upon ICU admission, the patient was intubated for respiratory failure and initially received propofol and fentanyl for sedation and analgesia but

was switched to dexmedetomidine alone due to hypotension. Throughout his ICU course, he required continuous renal replacement therapy and total parenteral nutrition. An echocardiogram from two months prior demonstrated an ejection fraction of 50% and normal diastolic function. Dexmedetomidine was titrated up to 0.7 mcg/kg/hour to achieve a goal RASS of −2 with no hemodynamic complications.

After two days of dexmedetomidine therapy, an intravenous bolus dose of fentanyl 50 mcg was given for acute pain, followed by an intravenous bolus dose of metoclopramide 5 mg given 30 minutes later. Within one hour, the patient's heart rate rapidly decreased, leading to a six-second asystolic pause. The pulse spontaneously returned, but the heart rate remained between 30 and 35 bpm for 15 minutes. Dexmedetomidine infusion was immediately discontinued, and the heart rate ultimately improved to normal without intervention. The patient was switched to midazolam infusion, and there were no further episodes. During the time of the asystole, the patient was also receiving rifaximin for a resolving hyperammonemia, famotidine, heparin, cefazolin, insulin, methimazole, metoclopramide, and norepinephrine. Select labs at this time are provided in Table 1. The patient ultimately expired on hospital day 21 due to cardiac arrest following a prolonged course.

2.3. Case 3. A 73-year-old male admitted with myasthenia gravis, benign prostate hypertrophy, and hyperlipidemia was admitted with myasthenia gravis crisis. He was initially treated with intravenous immunoglobulin but required intubation on day 2 for airway management and was later treated with plasmapheresis. During his intubation, he was initially sedated with continuous infusions of fentanyl and propofol. On day 4 of his hospital course, he was switched from propofol and fentanyl to dexmedetomidine monotherapy at doses between 0.1 and 0.4 mcg/kg/hr, and his heart rate ranged from 55 to 82 during this time. Due to agitation, he was then switched back to continuous infusions of fentanyl, and propofol was used for sedation and analgesia to maintain a RASS of −2. During this period, his fentanyl ranged from 50 to 150 mcg/hour, and his propofol ranged from 5 to 45 mcg/kg/min. His heart rate throughout this time ranged mainly between 55 and 110 bpm, with multiple excursions to 140 bpm due to severe agitation, for which he was started on quetiapine.

On day 9, dexmedetomidine was again added to his sedation regimen to facilitate extubation and titrated slowly to 0.4 mcg/kg/hour. On day 11 of his hospitalization, while receiving fentanyl 50 mcg/hour, dexmedetomidine 0.3 mcg/kg/hour, and propofol 20 mcg/kg/minute, his heart rate decreased to the mid-40s and ranged between 44 and 51 bpm. In response to the heart rate, fentanyl was discontinued, followed by dexmedetomidine, and finally propofol, all within two hours of each other. The heart rate began to increase back to normal within 30 minutes of discontinuing all three infusions. No other sedative agent was added after this, and the patient was successfully extubated the next day with no further hemodynamic complications and was discharged to a rehabilitation center after a prolonged hospital course. During the bradycardia episode, the patient was receiving methylprednisolone, quetiapine (started four days earlier for agitation), heparin, famotidine, and ceftriaxone and was on his fifth day of plasmapheresis therapy. He did not receive pyridostigmine until the last day of his hospitalization and had no other precipitating factors for bradycardia.

3. Discussion

Dexmedetomidine is an α_2 adrenergic receptor agonist, with studies demonstrating a high ratio of α_2/α_1-activity (1620 : 1) [3]. It is selective for G protein-binding adrenergic receptors, including α_{2A}-, α_{2B}-, and α_{2C}- adrenoceptor subtypes. α_{2A}-Adrenergic receptor agonism provides sedative and antinociceptive properties, while α_{2B}-adrenergic receptor has vasoconstrictive properties. α_{2C}-Adrenoceptor agonism has a variety of effects such as regulating dopaminergic and behavioral responses [4]. The presence of α_2 adrenergic receptors in the presynaptic and postsynaptic terminals contributes to its sedative and analgesic properties. The activation of the presynaptic terminal leads to decreased transmission of pain signals, and activation of the postsynaptic terminal inhibits the sympathetic nervous system, elucidating its hypotensive and bradycardic effects [5]. The activation of α adrenergic receptors causes hyperpolarization of membranes from potassium channel activation, which decreases norepinephrine release. This is significant in the locus coeruleus, which provides adrenergic innervation to the brain and associated with brain functions such as arousal and sleep [4].

Data regarding the association between dose of dexmedetomidine and the incidence of bradycardia seem inconclusive. One retrospective study that compared low- and high-dose dexmedetomidine in ICU patients showed no significant difference in the incidence of hypotension and bradycardia [6]. Another study that measured plasma concentrations of dexmedetomidine demonstrated an indirect relationship between concentration and heart rate [7]. Lastly, a retrospective cohort study identified risk factors such as advanced age and low baseline arterial blood pressure to be associated with hemodynamic instability with dexmedetomidine but did not identify doses greater than 0.7 mcg/kg/hour to be an independent risk factor [8]. Interestingly, cardiac or sedative medications given concurrently with dexmedetomidine were also not associated with higher rates of instability [8].

Fentanyl exerts its effects by binding to opioid receptors in the brain and spinal cord [9]. Fentanyl is known for its relatively favorable hemodynamic profile, especially in the critically ill when cardiovascular depression is undesired [10]. Although uncommon, fentanyl-induced bradycardia is a known adverse effect, yet the exact mechanism is unknown. A proposed mechanism involves the indirect increase of parasympathetic activity in the cardiac vagal neurons in the nucleus ambiguus. The stimulation of μ-opioid receptors in rats by endomorphin-1 postsynaptically via the G protein pathway inhibits calcium currents, leading to increased vagal stimulation to the heart [11]. In addition, fentanyl specifically has been suggested to have an inhibitory role in GABAergic

neurotransmission in cardiac vagal neurons, thus increasing parasympathetic activity with induced bradycardia [12].

This case series highlights three critically ill patients who developed significant bradycardia while receiving the combination of dexmedetomidine and fentanyl for sedation and analgesia. According to the Drug Interaction Probability Scale (DIPS), all three cases can be classified as probable drug interactions [13]. Although these drugs individually exert their effects via different pathways, little is known regarding a synergistic or additive effect on heart rate reduction. In 1994, Salmenperä and colleagues postulated that fentanyl may augment the bradycardic effects of dexmedetomidine in a dog model [14]. A shared pathway of μ-opioid and α_2 adrenergic receptors is the stimulation of the guanine nucleotide regulatory protein, leading to the decreased levels of adenylate cyclase. The downstream effects include hyperpolarization of the membranes secondary to the efflux of potassium ions [14, 15]. This may explain the additive or synergistic effects of bradycardia.

To our knowledge, this is the first such case series reporting clinically significant bradycardia among humans that appeared to be worsened when fentanyl and dexmedetomidine were given concomitantly. This finding is contradictory to previous reports that concomitant use of sedatives with dexmedetomidine does not increase the risk of hemodynamic instability [8]. Our findings warrant several considerations for the ICU clinician. First, as dexmedetomidine use in critically ill patients continues to expand, clinicians should be aware that significant bradycardia can develop when dexmedetomidine is used in combination with fentanyl, a commonly used analgesic in the ICU. This effect may be exaggerated in patients with liver dysfunction, as both medications are metabolized primarily via the liver. This effect may also be more pronounced in patients receiving prolonged infusions of dexmedetomidine. Although the Food and Drug Administration suggests that continuous infusions of dexmedetomidine should not exceed 24 hours [16], current practice often requires extension of the infusion duration beyond this recommendation. Indeed, for all three cases reported here, significant bradycardia or asystole occurred after dexmedetomidine was used for greater than 24 hours. Lastly, patients receiving fentanyl and dexmedetomidine may also be at an increased risk if they receive other agents that can cause bradycardia, including propofol and metoclopramide, both of which are frequently used in the ICU. Further research is warranted to identify risk factors and elucidate the mechanisms that result in life-threatening bradycardia.

References

[1] J. Barr, G. L. Fraser, K. Puntillo et al., "Clinical practice guidelines for the management of pain, agitation, and delirium in adult patients in the intensive care unit," Critical Care Medicine, vol. 41, no. 1, pp. 263–306, 2013.

[2] F. Yuan, H. Fu, P. Yang et al., "Dexmedetomidine-fentanyl versus propofol-fentanyl in flexible bronchoscopy: a randomized study," Experimental and Therapeutic Medicine, vol. 12, no. 1, pp. 506–512, 2016.

[3] R. Virtanen, J.-M. Savola, V. Saano, and L. Nyman, "Characterization of the selectivity, specificity and potency of medetomidine as an α2-adrenoceptor agonist," *European Journal of Pharmacology*, vol. 150, no. 1-2, pp. 9–14, 1988.

[4] S. M. Hoy and G. M. Keating, "Dexmedetomidine: A review of its use for sedation in mechanically ventilated patients in an intensive care setting and for procedural sedation," *Drugs*, vol. 71, no. 11, pp. 1481–1501, 2011.

[5] R. Gertler, HC. Brown, DH. Mitchell, and EN. Silvius, *Dexmedetomidine, a novel sedative-analgesic agent. Proc (Bayl Univ Med Cent)*, vol. 14, 14, 13–21, 2001.

[6] G. M. Jones, C. V. Murphy, A. T. Gerlach, E. M. Goodman, and L. J. Pell, "High-Dose Dexmedetomidine for Sedation in the Intensive Care Unit: An Evaluation of Clinical Efficacy and Safety," *Annals of Pharmacotherapy*, vol. 45, no. 6, pp. 740–747, 2011.

[7] T. J. Ebert, J. E. Hall, J. A. Barney, T. D. Uhrich, and M. D. Colinco, "The effects of increasing plasma concentrations of dexmedetomidine in humans," *Anesthesiology*, vol. 93, no. 2, pp. 382–394, 2000.

[8] C. J. Ice, H. A. Personett, E. N. Frazee, R. A. Dierkhising, R. Kashyap, and R. A. Oeckler, "Risk factors for dexmedetomidine-associated hemodynamic instability in noncardiac intensive care unit patients," *Anesthesia and Analgesia*, vol. 122, no. 2, pp. 462–469, 2016.

[9] P. W. H. Peng and A. N. Sandler, "A review of the use of fentanyl analgesia in the management of acute pain in adults," *Anesthesiology*, vol. 90, no. 2, pp. 576–599, 1999.

[10] P. S. Sebel, J. G. Bovill, R. A. A. Boekhorst, and N. Rog, "Cardiovascular effects of high-dose fentanyl anaesthesia," *Acta Anaesthesiologica Scandinavica*, vol. 26, no. 4, pp. 308–315, 1982.

[11] M. Irnaten, S. A. Aicher, J. Wang et al., "μ-opioid receptors are located postsynaptically and endomorphin-1 inhibits voltage-gated calcium currents in premotor cardiac parasympathetic neurons in the rat nucleus ambiguus," *Neuroscience*, vol. 116, no. 2, pp. 573–582, 2003.

[12] K. J. S. Griffioen, P. Venkatesan, Z.-G. Huang et al., "Fentanyl inhibits GABAergic neurotransmission to cardiac vagal neurons in the nucleus ambiguus," *Brain Research*, vol. 1007, no. 1-2, pp. 109–115, 2004.

[13] J. R. Horn, P. D. Hansten, and L. N. Chan, "Proposal for a new tool to evaluate drug interaction cases," *Annals of Pharmacotherapy*, vol. 41, no. 4, pp. 674–680, 2007.

[14] M. T. Salmenperä, F. Sziam, and C. C. Hug Jr., "Anesthetic and hemodynamic interactions of dexmedetomidine and fentanyl in dogs," *Anesthesiology*, vol. 80, no. 4, pp. 837–846, 1994.

[15] S. M. Crain, B. Crain, and M. H. Makman, "Pertussis toxin blocks depressant effects of opioid, monoaminergic and muscarinic agonists on dorsal-horn network responses in spinal cord-ganglion cultures," *Brain Research*, vol. 400, no. 1, pp. 185–190, 1987.

[16] Precedex, *Precedex™ [package insert]*, Hospira, Lake Forest, Ill, USA, 2016.

49

Adrenergic Inhibition with Dexmedetomidine to Treat Stress Cardiomyopathy during Alcohol Withdrawal

Zachary M. Harris,[1] Alvaro Alonso,[2] and Thomas P. Kennedy[3]

[1]*Tulane University Health Sciences Center, Department of Internal Medicine, New Orleans, LA 70112, USA*
[2]*Heart & Vascular Institute, Tulane University School of Medicine, New Orleans, LA 70112, USA*
[3]*Tulane University Health Sciences Center, Department of Medicine, Section of Pulmonary Diseases, Critical Care Medicine, and Environmental Medicine, New Orleans, LA 70112, USA*

Correspondence should be addressed to Zachary M. Harris; zharris@tulane.edu

Academic Editor: Chiara Lazzeri

Stress (Takotsubo) cardiomyopathy is a form of reversible left ventricular dysfunction with a heightened risk of ventricular arrhythmia thought to be caused by high circulating catecholamines. We report a case of stress cardiomyopathy that developed during severe alcohol withdrawal successfully treated with dexmedetomidine. The case involves a 53-year-old man with a significant history of alcohol abuse who presented to a teaching hospital with new-onset seizures. His symptoms of acute alcohol withdrawal were initially treated with benzodiazepines, but the patient later developed hypotension, and stress cardiomyopathy was suspected based on ECG and echocardiographic findings. Adjunctive treatment with the alpha-2-adrenergic agonist, dexmedetomidine, was initiated to curtail excessive sympathetic outflow of the withdrawal syndrome, thereby targeting the presumed pathophysiology of the cardiomyopathy. Significant clinical improvement was observed within one day of initiation of dexmedetomidine. These findings are consistent with other reports suggesting that sympathetic dysregulation during alcohol withdrawal produces ideal pathobiology for stress cardiomyopathy and leads to ventricular arrhythmogenicity. Stress cardiomyopathy should be recognized as a complication of alcohol withdrawal that significantly increases cardiac-related mortality. By helping to correct autonomic dysregulation of the withdrawal syndrome, dexmedetomidine may be useful in the treatment of stress-induced cardiomyopathy.

1. Background

In the United States, approximately 1.2 million patients are hospitalized annually for manifestations of alcohol abuse [1]. Of these patients, approximately 5%, or 60,000 patients, will develop delirium tremens. In the past, mortality for delirium tremens was as high as 20% [2]. Although current appropriate treatment may reduce mortality to a value as low as 1% [1], recent reports have quoted a mortality of 5–15%, or 3,000–9,000 deaths annually, from this condition [3].

During alcohol withdrawal, atrial and ventricular arrhythmia are common, reflecting the combined influence of direct alcoholic cardiac toxicity and the extreme elevations in circulating catecholamines [1]. In one study, 28% of rats undergoing an alcohol withdrawal protocol experienced spontaneous ventricular arrhythmia and related death [4]. Furthermore, 77% of animals undergoing withdrawal developed ventricular arrhythmia when exposed to exogenous epinephrine, and 31% of these animals died. Despite evidence of significant arrhythmogenicity during withdrawal in animal studies, our understanding of cardiac rhythm disturbance in patients actively withdrawing from alcohol remains limited.

Stress-induced (Takotsubo) cardiomyopathy, also known as transient apical ballooning or "broken heart" syndrome, is an increasingly recognized form of transient left ventricular dysfunction associated with emotional or physical stress. The syndrome was first recognized in a review of five cases and named Takotsubo because the left ventricle at end-systole assumes the shape of the octopus pots of Japanese fishermen in the Hiroshima fish markets, with a round bottom and narrow neck [5]. The syndrome predominantly affects postmenopausal woman (90% of cases) [6] with estimated prevalence of 0.7–2.5% [7]. Emerging evidence supports that adverse myocardial effects of high circulating catecholamines underlie the pathophysiology of stress cardiomyopathy [8]. Because symptoms are similar to those of acute myocardial infarction (e.g., sudden onset of chest pain, moderate increase in troponin levels, and electrocardiographic changes suggestive of ischemia), confirmed absence of coronary artery disease is necessary to establish the diagnosis. In contradistinction to acute plaque rupture, echocardiographic wall motion abnormalities in stress cardiomyopathy typically extend beyond the vascular distribution of a single epicardial artery [9].

Despite an excellent long-term prognosis of afflicted patients, stress cardiomyopathy carries a significant mortality rate in the acute setting (i.e., in-hospital mortality rate of 2%) [10]. Importantly, patients with stress cardiomyopathy have an increased rate of ventricular arrhythmia [11]. We report a case of stress cardiomyopathy occurring during severe alcohol withdrawal that was successfully treated with adjunctive dexmedetomidine and review the literature of stress cardiomyopathy associated with alcohol withdrawal.

2. Case Presentation

A 53-year-old African American man was brought in by his wife with new-onset seizures. The patient was unable to provide an accurate history due to altered mental status. Per the patient's wife, the patient had stopped drinking alcohol 24–48 hours prior to admission due to financial constraints, after consuming two pints of whiskey per day for the previous 10 years. The seizures began the evening prior to admission and continued throughout the night. These episodes lasted 1-2 seconds, were tonic-clonic in nature, and were associated with urinary incontinence and foaming at the mouth. His past medical history was significant only for hypertension. He had smoked one pack of cigarettes per day for the past 48 years. Upon arrival, his temperature was 37.1 degrees Celsius, pulse was 94 beats per minute, and blood pressure was 160/98 mmHg. Cardiovascular exam revealed a regular rate and rhythm with normal S1 and S2, abdominal exam disclosed hepatosplenomegaly, and neurologic exam was significant for tremulousness. The patient was disoriented on mental status exam. Mean corpuscular volume was 92.3 fL, platelet count was 58×10^3 per μL, AST was 199 units/L, and ALT was 89 units/L. An ECG done upon arrival revealed a normal sinus rhythm and QTc interval of 546 ms.

Given the recent onset of seizure-like episodes, history of abrupt discontinuation of chronic alcohol use, exam findings, and lab values consistent with ethanol abuse, a diagnosis of acute alcohol withdrawal was suspected. The patient was admitted to the medical intensive care unit. Treatment was initiated with diazepam 5 mg IV every 8 hours and lorazepam 2 mg IV every 1 hour as needed for agitation and anxiety. The

patient was also given 100 mg of thiamine, 1 mg of folic acid, and 2 gm of magnesium sulfate IV every 24 hours.

During the 1st hospital day, the patient exhibited witnessed tonic-clonic seizure activity, as well as significant anxiety and agitation. During the 2nd and 3rd hospital day, the patient's mental status fluctuated significantly. Intermittently, the patient was severely agitated, attempting to dislodge his indwelling urinary catheter and requiring 4-point soft restraints. Throughout this period, temperature peaked at 37.4 degrees Celsius, pulse ranged from 71 to 99 beats/minute, and blood pressure ranged from 118 to 154/88–103 mmHg. Diazepam was changed to 7.5 mg PO every 6 hours; however the patient still required lorazepam 2 mg IV every 4 hours for anxiety and agitation.

On the 4th hospital day, the patient developed hypotension. Blood pressure was 90–100/70–80 mmHg, and pulse was 82–99 beats/minute. The patient was significantly altered and was therefore unable to report subjective symptoms. ECG disclosed symmetric deep coving T waves in leads II, III, aVF, and V2–V6, as well as a prolonged QTc interval of 645 ms. Serum troponin I was elevated at 1.25 ng/mL. Repeat ECGs continued to show symmetric T wave inversions in the inferior limb and lateral chest leads. Serial troponin levels, however, trended downward. An urgent transthoracic echocardiogram revealed multiple left ventricular regional wall motion abnormalities, notably akinesis of the mid-distal anteroseptal, mid-distal anterolateral, mid-distal inferoseptal, mid-distal inferolateral, and apical segments (Figure 1). Of note, right ventricular systolic function was normal, and there was no mitral regurgitation. The left ventricular ejection fraction was estimated to be 40–45%. The clinical instability of the patient precluded emergent coronary angiography. Given the widespread repolarization abnormalities by ECG, diffuse wall motion abnormalities involving myocardial segments circumferentially throughout the entire cardiac apex, presence of an identifiable stressor, and downward trend of cardiac troponins, the diagnosis of stress cardiomyopathy was suspected. The patient continued to require additional doses of lorazepam 2 mg every 2 hours due to agitation and anxiety. On the 5th hospital day, adjunctive treatment with the alpha-2-adrenoreceptor agonist dexmedetomidine was initiated to reduce central sympathetic outflow, directly targeting the presumed pathobiology of the stress cardiomyopathy. A loading dose of 1 μg/kg IV was given over 10 minutes, followed by a maintenance infusion of 0.2 μg/kg/hr titrated by 0.1 μg/kg/hr every 15 minutes to maintain a Richmond Agitation-Sedation Scale of −1. The mean infusion rate was 0.31 μg/kg/hr, administered over a period of 23.93 hours (Figure 2).

On the 6th hospital day, the patient showed marked clinical improvement. Per the patient's family, mental status was at baseline. The patient denied shortness of breath or chest pain. Cardiovascular and pulmonary examinations were unchanged, and neurologic examination revealed no agitation, anxiety, or tremulousness. The patient was awake, alert, and oriented to person, place, and time. Dexmedetomidine therapy was weaned by 0.1 μg/kg/hr every 15 minutes. The patient was treated thereafter with tapering doses of diazepam PO, and no additional doses of lorazepam were

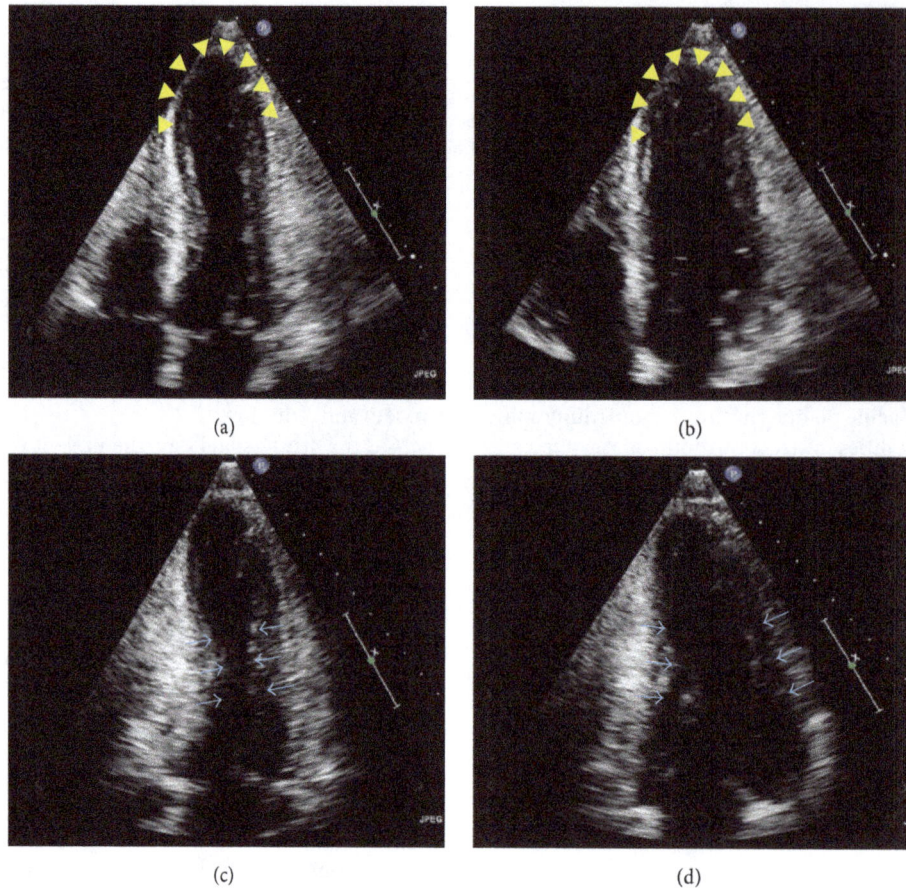

FIGURE 1: Initial transthoracic echocardiogram in the acute setting revealing features suggestive of stress cardiomyopathy. Systolic (a) and diastolic (b) apical 4-chamber views reveal akinetic apical and mid-anteroseptal segments (arrowheads) with hyperdynamic middle segments. Systolic (c) and diastolic (d) apical 2-chamber views disclose normal wall motion of the mid-cavity (arrows). The circumferential pattern of left ventricular myocardial dysfunction characterized by symmetric wall motion abnormalities involving the septal, anterior, and lateral walls is highly suggestive of stress cardiomyopathy.

required. A coronary angiogram was offered to the patient to rule out coronary artery obstruction; however the patient refused the procedure. One month after hospitalization, repeat ECG revealed improvement of the T wave inversions when compared to the ECGs during the event. The QTc was shortened to 495 ms. Coronary CT angiography was performed, which revealed absence of coronary artery disease. Repeat ECG two months later revealed a normal sinus rhythm with no significant T wave inversions. Subsequent echocardiography performed 14 months after the event revealed resolution of the acute regional wall abnormalities and confirmed a full recovery of ventricular systolic function, further supporting the diagnosis of stress cardiomyopathy (Figure 3).

3. Discussion

This case report describes a patient who developed stress cardiomyopathy during severe alcohol withdrawal. For this patient, we reasoned that high sympathetic outflow from the withdrawal syndrome caused stress cardiomyopathy. Although we were unable to angiographically confirm absence of acute plaque rupture at the time of the event due to clinical instability, we believe that the diffuse circumferential pattern of ventricular wall motion abnormalities extending beyond a single epicardial vascular territory as revealed by transthoracic echocardiography and global ECG abnormalities not confined to a particular anatomic distribution strongly argue against myocardial ischemia as the cause of the patient's presentation. Moreover, the coronary CT angiogram excluding the presence of coronary artery disease and the resolution of ECG changes further support the diagnosis and fulfill the proposed Mayo Clinic criteria for stress-induced cardiomyopathy [21]. Although repeat echocardiography was not obtained until 14 months after the event, demonstration of full recovery of ventricular function and complete resolution of the acute wall motion abnormalities strongly support the diagnosis according to the recent diagnostic criteria proposed by the Heart Failure Association of the European

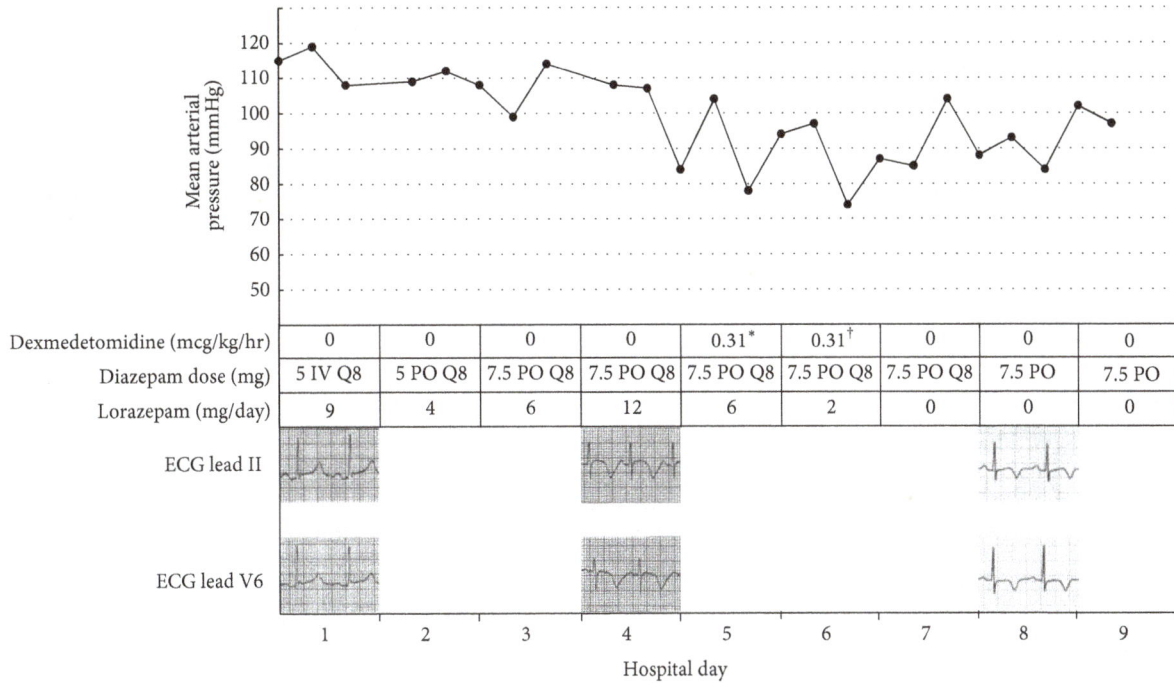

	1	2	3	4	5	6	7	8	9
Dexmedetomidine (mcg/kg/hr)	0	0	0	0	0.31*	0.31†	0	0	0
Diazepam dose (mg)	5 IV Q8	5 PO Q8	7.5 PO Q8	7.5 PO Q8	7.5 PO Q8	7.5 PO Q8	7.5 PO Q8	7.5 PO	7.5 PO
Lorazepam (mg/day)	9	4	6	12	6	2	0	0	0

FIGURE 2: Mean arterial pressure versus time; graph of mean arterial pressure readings against time with corresponding scheduled doses of diazepam, administration of lorazepam, infusion of dexmedetomidine, and ECG changes. *Infusion started at 11:15 AM. Does not include initial loading dose of 1 μg/kg over 10 minutes. †Infusion stopped at 11:11 AM.

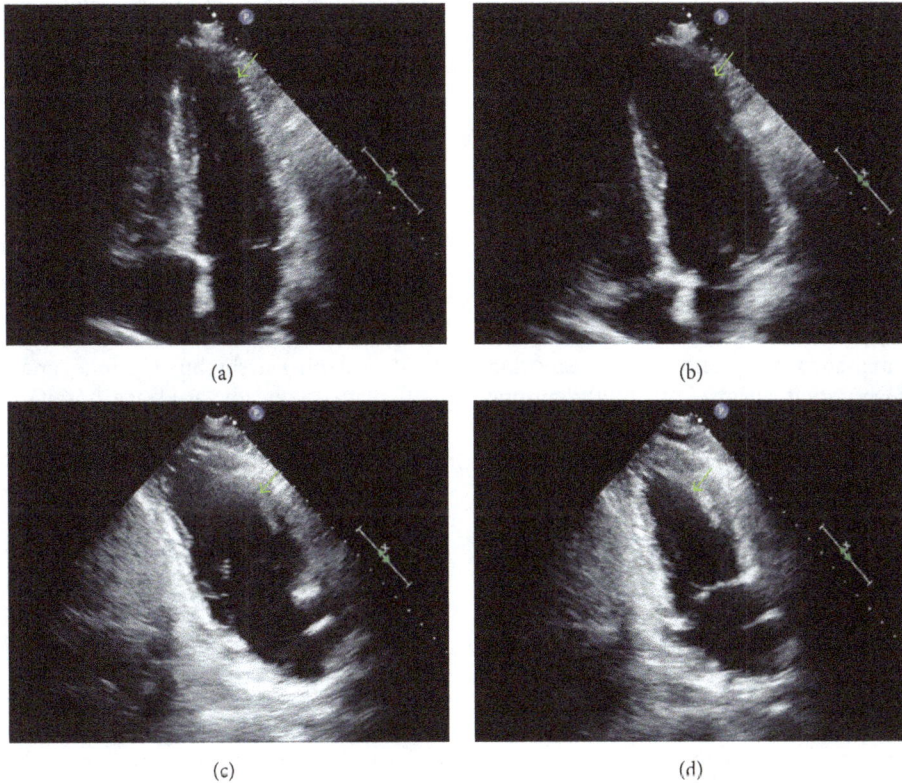

(a)

(b)

(c)

(d)

FIGURE 3: Repeat transthoracic echocardiogram confirming complete recovery of ventricular systolic function and resolution of the acute wall motion abnormalities, supporting the diagnosis of stress cardiomyopathy. Systolic (a) and diastolic (b) apical 4-chamber views and systolic (c) and diastolic (d) apical 2-chamber views reveal normal motion of the ventricular apex (arrows).

Society of Cardiology [22]. During the event, we targeted central alpha-2-adrenergic receptors with dexmedetomidine to curtail excessive catecholamine release, thereby disrupting the presumed pathophysiologic cause of the cardiomyopathy.

Increasing evidence suggests that catecholamine-mediated effects are responsible for the development of stress cardiomyopathy [8]. Exposure to endogenous (emotional, related to preexisting condition) or exogenous (trauma, surgical procedure, and exacerbation of preexisting condition) stress and increased sympathetic activity have been reported in most cases of stress cardiomyopathy. Reports have confirmed increased catecholamine levels in the serum of patients who developed stress cardiomyopathy [23, 24]. Stress cardiomyopathy is characterized by pathohistological changes similar to catecholamine cardiotoxic effects observed in animals and humans, including increased production of extracellular matrix proteins, contraction band necrosis (a unique form of myocyte injury highly specific for prolonged exposure to elevated levels of catecholamines), and mild neutrophil infiltration [25–27]. Furthermore, there is evidence that supraphysiologic catecholamine levels act through cardiomyocyte beta-adrenoreceptors to produce calcium-regulatory protein gene expression disturbances [28–31]. Calcium dysregulation has been demonstrated in stress cardiomyopathy, and increased densities of calcium-regulatory proteins, such as sarcolipin, have been found in cardiomyocytes of patients with stress cardiomyopathy [32]. The effects of catecholamine-induced calcium disturbances in the pathogenesis of stress cardiomyopathy are currently being explored.

Severe alcohol withdrawal is a hyperadrenergic state associated with elevated levels of circulating catecholamines and as such produces ideal pathobiology for the development of stress cardiomyopathy. The pathophysiology of acute alcohol withdrawal involves the compensatory neurobiological changes that occur in the setting of chronic alcohol ingestion [33]. Alcohol produces a generalized depressant effect on the central nervous system mainly through activation of the gamma aminobutyric acid (GABA) pathway. Acute ingestion of the drug boosts GABA activity, resulting in the anticonvulsant, sleep-inducing, antianxiety, and muscle relaxation effects of all GABA-boosting agents [34]. With chronic alcohol exposure, there is a compensatory upregulation of both $GABA_A$ receptors and excitatory glutamate N-methyl-D-aspartate (NMDA) receptor subunits. When alcohol is acutely withdrawn in the setting of long-term constant exposure (desistance), high NMDA and low GABA activity produce a state of central nervous system arousal. This molecular milieu is responsible for the initial clinical manifestations of acute alcohol withdrawal, including tremors, insomnia, vivid dreams, anorexia, anxiety, nausea and vomiting, paroxysmal sweating, weakness, and myalgia [1]. Notably, acute withdrawal produces unopposed catecholaminergic activation and decreased central inhibition that result in autonomic instability. Increased levels of urine, plasma, and cerebrospinal fluid norepinephrine and its metabolite, 3-methoxy-4-hydroxyphenylglycol (MHPG), are seen in alcoholics undergoing withdrawal [35–38]. Tachycardia, systolic hypertension, and a coarse tremor of the extended hands and tongue are common. Two–5% of patients in acute alcohol withdrawal will develop delirium tremens, a form of severe, late withdrawal lasting 5–7 days, which carries a high mortality rate [39]. During severe withdrawal and delirium tremens, elevated levels of circulating catecholamines are associated with increased cardiac output, stroke volume, and oxygen consumption [38, 40]. High circulating catecholamines and the resultant adverse effects on cardiomyocytes help explain the development of stress cardiomyopathy in patients undergoing severe withdrawal.

Although atrial and ventricular arrhythmia occur frequently during acute alcohol withdrawal, the pathophysiology of arrhythmogenesis during the withdrawal syndrome remains poorly understood [1, 4]. Stress cardiomyopathy may help explain increased arrhythmogenicity observed in alcohol withdrawal. Reports have demonstrated a significant (9%) incidence of ventricular arrhythmia during stress cardiomyopathy [11]. To the best of our knowledge, there have been at least nine published reports of stress cardiomyopathy occurring during acute alcohol withdrawal (Table 1) [12–20]. In our review of these cases, six out of the nine patients exhibited QT prolongation via ECG, and two of the patients developed ventricular arrhythmia (both degenerated to ventricular fibrillation). Two of the nine patients developed hypotension, which required vasopressor support. Confounding variables in these cases included recent usage of cocaine in one of the patients who developed ventricular fibrillation and major surgery requiring reintubation. Long-standing alcohol abuse by itself produces cardiotoxic effects and is a risk factor for sudden cardiac death [41]. Nonetheless, by increasing the likelihood of arrhythmia, stress cardiomyopathy may significantly contribute to mortality in acute alcohol withdrawal, especially in patients with a predisposition to cardiac arrhythmia from chronic alcohol abuse.

Emerging evidence supports that certain demographic and clinical features have significant prognostic implications on the clinical course of patients hospitalized for stress cardiomyopathy. According to one study, advanced age (≥75 years) appears to be an independent risk factor for major adverse events, including all-cause death, acute heart failure, life-threatening arrhythmia, stroke, and cardiogenic shock [42]. Patients of advanced age hospitalized for stress cardiomyopathy presented with significantly worse glomerular filtration rates, were more apt to receive inotropic agents during hospitalization, and did not recover cardiac systolic function at the time of discharge as efficiently when compared with younger patients.

Given its widespread availability and feasibility in the acute setting, echocardiography is frequently the first noninvasive imaging modality used to assess patients with stress cardiomyopathy [43]. In this case, transthoracic echocardiography played a central role in establishing the diagnosis of stress cardiomyopathy and furthermore provided important prognostic information in the acute setting. In contrast to acute myocardial infarction caused by occlusion of an epicardial artery, where wall motion abnormalities are typically limited to regions supplied by a single occluded vessel, the echocardiographic topography of left ventricular dysfunction in stress cardiomyopathy is characterized by

TABLE 1: Case reports of stress cardiomyopathy in patients with acute alcohol withdrawal. VTach, ventricular tachycardia; VFib, ventricular fibrillation; CXR, chest X-ray; CIWA, Clinical Institute Withdrawal Assessment of Alcohol scale.

Age/sex	Onset (from last drink)	Clinical features of withdrawal	Presenting features of stress cardiomyopathy	Notable case features	Reference
64/M	At least 5 days	Not described in case report	Decline in level of consciousness, sustained VTach with degeneration to VFib, cardiopulmonary arrest; subsequent ST segment elevation and later T wave inversion	QT prolongation on admission; patient required cardiopulmonary resuscitation	[12]
49/F	Not described in case report	Withdrawal seizure after episode of acute intoxication (time between events not described in case report)	Decreased level of consciousness, decreased O_2 saturation, rapid hypotension, infiltrate on CXR, ST elevation, and T wave inversion	—	[13]
25/F	Not described in case report	Seizure episode	Torsades de pointes with degeneration to VFib (in route to hospital), T wave inversion (3 hours after resuscitation) with QT prolongation	Cocaine use 3 days prior to seizure	[14]
61/M	36 hours	Not described in case report	Chest pain radiating to jaw, tachycardia, ST elevation, and T wave inversion	—	[15]
63/M	6-7 days	Grand mal seizure 3 days after alcohol cessation	Severe dyspnea, pulmonary edema, T wave inversion, QT prolongation	Resolution of stress cardiomyopathy confirmed at 10 weeks	[16]
56/M	5 days after hospitalization	Confusion, severe asthenia, anorexia, tremor	Tachycardia, decreased O_2 saturation, pulmonary edema, orthopnea, pathologic Q waves, elevated troponin I (1.08 ng/mL)	3 days after onset of stress cardiomyopathy, ECG showed diffuse T wave inversion and QT prolongation	[17]
57/F	<24 hours	2 episodes of seizures and confusion the morning after a night of binge drinking, fever, tachycardia, agitation, diaphoresis, tremulousness,	Hypotension, T wave inversion, QT prolongation, elevated troponin I (4.075 micrograms/L), subsequent elevated jugular venous pressure and peripheral edema	History of alcohol-related seizures; patient required vasopressor support; reversal of left ventricular wall motion abnormalities 12 days prior to admission	[18]
45/F	96–120 hours	Epigastric pain, nausea and vomiting 72 hours after discontinuation of alcohol, tremulousness, tachycardia, CIWA of 9	T wave inversion, troponin elevation (0.974 ng/mL)	—	[19]
57/F	>10 days	Intense agitation, tachycardia, tachypnea	Tachycardia, tachypnea, pulmonary edema, Q waves, ST elevation, T wave inversion, subsequent ECG revealed diffuse T wave inversion and QT prolongation	Patient admitted for elective thoracotomy; patient was reintubated after procedure due to hypoxemic respiratory failure; dexmedetomidine used in the treatment of withdrawal symptoms; patient later developed cardiogenic shock and required vasopressors and intra-aortic balloon pump	[20]

a diffuse, circumferential wall motion abnormality pattern typically involving myocardial segments spanning multiple vascular territories [43, 44]. Furthermore, there is evidence that regional wall motion abnormalities in stress cardiomyopathy tend to involve territories partially supplied by the right coronary artery to a significantly greater extent compared with anterior ST-elevation myocardial infarction [44]. Echocardiographic parameters used to quantify the anatomic extent of regional wall motion abnormalities, such as the left ventricular wall motion score index and the number of territories with regional wall motion abnormalities, are useful correlates with high sensitivities and specificities in the prediction of stress cardiomyopathy [44]. Immediate and accurate echocardiographic assessment of regional wall motion abnormalities is therefore crucially important in the differential diagnostic algorithm of patients presenting with clinical features suggestive of stress cardiomyopathy. In the presented case, transthoracic echocardiography revealed a distinctive pattern of contractility characterized by symmetrical regional wall motion abnormalities extending into the territory of multiple epicardial arteries and hypercontractility of the basal segments of the heart. This pattern was sufficiently characteristic to significantly raise the diagnostic pretest probability of stress cardiomyopathy, especially given the surrounding demographic and clinical context.

Moreover, a number of echocardiographic correlates provide prognostic information important in the clinical management of patients with stress cardiomyopathy [45]. In a recent multicenter prospective study, echocardiographic correlates including ventricular ejection fraction, wall motion score index, E/e' ratio, left ventricular outflow obstruction, pulmonary artery systolic pressure, right ventricular involvement, and reversible moderate-to-severe mitral regurgitation were associated with adverse hospitalization events (e.g., acute heart failure, cardiogenic shock, and in-hospital mortality) in patients diagnosed with stress cardiomyopathy [45]. At multivariate analysis, left ventricular ejection fraction (HR: 0.92; 95% CI: 0.89–0.95; $p < 0.001$), E/e' ratio (HR 1.13; 95% CI: 1.02–1.24; $p = 0.011$), and reversible moderate-to-severe mitral regurgitation (HR: 3.25; 95% CI 1.16–9.10; $p = 0.025$) were independent correlates of major adverse events. These features on initial echocardiogram in the acute setting should therefore raise clinician alertness to patients at risk of the development of major in-hospital adverse events, ultimately affecting clinical management of this high-risk patient subset. Right ventricular involvement is an echocardiographic correlate of stress cardiomyopathy syndrome severity that deserves special emphasis. In a study of 339 primarily female patients with stress cardiomyopathy, the presence of right ventricular involvement within 24 hours of symptom onset was an independent predictor of adverse events (HR: 2.327; 95% CI: 1.151–4.706; $p = 0.019$), albeit the prevalence of extensive right ventricular involvement was relatively low (<17%) [46]. In the presented case, the absence of specific features on the initial echocardiogram (e.g., left ventricular outflow obstruction, reversible moderate-to-severe mitral regurgitation, and right ventricular involvement) portended a favorable clinical prognosis.

Benzodiazepine therapy targeting $GABA_A$ receptors is the mainstay of treatment for acute alcohol withdrawal. This treatment strategy targets the imbalance between GABA neuroinhibitory activity and NMDA neuroexcitatory activity observed in alcohol withdrawal. In severe cases unmitigated by GABA-targeted agents, therapy directed toward dysautonomia may be beneficial [47]. Normally, central alpha-2-adrenoreceptors inhibit the firing of presynaptic norepinephrine neurons. In chronic alcohol users and in actively withdrawing patients, alpha-2-adrenergic receptor signaling may become less sensitive, resulting in dysregulation of norepinephrine and epinephrine release. This mechanism was identified in studies showing decreased blood pressure response to alpha-2-adrenoreceptor agonist therapy in patients actively withdrawing from alcohol [47]. Alpha-2-adrenergic agonists, such as clonidine, have been used to treat alcohol withdrawal, although their use has fallen off with the rise of the benzodiazepines. The alpha-2-adrenergic agonist dexmedetomidine, a novel agent with receptor specificity 8 times that of clonidine, has stimulated interest for its potential use in the treatment of acute alcohol withdrawal [48]. Dexmedetomidine aids in the treatment of active withdrawal by restoring alpha-2-adrenergic modulation, thus helping to correct catecholamine overproduction. Because it does not act on $GABA_A$ or opioid receptors, dexmedetomidine has the added benefit of conferring sedation without respiratory compromise [49], an effect that helped lead to the agent's approval for sedation by the Federal Drug Administration. Randomized clinical trials studying the utility of dexmedetomidine in the treatment of patients undergoing severe withdrawal are currently in effect. As in the presented case, the treatment of stress cardiomyopathy and prevention of subsequent cardiac complications may represent a beneficial, potentially unrecognized role of central alpha-2-adrenergic agonists like dexmedetomidine in acute alcohol withdrawal.

4. Conclusions

Despite our knowledge of cardiovascular dysregulation with abrupt cessation of alcohol, the pathophysiology of arrhythmogenesis in alcohol withdrawal remains poorly understood. In the case presented, the patient developed stress cardiomyopathy during acute alcohol withdrawal and was successfully treated with adjunctive dexmedetomidine. Our literature review supports the concept that supraphysiologic levels of catecholamines lead to the development of stress cardiomyopathy in alcohol withdrawal and that modulation of disorganized catecholamine release with alpha-2-adrenergic agonists may have an important role in treatment. Our review of nine published cases indicates that stress cardiomyopathy may be an important determinant of malignant arrhythmia in patients actively withdrawing from alcohol. Furthermore, this case demonstrates the central role of transthoracic echocardiography in the diagnostic workup and prognosis of patients suspected to have stress cardiomyopathy. Clinicians should be aware of stress cardiomyopathy as a complication of alcohol withdrawal that may significantly increase cardiac-related mortality. Studies examining the cardioprotective role of alpha-2-adrenoreceptor agonists in the treatment of alcohol withdrawal are warranted.

Authors' Contribution

The authors contributed equally to the preparation of the paper.

References

[1] R. C. Turner, P. R. Lichstein, J. G. Peden Jr., J. T. Busher, and L. E. Waivers, "Alcohol withdrawal syndromes: a review of pathophysiology, clinical presentation, and treatment," *Journal of General Internal Medicine*, vol. 4, no. 5, pp. 432–444, 1989.

[2] M. E. Tavel, W. Davidson, and T. D. Batterton, "A critical analysis of mortality associated with delirium tremens. Review of 39 fatalities in a 9-year period," *The American Journal of the Medical Sciences*, vol. 242, no. 2, pp. 18–29, 1961.

[3] M. de Wit, D. G. Jones, C. N. Sessler, M. D. Zilberberg, and M. F. Weaver, "Alcohol-use disorders in the critically ill patient," *Chest*, vol. 138, no. 4, pp. 994–1003, 2010.

[4] J. Liu and T. Fujimiya, "Abrupt termination of an ethanol regimen provokes ventricular arrhythmia and enhances susceptibility to the arrhythmogenic effects of epinephrine in rats," *Alcoholism: Clinical and Experimental Research*, vol. 34, supplement 1, pp. S45–S53, 2010.

[5] K. Dote, H. Sato, H. Tateishi, T. Uchida, and M. Ishihara, "Myocardial stunning due to simultaneous multivessel coronary spasms: a review of 5 cases," *Journal of Cardiology*, vol. 21, no. 2, pp. 203–214, 1991.

[6] A. Prasad, "Apical ballooning syndrome: an important differential diagnosis of acute myocardial infarction," *Circulation*, vol. 115, no. 5, pp. e56–e59, 2007.

[7] M. Gianni, F. Dentali, A. M. Grandi, G. Sumner, R. Hiralal, and E. Lonn, "Apical ballooning syndrome or takotsubo cardiomyopathy: a systematic review," *European Heart Journal*, vol. 27, no. 13, pp. 1523–1529, 2006.

[8] H. M. Nef, H. Möllmann, Y. J. Akashi, and C. W. Hamm, "Mechanisms of stress (Takotsubo) cardiomyopathy," *Nature Reviews Cardiology*, vol. 7, no. 4, pp. 187–193, 2010.

[9] L. Ng, J. Wang, L. Altaweel, and M. K. Athar, "Neurologic aspects of cardiac emergencies," *Critical Care Clinics*, vol. 30, no. 3, pp. 557–584, 2014.

[10] A. A. Elesber, A. Prasad, R. J. Lennon, R. S. Wright, A. Lerman, and C. S. Rihal, "Four-year recurrence rate and prognosis of the apical ballooning syndrome," *Journal of the American College of Cardiology*, vol. 50, no. 5, pp. 448–452, 2007.

[11] K. Tsuchihashi, K. Ueshima, T. Uchida et al., "Transient left ventricular apical ballooning without coronary artery stenosis: a novel heart syndrome mimicking acute myocardial infarction," *Journal of the American College of Cardiology*, vol. 38, no. 1, pp. 11–18, 2001.

[12] K. Suzuki, N. Osada, Y. J. Akasi et al., "An atypical case of 'Takotsubo cardiomyopathy' during alcohol withdrawal: abnormality in the transient left ventricular wall motion and a remarkable elevation in the ST segment," *Internal Medicine*, vol. 43, no. 4, pp. 300–305, 2004.

[13] S. A. Mitchell and R. A. Crone, "Takotsubo cardiomyopathy: a case report," *Journal of the American Society of Echocardiography*, vol. 19, no. 9, pp. 1190.e9–1190.e10, 2006.

[14] N. Kalra, P. Khetpal, and V. L. Sorrell, "Seriously stressed," *The American Journal of Medicine*, vol. 122, no. 8, pp. 735–737, 2009.

[15] A. G. Thompson and J. H. Hung, "Takotsubo cardiomyopathy associated with alcohol withdrawal," *Medical Journal of Australia*, vol. 194, no. 7, article 373, 2011.

[16] C. Stöllberger, H. Fischer, A. Pratter, and J. Finsterer, "Seizure-induced Takotsubo cardiomyopathy and thrombocytopenia," *European Journal of Neurology*, vol. 18, no. 6, pp. e68–e69, 2011.

[17] J. Alexandre, L. Benouda, L. Champ-Rigot, and F. Labombarda, "Takotsubo cardiomyopathy triggered by alcohol withdrawal," *Drug and Alcohol Review*, vol. 30, no. 4, pp. 434–437, 2011.

[18] P. Yazdan-Ashoori, R. Nichols, and A. Baranchuk, "Tako-tsubo cardiomyopathy precipitated by alcohol withdrawal," *Cardiology Journal*, vol. 19, no. 1, pp. 81–85, 2012.

[19] B. J. Stout, R. Hoshide, and D. S. Vincent, "Takotsubo cardiomyopathy in the setting of acute alcohol withdrawal," *Hawaii Journal of Medicine & Public Health*, vol. 71, no. 7, pp. 193–194, 2012.

[20] H. R. Omar, H. D. Abdelmalak, I. Komorova, E. Helal, and E. M. Camporesi, "Alcohol withdrawal-induced Takotsubo," *Internal and Emergency Medicine*, vol. 7, no. 2, pp. 107–108, 2012.

[21] M. Madhavan and A. Prasad, "Proposed Mayo Clinic criteria for the diagnosis of Tako-Tsubo cardiomyopathy and long-term prognosis," *Herz*, vol. 35, no. 4, pp. 240–244, 2010.

[22] A. R. Lyon, E. Bossone, B. Schneider et al., "Current state of knowledge on takotsubo syndrome: a position statement from the taskforce on takotsubo syndrome of the heart failure Association of the European Society of Cardiology," *European Journal of Heart Failure*, vol. 18, no. 1, pp. 8–27, 2015.

[23] Y. J. Akashi, K. Nakazawa, M. Sakakibara, F. Miyake, H. Koike, and K. Sasaka, "The clinical features of takotsubo cardiomyopathy," *Quarterly Journal of Medicine*, vol. 96, no. 8, pp. 563–573, 2003.

[24] J.-H. Park, S.-J. Kang, J.-K. Song et al., "Left ventricular apical ballooning due to severe physical stress in patients admitted to the medical ICU," *Chest*, vol. 128, no. 1, pp. 296–302, 2005.

[25] A. Movahed, W. C. Reeves, P. M. Mehta, M. G. F. Gilliland, S. L. Mozingo, and S. R. Jolly, "Norepinephrine-induced left ventricular dysfunction in anesthetized and conscious, sedated dogs," *International Journal of Cardiology*, vol. 45, no. 1, pp. 23–33, 1994.

[26] O. Yamanaka, F. Yasumasa, T. Nakamura et al., "'Myocardial stunning'-like phenomenon during a crisis of pheochromocytoma," *Japanese Circulation Journal*, vol. 58, no. 9, pp. 737–742, 1994.

[27] H. M. Nef, H. Möllmann, S. Kostin et al., "Tako-Tsubo cardiomyopathy: intraindividual structural analysis in the acute phase and after functional recovery," *European Heart Journal*, vol. 28, no. 20, pp. 2456–2464, 2007.

[28] B. Stein, S. Bartel, U. Kirchhefer et al., "Relation between contractile function and regulatory cardiac proteins in hypertrophied hearts," *The American Journal of Physiology—Heart and Circulatory Physiology*, vol. 270, no. 6, part 2, pp. H2021–H2028, 1996.

[29] M. O. Boluyt, X. Long, T. Eschenhagen et al., "Isoproterenol infusion induces alterations in expression of hypertrophy-associated genes in rat heart," *American Journal of Physiology—*

Heart and Circulatory Physiology, vol. 269, no. 2, part 2, pp. H638–H647, 1995.

[30] B. Linck, P. Bokník, H. A. Baba et al., "Long-term beta adrenoceptor-mediated alteration in contractility and expression of phospholamban and sarcoplasmic reticulum Ca(++)-ATPase in mammalian ventricle," *Journal of Pharmacology and Experimental Therapeutics*, vol. 286, no. 1, pp. 531–538, 1998.

[31] L. Lipskaia and A.-M. Lompré, "Alteration in temporal kinetics of Ca^{2+} signaling and control of growth and proliferation," *Biology of the Cell*, vol. 96, no. 1, pp. 55–68, 2004.

[32] H. M. Nef, H. Möllmann, C. Troidl et al., "Abnormalities in intracellular Ca^{2+} regulation contribute to the pathomechanism of Tako-Tsubo cardiomyopathy," *European Heart Journal*, vol. 30, no. 17, pp. 2155–2164, 2009.

[33] D. L. Longo, A. S. Fauci, D. L. Kasper, S. K. Hauser, J. L. Jameson, and J. Loscalzo, Eds., *Harrison's Principles of Internal Medicine*, vol. 2, McGraw-Hill, New York, NY, USA, 2012.

[34] H. Kalant, "Comparative aspects of tolerance to, and dependence on, alcohol, barbiturates and opiates," *Advances in Experimental Medicine and Biology*, vol. 85, pp. 169–186, 1977.

[35] D. A. Yost, "Alcohol withdrawal syndrome," *American Family Physician*, vol. 54, no. 2, pp. 657–669, 1996, Erratum in: *American Family Physician*, vol. 54, no. 8, p. 2377, 1996.

[36] R. J. Hawley, L. F. Major, E. A. Schulman, and M. Linnoila, "Cerebrospinal fluid 3-methoxy-4-hydroxyphenylglycol and norepinephrine levels in alcohol withdrawal. Correlations with clinical signs," *Archives of General Psychiatry*, vol. 42, no. 11, pp. 1056–1062, 1985.

[37] S. Borg, A. Czarnecka, H. Kvande, D. Mossberg, and G. Sedvall, "Clinical conditions and concentrations of MOPEG in the cerebrospinal fluid and urine of male alcoholic patients during withdrawal," *Alcoholism: Clinical and Experimental Research*, vol. 7, no. 4, pp. 411–415, 1983.

[38] J. F. Potter and D. G. Beevers, "Pseudo-phaeochromocytoma due to alcohol withdrawal," *Postgraduate Medical Journal*, vol. 61, no. 718, pp. 721–723, 1985.

[39] R. W. Carlson, N. N. Kumar, E. Wong-Mckinstry et al., "Alcohol withdrawal syndrome," *Critical Care Clinics*, vol. 28, no. 4, pp. 549–585, 2012.

[40] E. Abraham, W. C. Shoemaker, and S. F. McCartney, "Cardiorespiratory patterns in severe delirium tremens," *Archives of Internal Medicine*, vol. 145, no. 6, pp. 1057–1059, 1985.

[41] G. Wannamethee and A. G. Shaper, "Alcohol and sudden cardiac death," *British Heart Journal*, vol. 68, no. 5, pp. 443–448, 1992.

[42] R. Citro, F. Rigo, M. Previtali et al., "Differences in clinical features and in-hospital outcomes of older adults with tako-tsubo cardiomyopathy," *Journal of the American Geriatrics Society*, vol. 60, no. 1, pp. 93–98, 2012.

[43] R. Citro, A. R. Lyon, P. Meimoun et al., "Standard and advanced echocardiography in takotsubo (stress) cardiomyopathy: clinical and prognostic implications," *Journal of the American Society of Echocardiography*, vol. 28, no. 1, pp. 57–74, 2015.

[44] R. Citro, F. Rigo, Q. Ciampi et al., "Echocardiographic assessment of regional left ventricular wall motion abnormalities in patients with tako-tsubo cardiomyopathy: comparison with anterior myocardial infarction," *European Journal of Echocardiography*, vol. 12, no. 7, pp. 542–549, 2011.

[45] R. Citro, F. Rigo, A. D'Andrea et al., "Echocardiographic correlates of acute heart failure, cardiogenic shock, and in-hospital mortality in tako-tsubo cardiomyopathy," *JACC: Cardiovascular Imaging*, vol. 7, no. 2, pp. 119–129, 2014.

[46] R. Citro, E. Bossone, G. Parodi et al., "Independent impact of RV involvement on in-hospital outcome of patients with Takotsubo syndrome," *JACC: Cardiovascular Imaging*, 2015.

[47] M. Linnoila, I. Mefford, D. Nutt, and B. Adinoff, "NIH conference. Alcohol withdrawal and noradrenergic function," *Annals of Internal Medicine*, vol. 107, no. 6, pp. 875–889, 1987.

[48] A. J. Muzyk, J. A. Fowler, D. K. Norwood, and A. Chilipko, "Role of α2-agonists in the treatment of acute alcohol withdrawal," *Annals of Pharmacotherapy*, vol. 45, no. 5, pp. 649–657, 2011.

[49] R. R. Riker, Y. Shehabi, P. M. Bokesch et al. et al., "SEDCOM (Safety and Efficacy of Dexmedetomidine Compared With Midazolam) Study Group. Dexmedetomidine vs midazolam for sedation of critically ill patients: a randomized trial," *The Journal of the American Medical Association*, vol. 301, no. 5, pp. 489–499, 2009.

50

Chronic Skull Base Erosion from Temporomandibular Joint Disease Causes Generalized Seizure and Profound Lactic Acidosis

Mark A. Dobish ⓘ,[1] David A. Wyler,[2,3] Christopher J. Farrell,[3] Hermandeep S. Dhami,[4] Victor M. Romo,[5] Daniel D. Choi,[6] Travis Reed,[7] and Michael E. Mahla[8]

[1]Anesthesiology Resident, Department of Anesthesiology, Thomas Jefferson University Hospital, Philadelphia, PA, USA
[2]Assistant Professor of Anesthesiology and Critical Care Medicine, Department of Anesthesiology,
  Thomas Jefferson University Hospital, Philadelphia, PA, USA
[3]Assistant Professor of Neurological Surgery, Department of Neurosurgery, Thomas Jefferson University Hospital,
  Philadelphia, PA, USA
[4]Medical Student, Sidney Kimmel Medical College, Thomas Jefferson University Hospital, Philadelphia, PA, USA
[5]Assistant Professor of Anesthesiology, Department of Anesthesiology, Thomas Jefferson University Hospital, Philadelphia, PA, USA
[6]Assistant Professor of Oral and Maxillofacial Surgery, Department of Oral and Maxillofacial Surgery,
  Thomas Jefferson University Hospital, Philadelphia, PA, USA
[7]Resident, Department of Oral and Maxillofacial Surgery, Thomas Jefferson University Hospital, Philadelphia, PA, USA
[8]Professor and Executive Vice Chair of Anesthesiology, Department of Anesthesiology,
  Thomas Jefferson University Hospital, Philadelphia, PA, USA

Correspondence should be addressed to Mark A. Dobish; mad83@georgetown.edu

Academic Editor: Anita J. Reddy

This report displays a rare presentation of lactic acidosis in the setting of status epilepticus (SE). The differential diagnosis of lactic acidosis is broad and typically originates from states of shock; however, this report highlights an alternative and rare etiology, SE, due to chronic skull base erosion from temporomandibular joint (TMJ) disease. Lactic acidosis is defined by a pH below 7.35 in the setting of lactate values greater than 5 mmol/L. Two broad classifications of lactic acidosis exist: a type A lactic acidosis which stems from global or localized tissue hypoxia or a type B lactic acidosis which occurs once mitochondrial oxidative capacity is unable to match glucose metabolism. SE is an example of a type A lactic acidosis in which oxygen delivery is unable to meet increased cellular energy requirements. This report is consistent with a prior case series that consists of five patients experiencing generalized tonic-clonic (GTC) seizures and lactic acidosis. These patients presented with a pH range of 6.8-7.41 and lactate range of 3.8-22.4 mmol/L. Although severe lactic acidosis following GTC has been described, this is the first report in the literature of chronic skull base erosion from TMJ disease causing SE.

1. Introduction

Status epilepticus (SE) is a neurological emergency with a reported mortality rate between 7.6% and 43% [1]. The three most common etiologies of SE in adults are anticonvulsant noncompliance, alcohol withdrawal, and central nervous system infections which have a reported incidence of 29%, 26%, and 8%, respectively [2]. Other less common etiologies of seizures and SE are rare autoimmune and paraneoplastic disorders, hereditary mitochondrial disease, and rare chromosomal disorders [3]. Trauma is a common source of SE and is attributed as the causative factor in approximately 8% of cases [4].

Lactic acidosis commonly accompanies status epilepticus and is recognized as a transient phenomenon. This is due to over-activity of both neurons and skeletal muscle leading to anaerobic metabolism and the production of lactic acid. Concentrations of lactic acid have been shown to decrease

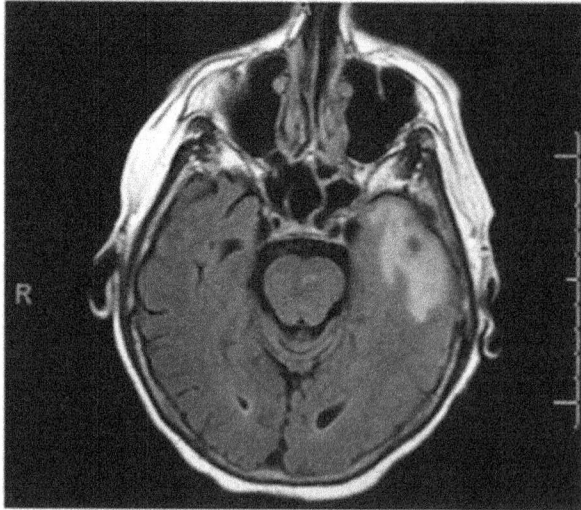

FIGURE 1: Axial flair MRI showing vasogenic edema of the temporal lobe.

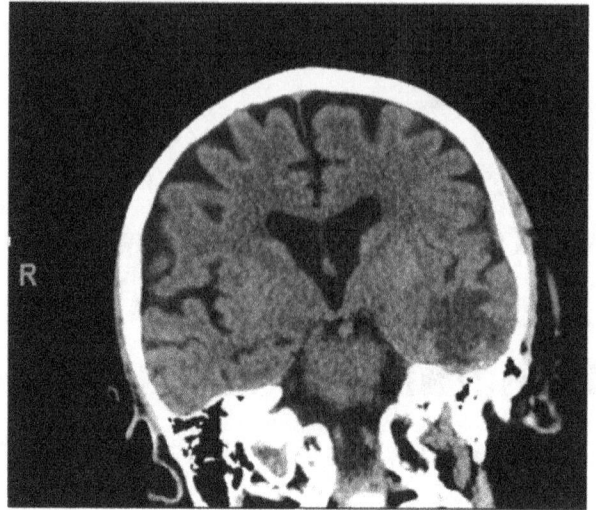

FIGURE 2: Coronal CT demonstrates hypodense left temporal lobe vasogenic edema.

rapidly following SE [5], such that other etiologies should be investigated if this does not occur. Other common sources of lactic acidosis include shock, sepsis, occult malignancy, liver disease, genetic conditions, and medication side effects.

Displacement of the condylar head into the middle cranial fossa is an extremely rare event. A literature review reveals 55 cases of displaced condyles into the middle cranial fossa, all the result of trauma [6, 7]. We describe a case report of chronic temporomandibular joint (TMJ) osteoarthritis causing severe erosive changes in the glenoid fossa leading to intracranial edema, new onset SE, and intracranial displacement of the mandibular condyle.

2. Case Report

A 65-year-old patient developed acute onset aphasia at her home followed by SE while conversing with her sister on the phone. Seizure activity was witnessed by paramedics upon arrival. Due to the inability to open the patient's oral cavity, a blind nasal intubation was performed at the scene.

Upon arrival to the emergency department, SE was treated with bolus doses of midazolam followed by a levetiracetam load. A propofol infusion was started for sedation. Initial laboratory findings were significant for a metabolic acidosis with pH 6.9, CO_2 80 mEq/L, and lactate 11.0 mmol/L. Computed tomography (CT) imaging showed vasogenic edema in the left temporal lobe secondary to intracranial displacement of the left mandibular condyle through a 1.3 × 0.7 cm defect of the glenoid fossa of the temporal bone. Advanced osteoarthritic changes were noted in bilateral TMJ spaces as well as asymptomatic thinning and perforation of the contralateral glenoid fossa. MRI confirmed these findings and further portrayed abnormally enhancing soft tissue that surrounded the mandibular condyle that likely represented fragmented pieces of the glenoid fossa (Figures 1–4).

Three days following admission, the patient was extubated without complication and plans were arranged for

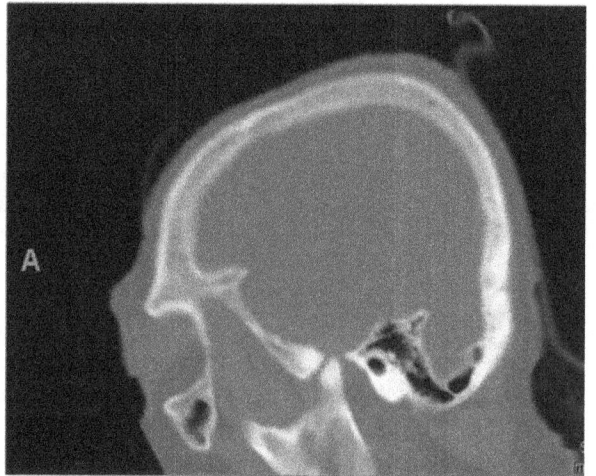

FIGURE 3: Sagittal CT demonstrates erosion of the skull base and protrusion of the TMJ.

surgical repositioning of the mandibular condyle and skull base reconstruction. The patient reported a history of chronic TMJ osteoarthrosis for more than twenty years with a progressive shift in occlusion over the past several years. The patient denied any previous history of seizures, traumatic incidents or TMJ surgical interventions. On exam, there was significant trismus, a mildly canted mandible, and over-collapsed left posterior dentition consistent with an intracranially displaced mandibular condyle.

Based on this preoperative assessment, a difficult airway was anticipated. Furthermore, all jaw manipulation was avoided due to the temporal glenoid defect. An asleep nasal intubation was planned and the patient was brought to the operating room. Standard monitors were applied and each nare was premedicated with two sprays of oxymetazoline in the sitting position. Following pre-oxygenation, general anesthesia was induced with fentanyl, lidocaine, propofol,

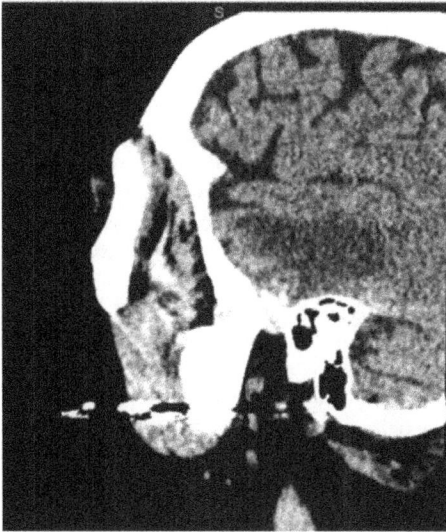

FIGURE 4: Soft tissue window sagittal CT illustrating intracranial edema surrounding the glenoid fossa.

and rocuronium. The right nare was then dilated using 28, 30, and 32 French lubricated nasal airways. A 6.5 mm nasal endotracheal tube (ETT) was advanced atraumatically into the posterior oropharynx and ventilation at this position was confirmed prior to further airway instrumentation. Next, a McGrath 3 blade was carefully inserted into the vallecula and a Cormack-Lehane Grade I view of the laryngeal inlet was obtained with minimal jaw manipulation. The ETT passed through the cords atraumatically. Following positioning and mayfield pinning, a portable bronchoscope was used to confirm final ETT location and the tube was secured at 26 cm at the right nare.

The patient's intraoperative course lasted approximately eleven hours during which time the patient underwent a left middle fossa craniotomy, TMJ arthroplasty, glenoid fossa reconstruction with split-thickness calvarial bone graft, and maxillomandibular fixation. The surgery was performed by a team of neurosurgeons and oral and maxillofacial surgeons. Prior to incision, the patient received mannitol 1 g/kg, dexamethasone 10 mg, and furosemide 20 mg to reduce cerebral edema and optimize surgical conditions. Urine output was replaced in a 1:1 fashion with 0.9% normal saline. Maintenance of anesthesia was accomplished with a total intravenous technique consisting of propofol, remifentanil, and phenylephrine to support blood pressure as needed. At the conclusion of the procedure, the patient's neuromuscular blockade was fully reversed. She was awakened for a "neurologic wake-up test" which was normal. This was accomplished on dexmedetomidine 0.5 mcg/kg/hr and remifentanil 0.05 mcg/kg/min. The patient remained intubated due to a concern for glottic swelling and was taken to the ICU where she was extubated two days later. The patient was seizure free for the remainder of the hospitalization and was discharged on postoperative day five. At 6 months follow up, the patient continues to do well with resolution of aphasia, no residual weaknesses, and no further episodes of seizures.

3. Discussion

To our knowledge, this is the first case that presents SE caused by skull base erosion of the TMJ. The presumed etiology, supported by imaging, is an arthropathy that slowly weakened the TMJ causing progressive intracranial swelling and edema deep to the glenoid fossa. Intraoperative pathology indicated non-inflammatory degenerative joint pathology without cellular infiltrates, indicating a diagnosis of TMJ osteoarthritis. This ultimately caused SE, and the motor involvement caused the mandibular condyle to protrude intracranially through the perforated glenoid fossa.

Displacement of the mandibular condyle into the middle cranial fossa is an extremely rare finding due to the unique and protective anatomy of the TMJ complex. The glenoid fossa, although often as thin as 1 mm, rarely receives a large impactful force in its central portion due to the rounded nature of the condylar head. Additionally, any traumatic force distributed through the mandible has a tendency to fracture at the condylar neck as a protective measure. The patient was found sitting in a chair by EMS; therefore a fall or mechanical trauma was unlikely to have accounted for this finding. Additionally, an asymptomatic perforation of the contralateral glenoid fossa and progressive shift in occlusion support the chronic nature TMJ osteoarthritis.

The severity of this seizure is further illustrated by the lactic acidosis found on arrival - pH 6.9 and lactate 11.0 mmol/L. Since EMS responded immediately, these values are unlikely to have resulted from prolonged muscle breakdown. Initial creatinine phosphokinase value was normal, 166 U/L.

The differential diagnosis of lactic acidosis is broad and can occur as a result of genetic conditions, medication side effects, malignancy, or pathologic conditions that cause sepsis, anemia, liver dysfunction, or decreased cardiac output. Basal lactate production is about 0.8 mmol/kg/hour [8], and a normal reference range is typically 2 mmol/L or less [9]. Lactic acidosis is defined by a pH below 7.35 in the setting of lactate values greater than 5 mmol/L [10]. Lactate levels are routinely used as a marker for tissue hypoperfusion, and in cases of septic shock values greater than 4 mmol/L have been used as a threshold for aggressive fluid therapy [11]. Two broad classifications of lactic acidosis exist: a type A lactic acidosis which stems from global or localized tissue hypoxia or a type B lactic acidosis which occurs once mitochondrial oxidative capacity is unable to match glucose metabolism [12]. Causes of a type B lactic acidosis occur due to mitochondrial dysfunction and include, but are not limited to, malignancy, trauma, medication side effects, thiamine deficiency, or mitochondrial myopathy [13]. SE is an example of a type A lactic acidosis in which oxygen delivery is unable to meet increased cellular energy requirements, leading to anaerobic metabolism. In this state of localized hypoxia in the brain, pyruvate from cellular glycolysis is converted into lactate in the liver where it is metabolized back to glucose by the Cori cycle.

This case is consistent with two prior case series. The first case series consists of five patients experiencing SE in Scandinavia - these patients presented with a pH range of 6.8-7.41 and lactate range of 3.8-22.4 mmol/L [14]. The second case series of 8 patients, published in 1977, found an average pH of 7.14 (6.86-7.36mmol/L) and an average lactate of 6.6 mmol/L (4.2-10.7 mmol/L) [15].

Treatment options of intracranial condylar dislocation consist of closed reduction and open reduction, with or without reconstruction of the glenoid fossa. Decision making depends on timing of presentation and presence of neurologic symptoms. In the acute setting, an attempt should be made to manually reduce the displaced condyle followed by a period of MMF. However, when there is delayed presentation, it often necessitates an open approach to free the fibrosed mandibular condyle. Fossa reconstruction options described in the literature include autogenous grafts (cartilage or bone), titanium mesh, and alloplastic materials [16–18].

In conclusion, the most common causes of SE are anticonvulsant noncompliance, alcohol withdrawal, and nervous system infections. While seizures can result from traumatic intracranial dislocation of the mandibular condyle, this is the first known report describing long-standing TMJ disease leading to intracranial swelling and edema followed by new onset SE.

Disclosure

This abstract and manuscript was presented in poster form at the Society of Critical Care and Anesthesiology annual conference in Chicago in April 2018.

Acknowledgments

David A. Wyler receives funding from the company ArtMedical Safety Technology.

References

[1] R. F. M. Chin, B. G. R. Neville, and R. C. Scott, "A systematic review of the epidemiology of status epilepticus," *European Journal of Neurology*, vol. 11, no. 12, pp. 800–810, 2004.

[2] M. J. Aminoff and R. P. Simon, "Status epilepticus. Causes, clinical features and consequences in 98 patients," *American Journal of Medicine*, vol. 69, no. 5, pp. 657–666, 1980.

[3] R. Y. L. Tan, A. Neligan, and S. D. Shorvon, "The uncommon causes of status epilepticus: A Systematic Review," *Epilepsy Research*, vol. 91, no. 2-3, pp. 111–122, 2010.

[4] D. H. Lowenstein and B. K. Alldredge, "Status epilepticus at an urban public hospital in the 1980s," *Neurology*, vol. 43, no. 3, pp. 483–488, 1993.

[5] C. E. Orringer, J. C. Eustace, C. D. Wunsch, and L. B. Gardner, "Natural History of Lactic Acidosis after Grand-Mal Seizures: A Model for the Study of an Anion-Gap Acidosis Not Associated with Hyperkalemia," *The New England Journal of Medicine*, vol. 297, no. 15, pp. 796–799, 1977.

[6] M. Zhang, A. L. Alexander, S. P. Most, G. Li, and O. A. Harris, "Intracranial Dislocation of the Mandibular Condyle: A Case Report and Literature Review," *World Neurosurgery*, vol. 86, pp. 514.e1–514.e11, 2016.

[7] E. R. Rikhotso and M. A. Bobat, "Total Alloplastic Joint Reconstruction in a Patient With Temporomandibular Joint Ankylosis Following Condylar Dislocation Into the Middle Cranial Fossa," *Journal of Oral and Maxillofacial Surgery*, vol. 74, no. 12, pp. 2378–2378.e5, 2016.

[8] P. J. Fall and H. M. Szerlip, "Lactic acidosis: From sour milk to septic shock," *Journal of Intensive Care Medicine*, vol. 20, no. 5, pp. 255–271, 2005.

[9] O. Kruse, N. Grunnet, and C. Barfod, "Blood lactate as a predictor for in-hospital mortality in patients admitted acutely to hospital: a systematic review," *Scandinavian Journal of Trauma, Resuscitation and Emergency Medicine* , vol. 19, article 74, 2011.

[10] S. M. Forsythe and G. A. Schmidt, "Sodium bicarbonate for the treatment of lactic acidosis," *CHEST*, vol. 117, no. 1, pp. 260–267, 2000.

[11] E. Rivers, B. Nguyen, S. Havstad et al., "Early goal-directed therapy in the treatment of severe sepsis and septic shock," *The New England Journal of Medicine*, vol. 345, no. 19, pp. 1368–1377, 2001.

[12] M. Scrutton, "Clinical and biochemical aspects of lactic acidosis," *FEBS Letters*, vol. 70, no. 1-2, pp. 294-295, 1976.

[13] A. J. Reddy, S. W. Lam, S. R. Bauer, and J. A. Guzman, "Lactic acidosis: Clinical implications and management strategies," *Cleveland Clinic Journal of Medicine*, vol. 82, no. 9, pp. 615–624, 2015.

[14] K. Lipka and H.-H. Bülow, "Lactic acidosis following convulsions," *Acta Anaesthesiologica Scandinavica*, vol. 47, no. 5, pp. 616–618, 2003.

[15] C. E. Orringer, J. C. Eustace, C. D. Wunsch, and L. B. Gardner, "Natural History of Lactic Acidosis after Grand-Mal Seizures," *The New England Journal of Medicine*, vol. 297, no. 15, pp. 796–799, 1977.

[16] Y. He, Y. Zhang, Z.-L. Li, J.-G. An, Z.-Q. Yi, and S.-D. Bao, "Treatment of traumatic dislocation of the mandibular condyle into the cranial fossa: Development of a probable treatment algorithm," *International Journal of Oral and Maxillofacial Surgery*, vol. 44, no. 7, pp. 864–870, 2015.

[17] N. Ohura, S. Ichioka, T. Sudo, M. Nakagawa, K. Kumaido, and T. Nakatsuka, "Dislocation of the Bilateral Mandibular Condyle Into the Middle Cranial Fossa: Review of the Literature and Clinical Experience," *Journal of Oral and Maxillofacial Surgery*, vol. 64, no. 7, pp. 1165–1172, 2006.

[18] V. Arya and R. Chigurupati, "Treatment Algorithm for Intracranial Intrusion Injuries of the Mandibular Condyle," *Journal of Oral and Maxillofacial Surgery*, vol. 74, no. 3, pp. 569–581, 2016.

51

Inspiratory Muscle Training with Isokinetic Device to Help Ventilatory Weaning in a Patient with Guillain-Barré Syndrome by Zika Virus

Leonardo Cordeiro de Souza ⓘ,[1,2] **Amarildo Abreu de Souza,**[2] **Eric Eduardo Pinto de Almeida,**[2] **Leo Honse Ribeiro,**[2] **Marcos David Parada Godoy,**[1,2] **Wanderlei Augusto Junior,**[2] **and Jocemir Ronaldo Lugon**[3]

Medical Science Post-Graduation Program, Universidade Federal Fluminense, Niterói, RJ, Brazil
[2]*Intensive Care Division, Hospital e Clínica São Gonçalo, São Gonçalo, RJ, Brazil*
[3]*Nephrology Division, Universidade Federal Fluminense, Niterói, RJ, Brazil*

Correspondence should be addressed to Leonardo Cordeiro de Souza; leonardo.uti@gmail.com

Academic Editor: Petros Kopterides

Zika is an arbovirus infection mainly transmitted by the mosquito *Aedes aegypti*. In 2016, the burden of Zika epidemic in Brazil was significant. Patients affected by Zika virus can develop Guillain-Barré syndrome, evolving to muscle respiratory failure requiring mechanical ventilation. In this setting, delayed recovery of the muscle weakness can result in prolonged weaning, a condition that by itself is related to a high mortality rate. The study is reporting a case of a patient with Zika and Guillain-Barré syndrome who underwent an inspiratory muscle training program starting after twenty-five days of mechanical ventilation and guided by serial measurements of the timed inspiratory effort (TIE) index. The patient was successfully weaned in two weeks and discharged from the hospital 30 days after extubation.

1. Introduction

In recent years, Brazil has witnessed an outbreak of new diseases transmitted by the mosquito *Aedes aegypti*. The emergence of Zika virus (an arbovirus of the Flavivirus genus) took place in northeast part of Brazil in 2015 and was followed by a rapid countrywide spread. By 2016, the numbers of Zika epidemics in Brazil were alarming: according to the Ministry of Health, the Zika virus reached more than 200 thousand people [1].

Guillain-Barré syndrome (GBS) is a neurological syndrome of autoimmune origin, characterized by an acute inflammatory polyradiculoneuropathy, which progresses rapidly, triggering an ascending symmetrical muscular weakness. This acute demyelinating neuropathy, which comprehensively affects the peripheral nervous system, carries a potentially fatal course [1].

Patients with Guillain-Barré syndrome related to the Zika virus may have respiratory muscle dysfunction, rapidly evolving to acute respiratory failure requiring the use of mechanical ventilation (MV). The delayed recovery of the muscle weakness can result in prolonged weaning, a condition that by itself is associated with a high mortality rate [1–3].

Inspiratory muscle training (IMT) with linear pressure loading devices is the major current therapeutic expectation in the quest for ventilator independence. Since 2002, several studies have demonstrated that the use of IMT may increase the success rate of the weaning process [2, 4]. To improve these numbers the timed inspiratory effort (TIE) index was incorporated to compose the tools used to assess and guide the recovery of respiratory muscle dysfunction.

This is a report of a case of a Zika-related Guillain-Barré syndrome in prolonged mechanical ventilation that underwent an IMT program with an isokinetic electronic load device. The adequacy of the inspiratory muscle strength was assessed and guided by serial measurements of the timed inspiratory effort (TIE) index, recently reported as a useful tool to help in the mechanical ventilation weaning.

2. Methods

The patient was cared for in a hospital located in the city of São Gonçalo, in the state of Rio de Janeiro, Brazil, from June 28th, 2017, to August 22nd, 2017. A free and informed signed consent form was obtained for the study.

2.1. Measurement of the TIE Index. A recently proposed timed inspiratory effort (TIE) index, which integrates the PImax with the time to reach it, showed better performance than the rapid and superficial respiration index (f/Vt), maximal inspiratory pressure (PImax), respiratory drive (P0.1), and integrative weaning index (IWI). The TIE index is calculated as the ratio of the PImax registered after the first 30 seconds of observation by the corresponding time to reach it while keeping the airways occluded with a unidirectional valve for up to 60 seconds [2].

For the measurement of maximal inspiratory pressure (MIP) and TIE index we used a prototype of a digital vacuometer called MagnaTIE (Magnamed, São Paulo, SP, Brazil), with a scale of 300 cmH_2O and an increment of 0.1 cmH_2O and a time interval of 100 ms for each pressure.

As a safety measure during the use of the TIE index, the subject of the study was kept under continuous surveillance through the multiparameter monitor (Dixtal, São Paulo, SP, Brazil); if any sign of instability was noticed by the examiner, the test was stopped and the patient returned to MV.

The method used was the occlusion of the airway with the unidirectional valve. The patient was positioned in dorsal decubitus, with the head elevated to 45 degrees. The cuff was hyperinflated to prevent leakage during measurement. After tracheal aspiration, patient remains connected to the mechanical ventilator for rest for two minutes with 100% oxygen inspired fraction (FiO2).

After the hyperoxygenation, mechanical ventilator disconnection was performed and after 10 seconds of spontaneous breathing, the digital vacuometer was connected manually in the end of an expiration to the artificial airway, keeping the airways occluded for up to 60 seconds and recording the values corresponding to each inspiratory effort. Thereby, the TIE index was calculated with the ratio of the maximum inspiratory pressure registered after the first 30 seconds of observation and the corresponding time to reach it [2].

Weaning success was predicted by values of the TIE index ≥1.0 cmH_2O/s, and the patient uninterruptedly remained on spontaneous breathing for 5 days [5]. The decision to return to mechanical ventilation was made by a respiratory physiotherapist and the physician in charge, based on the signs of poor tolerance used routinely in the hospital [2].

The IMT was conducted daily between 08:00 and 10:00 am. The established intermittent protocol consisted of imposing an inspiratory load for 30 breath cycles in three periods

(Figure 1). Each period of 10 breath cycles was divided two steps: in the first, the load was gradually increased until the target was reached (45% of the MIP); in the second, the remaining 5 breath cycles of the period were run under the target load. At the end of the third period, patients had one period of rest (breathing without inspiratory load) of 2-3 minutes and underwent three more periods of training totaling 6 periods (60 breath cycles) of training each time. If signs of intolerance were observed during the IMT the patient was returned to MV. After each training session, the patient was returned to the MV in PSV mode for two hours to rest, a protocol of progressively lengthening tracheal collar trials, which increased in length each day [5]. The patient was reassessed weekly for the TIE index.

3. Case Report

A 33-year-old male, without comorbidities, was admitted to the hospital on June 28th, 2017, reporting fever (39.5°C) and paresthesia in the feet upwards. He had difficulty in walking and speaking; he also related episode of the fall from his own height. He was admitted to the intensive care unit (ICU) with dyspnea, pneumonia, and complaints of persistent muscular pain. His initial laboratory tests showed hemoglobin 14.0 g/dL, white blood count 6.780/mm³, BUN 8.4 mg/dL, creatinine 0.72 mg/dL, Na 143mEq/L, K 4.2 mEq/L, CK 138U/L, and PCR 10.1mg/dL. On the second day of admission, serology was positive for Zika virus (IgG antibodies).

On June/30/2017, he developed acute respiratory insufficiency type II, requiring sedation and orotracheal intubation and was placed on mechanical ventilation with pressure controlled mode (PCV). Due to the severity of his clinical condition, he was maintained with this regimen until the beginning of the weaning process. His cerebrospinal fluid showed an increased presence of proteins (191mg/dL) with a normal cell count consistent with Guillain-Barré syndrome. Blood cultures for bacteria or fungi and serological tests for toxoplasmosis, herpes, varicella, and HIV were all negative. During his stay in the ICU, 0.4g/kg intravenous immunoglobulin was administered for 5 days without improvement. In the same period, the patient developed septic shock of undetermined focus, with vasoactive amines and intravenous antimicrobial agents being administered for 10 days (Meropenem combined with Fluconazole) according to the Campaign Surviving Sepsis and Latin America Sepsis Institute, ILAS.

The 840TM mechanical ventilator (Covidien-Nellcor and Puritan Bennett, Boulder, Colorado, USA) was used. The patient was tracheostomized after 48 hours of intubation, remaining for 25 days on mechanical ventilation in the ICU; after that, he was transferred to the prolonged ventilation unit after three unsuccessful attempts at conventional weaning trial with trach collar, in which he did not reach a spontaneous breathing higher than 15 minutes. At that time, the patient was awake, cooperative, hemodynamically stable, and free of infection. The IMT program using the electronic isokinetic loading device (POWERbreathe KH-2, London, UK) was started on day 26 of MV, in which 6 sets

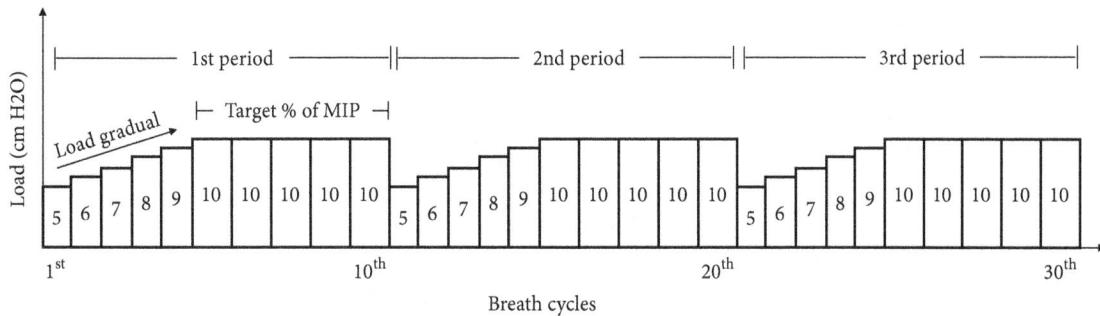

FIGURE 1: Diagram of the protocol in 3 load cycles each (in each inspiratory muscle training session the procedures were performed twice).

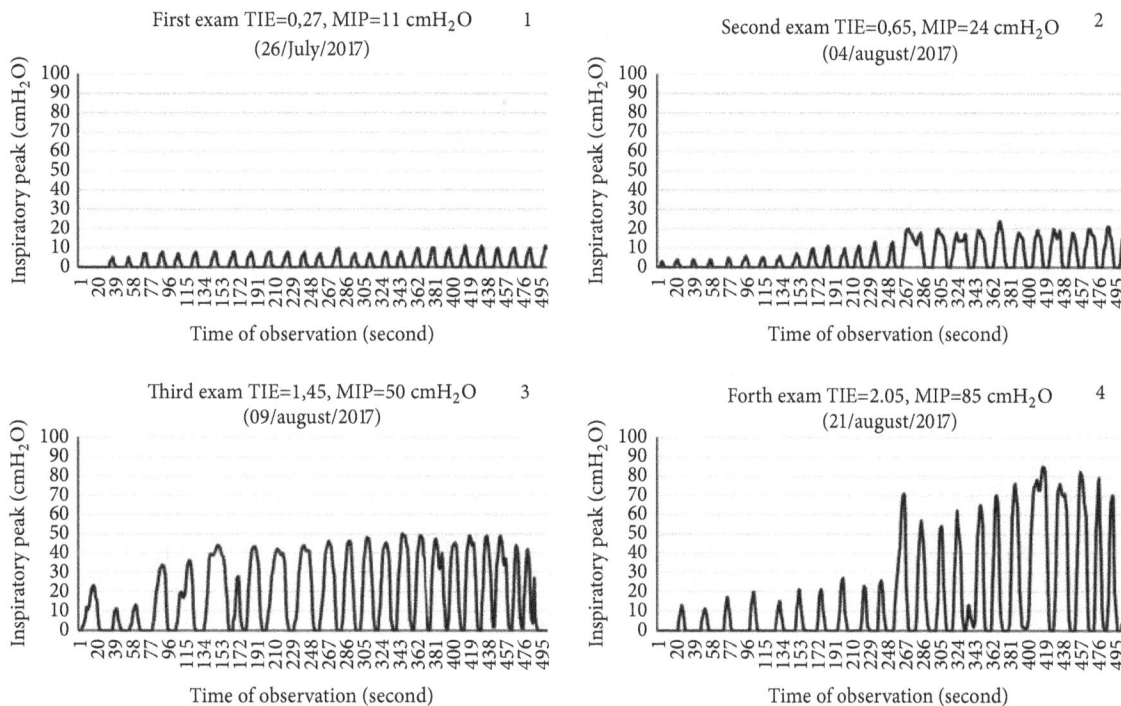

FIGURE 2: Graphics of inspiratory peaks in the serial weekly measurement of TIE index from the first until the last measurement along inspiratory muscle training program.

were done with 10 repetitions to achieve the 60 efforts daily intermittently and incrementally; see Figure 1.

The muscle function of the patient at start of the training program evaluated by the Medical Research Council (MRC) scoring was 12 (20% of normal); the correspondent value using the functional status score (FSS-ICU) was 3 (8.6% of normal). By this time, his maximal inspiratory pressure (MIP) was 11cmH2O and the TIE index 0.27cmH$_2$O/s, when the training load was adjusted to a maximum of 5 cmH$_2$O (45% of the MIP). On day 36 of MV, his MIP had increased to 24 cmH$_2$O with a TIE index of 0.65 cmH$_2$O/s, a time when the training load was set to 12cmH$_2$O (50% of the MIP). In the following week, the MIP reached 50cmH2O, the TIE index was 1.45 cmH$_2$O/s, and the training load was set to 28cmH$_2$O (56% of the MIP). On day 14 after the start of IMT, the patient was successfully weaned off the ventilator. A daily training with a load of 30cmH$_2$O (60%) was maintained. On day 26 of

IMT, his MIP was 85cmH$_2$O and the TIE index 2.05cmH$_2$O/s (Figure 2). He was discharged from the ICU after 64 days.

The IMT program was accompanied by an early mobilization and physical therapy protocol, active member exercising in bed followed by resistance exercising against gravity at the bedside, evolving to moving to standing position. Hospital discharge took place on September 8th, 2017, totaling 71 days of hospitalization. By that time, the scoring values using the MRC assessment and the FSS-ICU scale were 34 (57% of normal) and 18 (51.4 of normal), respectively.

4. Discussion

Prolonged MV is associated with several complications, such as ventilator-associated pneumonia (VAP), ventilation-induced diaphragmatic dysfunction (VIDD), and critical patient polyneuropathy [3, 6]. Jubram et al., in 2013, published a prospective, randomized, blind study in which 312 patients on prolonged ventilation (median stay in MV of 34 days) were analyzed. The success rate of weaning was 49%, patients who returned to mechanical ventilation after weaning success were 12.1%, hospital mortality rate was 55%, and mortality after 1 year was 63% [5].

Numerous efforts have been made in the attempt to reduce MV time, ICU length of stay, and sequel of immobility. For this purpose, some studies have used IMT with encouraging results. The use of IMT is associated with an increase in the success rate of prolonged weaning (71% compared to 47% in the control group) [7]. In a systematic review, in which 10 studies were selected, it was clear that only patients with difficulty in ventilatory weaning benefited from inspiratory muscle training [4]. The training of inspiratory muscles seems to emerge as an important adjunctive therapeutic tool to address the failure of weaning of long-stay patients in MV. However, it is still unclear which type of protocol should be used: load, duration, intensity, and frequency. Regarding this, the team experience with measurement of the TIE index was the only resource used as a guide to prescribe the IMT [2, 8].

The TIE index was idealized by Souza and Lugon (2015) and considers the combination of respiratory center stimulation and muscle response time. In two publications this index presented better accuracy than the other ones to predict the outcome of ventilatory weaning [2, 8]. It is our view that this new tool allows quantitative assessment of the inspiratory muscles supplanting the clinical judgment toward the guiding of the prescription of the parameters, which could help the rehabilitation process.

The score of MRC assessment at ICU admission was 12 (20% of normal) indicating severe muscle weakness. In contrast, at hospital discharge the score was 34 (57% of normal). Findings were similar when using the FSS-ICU scale, with corresponding numbers of 3 (8.6% of normal) and 18 (51.4% of normal). Our findings are in agreement with other reports suggesting that interventions that aim to encourage activity and early mobilization in the ICU may reduce duration of MV, length of stay in ICU, and at the same time improve patients' physical function [9, 10]. Only one study was found using the same electronic isokinetic inspiratory loading device and an increase in inspiratory muscle strength resulting in a favorable outcome was also reported [10]. However, caution should be exercised regarding conclusions as to the definite role of this new device in this setting because the experience with it is very small.

In conclusion, the use of inspiratory muscle training (IMT) with electronic isokinetic loading guided by serial measurement of the TIE index was found to be instrumental to provide strength gain and resistance to respiratory muscles. As a result, a patient with Guillain-Barré syndrome related to Zika virus infection was successfully weaned off the ventilator and discharged from the ICU and from the hospital. Of interest, at 6 months of hospital discharge, the patient remains on a regular physical therapy program and is gradually coming back to his normal days activities, like driving a car.

Authors' Contributions

Leonardo Cordeiro de Souza and Jocemir Ronaldo Lugon contributed to the design and manuscript preparation. Leo Honse Ribeiro, Amarildo Abreu de Souza, Eric Eduardo Pinto de Almeida, Wanderlei Augusto Junior, and Marcos David Parada Godoy helped in the patient care and the case report.

Acknowledgments

The authors are thankful to all respiratory physiotherapists (in particular Raphaela Cristina Carvalho Cordeiro) and physicians of the intensive care unit of Hospital e Clínica São Gonçalo (RJ) for their collaboration in our study. Magnamed, São Paulo, Brazil, provided funding for publication and support. Toru Miyagi (Chief Engineer) was responsible for the project MagnaTIE. Support was also provided by POWERbreathe, London, UK. Harry Brar (President) was responsible for donation of the KH2.

References

[1] C. Filho, JIG et al., "Revisão da literatura: relação entre Zika vírus e síndrome de Guillain- Barré," *Revista Ciência e Estudos Acadêmicos de Medicina - Número 5*, Universidade do Estado de Mato Grosso - UNEMAT (Cáceres), pp. 22–29, 2016.

[2] L. C. de Souza, F. S. Guimarães, and J. R. Lugon, "Evaluation of a new index of mechanical ventilation weaning: the timed inspiratory effort," *Journal of Intensive Care Medicine*, vol. 30, pp. 37–43, 2013.

[3] M. Decramer and G. Gayan-Ramirez, "Ventilator-induced Diaphragmatic Dysfunction," *American Journal of Respiratory and Critical Care Medicine*, vol. 170, no. 11, pp. 1141-1142, 2004.

[4] M. Elkins and R. Dentice, "Inspiratory muscle training facilitates weaning from mechanical ventilation among patients in the intensive care unit: A systematic review," *Journal of Physiotherapy*, vol. 61, no. 3, pp. 125–134, 2015.

[5] A. Jubran, B. J. B. Grant, L. A. Duffner et al., "Effect of pressure support vs unassisted breathing through a tracheostomy collar on weaning duration in patients requiring prolonged mechanical ventilation: A randomized trial," *Journal of the American Medical Association*, vol. 309, no. 7, pp. 671–677, 2013.

[6] S. Levine, T. Nguyen, N. Taylor et al., "Rapid disuse atrophy of diaphragm fibers in mechanically ventilated humans," *The New England Journal of Medicine*, vol. 358, no. 13, pp. 1327–1335, 2008.

[7] A. D. Martin, B. K. Smith, P. D. Davenport et al., "Inspiratory muscle strength training improves weaning outcome in failure to wean patients: a randomized trial," *Critical Care*, vol. 15, no. 2, article R84, 2011.

[8] L. C. de Souza, F. S. Guimarães, and J. R. Lugon, "The timed inspiratory effort: A promising index of mechanical ventilation weaning for patients with neurologic or neuromuscular diseases," *Respiratory Care*, vol. 60, no. 2, pp. 231–238, 2015.

[9] V. Z. M. Silva, J. A. A. Neto, G. C. Junior, M. Pinedo, M. N. Dale, J. M. Zanni et al., "Versão brasileira da Escala de Estado Funcional em UTI: tradução e adaptação transcultural," *Revista Brasileira de Terapia Intensiva*, vol. 29, pp. 34–38, 2017.

[10] L. C. Souza, J. F. R. Campos, L. P. Daher, P. F. da Silva, A. Ventura et al., "Mechanical Ventilation Weaning in Inclusion Body Myositis: Feasibility of Isokinetic Inspiratory Muscle Training as an Adjunct Therapy," *Case Report in Critical Care*, Article ID 902541, 2014.

Permissions

List of Contributors

Braden Powers, Aditya Uppalapati, Sindhura Gogineni and Zafar Akram Jamkhana
Division of Pulmonary, Critical Care and Sleep Medicine, Saint Louis University 1402 South Grand Avenue, MC/SLUH/7 FDT, St. Louis, MO 63110-0250,USA

Jose Orsini, Christa Blaak, Eric Tam, Salil Rajayer, Joaquin Morante, Angela Yeh and Ashvin Butala
Department of Medicine, New York University School of Medicine,Woodhull Medical and Mental Health Center, 760 Broadway, Brooklyn, NY 11206, USA

M. P. Hennus
Department of Pediatric Intensive Care, Wilhelmina Children's Hospital, University Medical Center Utrecht, 3508 AB Utrecht, The Netherlands

L. Speleman
Department of Pediatric Otorhinolaryngology, Wilhelmina Children's Hospital, University Medical Center Utrecht, 3508 AB Utrecht, The Netherlands

Joana Miranda, Henrique Soares, Ana Vilan and Hercília Guimarães
Division of Neonatology, Hospital of São João, Faculty of Medicine, University of Porto, Porto, Portugal

Gustavo Rocha
Division of Neonatology, Hospital of São João, Faculty of Medicine, University of Porto, Porto, Portugal
Division of Neonatology, Hospital of São João, Piso 2, Alameda Professor Hernâni Monteiro, 4200-319 Porto, Portugal

Otília Brandão
Department of Pathology, Hospital of São João, Faculty of Medicine, University of Porto, Porto, Portugal

Arthur Shiyovich
Internal Medicine E, Soroka University Medical Center, 84101 Beer Sheva, Israel

Lior Nesher
Internal Medicine E, Soroka University Medical Center, P.O. Box 151, 84101 Beer Sheva, Israel
Department of Emergency Medicine, Rekanati School for Community Health Professions, Faculty of Health Sciences, Ben-Gurion University of the Negev, 84105 Beer Sheva, Israel

J. Spapen
Department of Internal Medicine, University Hospital, Vrije Universiteit Brussel, Laarbeeklaan 101, 1090 Brussels, Belgium

J. De Regt, P. M. Honoré and H. Spapen
Department of Intensive Care, University Hospital, Vrije Universiteit Brussel, Laarbeeklaan 101, 1090 Brussels, Belgium

K. Nieboer
Department of Radiology, University Hospital, Vrije Universiteit Brussel, Laarbeeklaan 101, 1090 Brussels, Belgium

G. Verfaillie
Department of Thoracic Surgery, University Hospital, Vrije Universiteit Brussel, Laarbeeklaan 101, 1090 Brussels, Belgium

Deepu Daniel
Broward Health Medical Center, Fort Lauderdale, FL 33316, USA

Sunil Kumar
Pulmonary/Critical Care Medicine, Broward Health Medical Center, Fort Lauderdale, FL 33316, USA

Gillian A. Beauchamp and Jason T. McMullan
Department of Emergency Medicine, University of Cincinnati, Cincinnati, OH 45267, USA

Jordan B. Bonomo
Department of Emergency Medicine, University of Cincinnati, Cincinnati, OH 45267, USA
Division of Neurocritical Care, Department of Neurosurgery, University of Cincinnati, 231 Albert Sabin Way, ML 0769, MSB 1654, Cincinnati, OH 45267, USA

José A. Fernández, Antonio Fernández-Valiñas, Daniel Hernández, Joel Orozco and Antonio Lugo
Hospital Ángeles Clínica Londres, Durango No. 50, Roma Norte, Cuauhtémoc, 06700 Ciudad de México, DF, Mexico

Irfanali R. Kugasia and Nehad Shabarek
Department of Internal Medicine, Lincoln Medical and Mental Health Center, 234 East 149th Street, Bronx, NY 10451, USA

Michele Umbrello, Davide Ottolina and Giancarlo Zanforlin
Unità Operativa di Anestesia e Rianimazione, Azienda Ospedaliera San Paolo, Polo Universitario, Via A. Di Rudinì 8, 20142Milano, Italy

Gaetano Iapichino
Unità Operativa di Anestesia e Rianimazione, Azienda Ospedaliera San Paolo, Polo Universitario, Via A. Di Rudinì 8, 20142Milano, Italy
Dipartimento di Fisiopatologia Medico-Chirurgica e dei Trapianti, Università degli Studi di Milano, Via F. Sforza 35, 20122 Milano, Italy

Marco Gardinali
Unità Operativa di Medicina IV, Azienda Ospedaliera San Paolo, Polo Universitario, Via A. Di Rudinì 8, 20142Milano, Italy

Ayelet Machtei
Neonatal Intensive Care Unit, Schneider Children's Medical Center of Israel, 14 Kaplan Street, 49202 Petah Tikva, Israel

Gil Klinger and Lea Sirota
Neonatal Intensive Care Unit, Schneider Children's Medical Center of Israel, 14 Kaplan Street, 49202 Petah Tikva, Israel
The Sackler School of Medicine, Tel Aviv University, Tel Aviv, Israel

Rivka Shapiro
The Sackler School of Medicine, Tel Aviv University, Tel Aviv, Israel
Institute of Gastroenterology, Nutrition and Liver Diseases, Schneider Children's Medical Center of Israel, Petah Tikva, Israel

Osnat Konen
The Sackler School of Medicine, Tel Aviv University, Tel Aviv, Israel
Radiology Department, Schneider Children's Medical Center of Israel, Petah Tikva, Israel

Muhammad Kashif and Hassan Tariq
Department ofMedicine, Bronx Lebanon Hospital Center, 1650 Selwyn Avenue, SuiteNo. 10 C, Bronx, NY 10457, USA

Mohsin Ijaz and Jose Gomez-Marquez
Division of Pulmonary and Critical Care Medicine, Department of Medicine, Bronx Lebanon Hospital Center, 1650 Selwyn Avenue, Suite No. 12 F, Bronx, NY 10457, USA

Nisha Rani Agrawal, Garima Gupta and Kusum Verma
Department of Obstetrics and Gynecology, Institute of Medical Sciences, Banaras Hindu University, Uttar Pradesh, Varanasi 221005, India

Neeraj Varyani
Department of General Medicine, Institute of Medical Sciences, Banaras Hindu University, Uttar Pradesh, Varanasi 221005, India

Daniel Vitorio
Intensimed Research Group, Adult Intensive Care Unit, Hospital São Camilo, Pompéia, 05024-000 São Paulo, SP, Brazil

Alexandre Toledo Maciel
Intensimed Research Group, Adult Intensive Care Unit, Hospital São Camilo, Pompéia, 05024-000 São Paulo, SP, Brazil
Intensive Care Unit, Department of Medical Emergencies, Hospital das Clinicas, 05403-001 São Paulo, SP, Brazil

Beatriz Wills-Sanin and Andrés F. Buitrago
Department of Critical Care, University Hospital Fundación Santa Fe de Bogotá, Calle 119 No. 7-75, A.A. 220246, Bogotá, Colombia

Yenny R. Cárdenas, Lucas Polanco, Oscar Rivero and Sebastian Suarez
University Hospital Fundación Santa Fe de Bogotá, Calle 119 No. 7-75, A.A. 220246, Bogotá, Colombia

Paul N. Hein and Munveer S. Bhangoo
Department of Internal Medicine, Scripps Green Hospital, 10666 N Torrey Pines Road (403C), La Jolla, CA 92037, USA

Maida V. Soghikian
Division of Chest and Critical Care Medicine, Scripps Green Hospital, La Jolla, CA 92037, USA

Haris Kalatoudis, Fuad Zeid and Yousef Shweihat
Pulmonary Department, Byrd Clinical Center, Marshall University School of Medicine, 1249 15th Street, Huntington, WV 25701, USA

Meena Nikhil
Internal Medicine Department, Marshall University School of Medicine, 1600 Medical Center Drive, Huntington, WV 25701, USA

Tohru Shiratori
Division of Intensive Care Unit, Ina Central Hospital, 1313-1 Koshiroukubo, Ina, Nagano 396-8555, Japan

Atsushi Sato
Department of Neurosurgery, Ina Central Hospital, 1313-1 Koshiroukubo, Ina, Nagano 396-8555, Japan

Masao Fukuzawa
Department of Dermatology, Ina Central Hospital, 1313-1 Koshiroukubo, Ina, Nagano 396-8555, Japan

Naoko Kondo
Department of Anesthesiology, Ina Central Hospital, 1313-1 Koshiroukubo, Ina, Nagano 396-8555, Japan

Shogo Tanno
Department of Emergency Medicine, Ina Central Hospital, 1313-1 Koshiroukubo, Ina, Nagano 396-8555, Japan

Oleg Stens
Department of Internal Medicine, Harbor-UCLA Medical Center, Torrance, CA, USA

Gabriel Wardi
Department of Emergency Medicine, University of California, San Diego, San Diego, CA, USA
Division of Pulmonary, Critical Care, and Sleep Medicine, University of California, San Diego, La Jolla, CA, USA

Demosthenes Papamatheakis
Division of Pulmonary, Critical Care, and Sleep Medicine, University of California, San Diego, La Jolla, CA, USA

Matthew Kinney
Department of Orthopedic Surgery, University of California, San Diego, San Diego, CA, USA

Stephanie Shin
Pulmonary and Critical Care Medicine, Sharp Memorial Hospital, San Diego, CA, USA

Stefan W. Malin
Department of Pediatrics, Indiana University School of Medicine, Indianapolis, IN, USA

Riad Lutfi, Matthew L. Friedman and Alicia M. Teagarden
Division of Pediatric Critical Care, Department of Pediatrics, Indiana University School of Medicine, Indianapolis, IN, USA

Nobuki Shioya, Shigehiro Shibata, Masahiro Kojika and Shigeatsu Endo
Department of Critical Care and Emergency, Iwate Prefectural Advanced Critical Care and Emergency Center, Iwate Medical University, 19-1 Uchimaru, Morioka 020-8505, Japan

J. Wallenborn
Department of Anesthesiology and Intensive Care Medicine, HELIOS Klinikum Aue, Gartenstraße 6, 08280 Aue, Germany
Department of Anesthesiology and Intensive Care Medicine, Universit'atsklinikumCarl Gustav Carus, Technische Universität Dresden, Fetscherstraße 74, 01307 Dresden, Germany

M. Fischer
Department of Dermatology and Venerology, HELIOS Klinikum Aue, Gartenstraße 6, 08280 Aue, Germany
Department of Dermatology and Venerology, Martin-Luther-Universität Halle-Wittenberg, Ernst-Grube-Straße 40, 06097 Halle, Germany

Pablo Lucero
Hospital Británico de Buenos Aires, Intensive Care Services, Argentina

Sebastián Chapela
Hospital Británico de Buenos Aires, Intensive Care Services, Argentina
Universidad de Buenos Aires, Facultad de Medicina, Departamento de Bioquimica Humana, Argentina

Rashmi Mishra and Misbahuddin Khaja
Division of Pulmonary and Critical Care Medicine, Bronx Lebanon Hospital Center Affiliated to Icahn School of Medicine at Mount Sinai, 1650 Grand Concourse, Bronx, NY 10457, USA

Pavithra Reddy
Department of Medicine, Bronx Lebanon Hospital Center Affiliated to Icahn School of Medicine at Mount Sinai, 1650 Grand Concourse, Bronx, NY 10457, USA

Guillermo J. Giangreco
Baltimore-Washington Medical Center, Glen Burnie, MD 21061, USA

Dean Campbell and Mark J. Cowan
University of Maryland School of Medicine, Baltimore, MD 21201, USA

Konstantinos Raymondos
Anaesthesiology and Intensive Care Medicine, Hannover Medical School, 30625 Hannover, Germany

Jörg Ahrens
Anaesthesiology and Intensive Care Medicine, Klinikum Links derWeser, 28277 Bremen, Germany

Ulrich Molitoris
Cardiothoracic, Transplantation and Vascular Surgery, Hannover Medical School, 30625 Hannover, Germany

Lee D. Murphy and Riad Lutfi
Division of Pediatric Critical Care Medicine, Department of Pediatrics, Indiana University School of Medicine, Indianapolis, IN, USA

Mouhammad Yabrodi
Division of Pediatric Critical Care Medicine, Department of Pediatrics, Indiana University School of Medicine, Indianapolis, IN, USA
Division of Pediatric Cardiology, Department of Pediatrics, Indiana University School of Medicine, Indianapolis, IN, USA

Francesca Leonardis, Viviana De Angelis, Francesca Frisardi and Chiara Pietrafitta
Intensive Care Unit, Fondazione Policlinico Tor Vergata, Viale Oxford 81, 00133 Roma RM, Italy

Ivano Riva, Tino Martino Valetti, Valentina Broletti and Gianmariano Marchesi
Intensive Care Unit 3, Department of Anesthesia and Intensive Care, ASST Papa Giovanni XXIII, Piazza OMS 1, 24127 Bergamo BG, Italy

Lorenza Menato, Roberto Nani, Franco Marson and Mirca Fabbris
Intensive Care Unit, Azienda ULSS 2 Marca Trevigiana, Presidio Ospedaliero di Treviso, Piazzale dell'Ospedale 1, 31100 Treviso TV, Italy

Luca Cabrini, Sergio Colombo and Alberto Zangrillo
Anesthesia and Intensive Care Unit, IRCSS San Raffaele, Via Olgettina 60, 20132 Milano MI, Italy

Carlo Coniglio and Giovanni Gordini
Resuscitation and Territorial Emergency Unit, Maggiore Hospital, Largo Nigrisoli 2, 40133 Bologna BO, Italy

Lucia Stalteri, Giovanni Giuliani, Vittorio Dalmastri and Gaetano La Manna
Nephrology, Dialysis and Transplantation Unit, Azienda Ospedaliera-Universitaria di Bologna, Via Massarenti 9, 40138 Bologna BO, Italy

María Jesús Gómez Ramos, Carmen Sánchez Álvarez and Lisa Ortin Katnich
Department of ICU, Reina Sofía General University Hospital, University of Murcia, 30.003 Murcia, Spain

Francisco Miguel González Valverde
Department of Surgery, Reina Sofía General University Hospital, University of Murcia, 30.003 Murcia, Spain

Francisco Pastor Quirante
Department of Pathology, Reina Sofía General University Hospital, University of Murcia, 30.003 Murcia, Spain

Ester Ilyayeva, Khaled Nada, Roxane Farahi Far, Kamal Albright, Manmeet Kaur Gujral and Menachem Gold
Lincoln Medical and Mental Health Center, 234 E 149Th St., Bronx, NY 10451, USA

Daniel Lachant and David Trawick
Division of Pulmonary and Critical Care Medicine, University of Rochester Medical Center, 601 Elmwood Avenue, Rochester, NY 14624, USA

Andrea Berkes, Edit Szikszay and Tamás Szabó
Department of Pediatrics, University of Debrecen, Debrecen 4012, Hungary

György Balla
Department of Pediatrics, University of Debrecen, Debrecen 4012, Hungary

HAS-UD Vascular Biology and Myocardial Pathophysiology Research Group, Hungarian Academy of Sciences, Debrecen 4012, Hungary

János Kappelmayer and Adrienne Kerényi
Institute of Laboratory Medicine, University of Debrecen, Debrecen 4012, Hungary

László Ujhelyi and József Balla
Department of Medicine, Faculty of Medicine, University of Debrecen, Debrecen 4012, Hungary

Krisztina Bari
Fresenius Medical Care, NephroCare University of Debrecen, Debrecen 4012, Hungary

Gurveen Malhotra and Tanjeev Kaur
University of Illinois at Chicago, Chicago, IL 60612, USA

Nitya Ramreddy
Internal Medicine, Mount Sinai Hospital, Chicago, IL 60608, USA

Serafin Chua
Rheumatology, Mount Sinai Hospital, Chicago, IL 60608, USA

Mira Iliescu
Pulmonary and Critical Care Medicine, Mount Sinai Hospital, Chicago, IL 60608, USA

Kazumasa Emori, Nobuhiro Takeuchi and Junichi Soneda
Department of Cardiovascular Surgery, Kobe Tokusyukai Hospital, 1-3-10 Kamitakamaru, Tarumi-ku, Kobe-shi, Hyogo 655-0017, Japan

Anton Lund, Ditte G. Strange and Kirsten Møller
Department of Neuroanaesthesiology, Rigshospitalet, University of Copenhagen, Copenhagen, Denmark

Mette B. Damholt
Department of Nephrology, Rigshospitalet, University of Copenhagen, Copenhagen, Denmark

Jesper Kelsen
Department of Neurosurgery, Rigshospitalet, University of Copenhagen, Copenhagen, Denmark

Hasse Møller-Sørensen
Department of Cardiothoracic Anaesthesiology, Rigshospitalet, University of Copenhagen, Copenhagen, Denmark

Mario Pezzi, Silvia Renda, Anna Maria Giglio, Anna Maria Scozzafava, Simona Paola Tiburzi, Patrizia Casella and Mario Verre
Anaesthesia and Intensive Care Unit, General Hospital "Pugliese-Ciaccio", Viale Pio X, 88100 Catanzaro, Italy

Fabrizio Iannelli
Bellco, 41037 Mirandola, Italy

Ayla Gordon, Gina LaCapra and Roberto Roberti
Overlook Medical Center, Summit, NJ, USA

Varalaxmi Bhavani Nannaka and Dmitry Lvovsky
Division of Pulmonary and Critical Care Medicine, Bronx Lebanon Hospital Center, Bronx, NY 10457, USA

Nihar Jani
Department of Internal Medicine, Bronx Lebanon Hospital Center, Bronx, NY 10457, USA

Masooma Niazi
Department of Pathology and Histology, Bronx Lebanon Hospital Center, Bronx, NY 10457, USA

Anusha Battineni, Naresh Mullaguri, Shail Thanki and Raghav Govindarajan
Department of Neurology, University of Missouri, 1 Hospital Drive, Columbia, MO 65212, USA

Anand Chockalingam
Department of Cardiology, University of Missouri, 1 Hospital Drive, Columbia, MO 65212, USA

Christan D. Santos and Robert A. Ratzlaff
Department of Critical Care Medicine, Mayo Clinic, Jacksonville, FL, USA

Jennifer C. Meder
Department of Nutritional Services, Mayo Clinic, Jacksonville, FL, USA

Paldeep S. Atwal
Department of Clinical Genomics, Mayo Clinic, Jacksonville, FL, USA

Nicole E. Joyce
Division of Hospital Internal Medicine, Mayo Clinic, Jacksonville, FL, USA

M. Fröhlich-Gildhoff, C. Berhold, U. Ketterer, S. Kische and H. Ince
Department of Cardiology and Intensive Care Medicine, Vivantes Klinikum im Friedrichshain, Landsberger Allee 49, 10249 Berlin, Germany

W. J. Jabs and M. K. Kuhlmann
Department of Nephrology, Vivantes Klinikum im Friedrichshain, Landsberger Allee 49, 10249 Berlin, Germany

Guillaume Morel
Service d'Hématologie, CHU de Strasbourg, 67000 Strasbourg, France

Joy Mootien, Philippe Guiot and Khaldoun Kuteifan
Service de Réanimation Médicale, GHRSMA, 68100 Mulhouse, France

Farheen Manji
University of Calgary and Alberta Health Services, Calgary, AB, Canada
Department of Medicine, University of Calgary, Calgary, AB, Canada

Benjamin Wierstra and Juan Posadas
University of Calgary and Alberta Health Services, Calgary, AB, Canada
Department of Critical Care, University of Calgary, Calgary, AB, Canada

Robin Paudel, Prerna Dogra and Saurav Suman
Department of Internal Medicine, University of Kentucky, Lexington, KY, USA

Saurav Acharya and Jyoti Matta
Department of Internal Medicine, Jersey City Medical Center, Jersey City, NJ, USA

Carlos Salazar
Department of Internal Medicine,Weiss Memorial Hospital, 4646 N. Marine Drive, Chicago, IL 60640, USA

Romeo A. Majano
Miami Cardiac and Vascular Institute, South Miami Hospital, Baptist Health, 6200 SW73 Street, South Miami, FL 33143, USA

Motohiro Asaki, Takamitsu Masuda and Yasuo Miki
Department of Emergency Medicine, Emergency and Critical Care Center, Fujieda Municipal General Hospital, Shizuoka, Japan

Channing Hui
Rutgers-RobertWood Johnson Medical School, Department of Emergency Medicine, One RobertWood Johnson Place, MEB 389, New Brunswick, NJ 08901, USA

Maria Cardinale
Ernest Mario School of Pharmacy, Rutgers University, 160 Frelinghuysen Rd., Piscataway Township, NJ 08854, USA

Balaji Yegneswaran
Saint Peter's University Hospital, 254 Easton Ave., New Brunswick, NJ 08901, USA

Zachary M. Harris
Tulane University Health Sciences Center, Department of Internal Medicine, New Orleans, LA 70112, USA

Alvaro Alonso
Heart and Vascular Institute, Tulane University School of Medicine, New Orleans, LA 70112, USA

Thomas P. Kennedy
Tulane University Health Sciences Center, Department of Medicine, Section of Pulmonary Diseases, Critical Care Medicine, and Environmental Medicine, New Orleans, LA 70112, USA

Mark A. Dobish
Anesthesiology Resident, Department of Anesthesiology, Thomas Jefferson University Hospital, Philadelphia, PA, USA

David A. Wyler
Assistant Professor of Anesthesiology and Critical Care Medicine, Department of Anesthesiology, Thomas Jefferson University Hospital, Philadelphia, PA, USA Assistant Professor of Neurological Surgery, Department of Neurosurgery, Thomas Jefferson University Hospital, Philadelphia, PA, USA

Christopher J. Farrell
Assistant Professor of Neurological Surgery, Department of Neurosurgery, Thomas Jefferson University Hospital, Philadelphia, PA, USA

Hermandeep S. Dhami
Medical Student, Sidney Kimmel Medical College,omas Jefferson University Hospital, Philadelphia, PA, USA

Victor M. Romo
Assistant Professor of Anesthesiology, Department of Anesthesiology, omas Jefferson University Hospital, Philadelphia, PA, USA

Daniel D. Choi
Assistant Professor of Oral and Maxillofacial Surgery, Department of Oral and Maxillofacial Surgery, Thomas Jefferson University Hospital, Philadelphia, PA, USA

Travis Reed
Resident, Department of Oral and Maxillofacial Surgery, Thomas Jefferson University Hospital, Philadelphia, PA, USA

Michael E. Mahla
Professor and Executive Vice Chair of Anesthesiology, Department of Anesthesiology,

Thomas Jefferson University Hospital, Philadelphia, PA, USA

Leonardo Cordeiro de Souza and Marcos David Parada Godoy
Medical Science Post-Graduation Program, Universidade Federal Fluminense, Niterói, RJ, Brazil Intensive Care Division, Hospital e Clínica São Gonçalo, São Gonçalo, RJ, Brazil

Abreu de Souza, Eric Eduardo Pinto de Almeida, Leo Honse Ribeiro and Wanderlei Augusto Junior
Intensive Care Division, Hospital e Clínica São Gonçalo, São Gonçalo, RJ, Brazil

Jocemir Ronaldo Lugon
Nephrology Division, Universidade Federal Fluminense, Niterói, RJ, Brazil

Index